CLUMSY CHILD SYNDROMES

CLUMSY CHILD SYNDROMES

Descriptions, Evaluation and Remediation

Bryant J. Cratty

University of California
Los Angeles, USA

harwood academic publishers
USA • Switzerland • Australia • Belgium
France • Germany • Great Britain • India • Japan
Malaysia • Netherlands • Russia • Singapore

Harwood Academic Publishers

820 Town Center Drive
Langhorne, Pennsylvania 19047
United States of America

Post Office Box 90
Reading, Berkshire RG1 8JL
Great Britain

Private Bag 8
Camberwell, Victoria 3124
Australia

3-14-9, Okubo
Shinjuku-ku, Tokyo 169
Japan

58, rue Lhomond
75005 Paris
France

Emmaplein 5
1075 AW Amsterdam
Netherlands

Christburger Str. 11
10405 Berlin
Germany

Library of Congress Cataloging-in-Publication Data

Cratty, Bryant J.
Clumsy child syndromes : descriptions, evaluation, and remediation / Bryant J. Cratty.
p. cm.
Includes bibliographical references.
ISBN 3-7186-0548-1 (hardcover) 3-7186-0575-9 (softcover)
1. Movement disorders in children. 2. Clumsiness in children. 3. Psychomotor disorders in children. I. Title.
RJ496.M68C73 1993
618.92'7—dc20 92-34999
CIP

THIS BOOK IS DEDICATED TO PERCEPTIVE EDUCATORS WHO DO NOT SAY "WE HAVE NO CHILDREN WITH PROBLEMS IN *OUR* SCHOOL!"

CONTENTS

CHAPTER 4 ORGANOGENESIS AND DEVELOPMENT DEFICITS

CHAPTER 5 SUB-SYNDROMES

CHAPTER 6 MOVEMENT CHARACTERISTICS

CHAPTER 7 DYSGRAPHIA

ILLUSTRATIONS

CHARTS

FIGURE

PLATES

TABLES

ACKNOWLEDGEMENTS

I am grateful for the continued inspiration I obtained from a large number of graduate and undergraduate students who, during the past three decades, have assisted us with our "kids program" at UCLA. Many seem to have been positively influenced by the experience and subsequently entered the fields of medicine, special education, occupational and physical therapy, and adapted physical education. Some now serve as clinicians, as while others occupy positions as faculty-researchers within professional schools, colleges and universities.

My close friend and colleague, Iraneide J. De Oliveira, has been a constant support this past ten years, both when conducting research and when serving as a competent administrator for the clinic program we conduct together. The clinical skills she exhibits when working with young children are truly remarkable, and I learn from her every day how to get the most out of youngsters who at times prove "difficult." Her work and dedication while achieving competencies in several languages and obtaining two university degrees has also inspired me to put forth extra effort.

Many colleagues from other countries have provided me with positive models of effort and achievement over the past several decades. These include Dr. Ernest Kiphard from Germany, Dr. Victor Matsudo and Dr. Dietmar Samulski from Brazil, Professor J. Bhullar from India, Dr. Fidelis Amuchie from Nigeria, Dr. Yuri Hanin from the former USSR, Dr. Vitor de Fonesca from Portugal, Professor Atsui Fujita from Japan, Dr. Guy Missoum from France, Professor Miroslav Vanek from Czechoslovakia, Dr. Jorge Gleser from Israel, Dr. Gunnar Borg from Sweden, and Professor Carlos Guardia from Venezuela, as well as others from China, The Netherlands, Norway, Belgium, Finland, Spain, Switzerland, and England.

My colleague Dr. Motohide Miyrahara has assisted me competently both in research with learning disabled children and also when serving as clinician in our children's program. The faculty of the Landmark West School, including its director Richard L. Goldman and Academic Dean Mary Ulasewitz, have been valued professional colleagues. They have assisted us in our recent research and clinical efforts that have included exploring the abilities of, and programming for, the improvement of the perceptual-motor abilities of learning disabled children.

Finally, I am most grateful for the trust of several thousand parents who, during the past thirty years, have shown confidence in me and my staff by placing their children in our charge. We have learned from these mothers and fathers about the difficult problems their awkward children encounter. From their children we have also obtained insights about how to rectify some of the practical, social and emotional effects of incoordination.

Chapter 1
Introduction

OVERVIEW

Awkward children are likely to elicit various reactions from those observing their struggles as they attempt to perform physical tasks. For example, they may be the victims of social derision from their brothers and sisters. Peers in school may also ridicule them, and ostracize incompetent performers from games and sports. Their teachers may become impatient as printed or written lessons are not copied neatly and rapidly enough to match the efforts of their physically more capable classmates.

Parents, when confronting evidence of incoordination in their offsprings, also have reactions that vary from household to household. Some accurately assess the nature of the problem and seek valid evaluations and professional help. Others may ignore the difficulties their children have when attempting physical skills. While still others may deny there is a problem present, often citing evidence of their child's intellectual social and/or creative prowess as ways to counter criticisms of their offspring's poor motor abilities.

Fathers may become tense while attempting to play ball with their poorly coordinated sons in the back yard, and later may withdraw from such potentially useful encounters. A mother, after receiving reports from a nursery school teacher that include the words "delayed development", may frantically begin to seek a solution to the problem by consulting the family pediatrician, and a number of other medical, educational and paramedical specialists.

IDENTIFICATION AND DEFINITIONS

Identification

Physically awkward children may pose evaluation and labeling problems to professionals assessing them. Some pediatricians, who may have only been exposed to youngsters with obvious symptoms of cerebral palsy, may shrug off symptoms of incoordination as simply a collection of unusual neurological 'soft signs'. Furthermore some may tell parents that the child may outgrow poor coordination, and thus the problem is not of importance. Many medical specialists, however, are becoming aware of the existence of the significant percentage of these children found within apparently normal populations. These doctors actively assist parents to seek remedial help for their youngster's problems.

Child psychologists, whose evaluation tools usually include collecting samples of printing and figure drawing, may correctly identify a graphic problem. However psychologists usually do not assess deficiencies reflecting the child's integration of the larger muscle groups. Some learning disability specialists, and educational therapists may mistakenly assume that because the child prints slowly and poorly, other academic difficulties must inevitably be present.

Definitions

Awkward children have been given various labels throughout the past several decades. They have sometimes been dubbed 'minimally brain damaged'. This type of definition infers that poor motor coordination is caused by easily identifiable neurological underpinnings.

Some have referred to physically awkward children as hyperactive, or possessing an "attentional deficit". Those formulating this type of label apparently ignore the premise that it is possible for a child to be hyperactive and well-coordinated, or to be uncoordinated and yet evidence good attention and impulse control.

Others have described awkward children as evidencing *developmental apraxia.* The prefix "developmental" usually means that the condition is apparent early in life, and that the awkwardness observed is reflected by the inability to integrate task's submovements into complex wholes. Furthermore "developmental apraxia" implies that youngsters given this label are not mastering appropriate physical skills at the ages expected by members of their sub-culture. Various forms of developmental dyspraxia and apraxia are discussed in chapter 6.

An early definition of incoordination was formulated by Gubbay (1975), who wrote that "the clumsy child is to be regarded as one who is mentally normal, without bodily deformity, and whose physical strength, sensation and coordination are virtually normal by the standards of routine conventional neurological assessment, but whose ability to perform skilled purposive movement is impaired." Gubbay's description poses several problems, however. For example, his definition suggested that the nervous system does not somehow mediate awkward motor behavior, as he pointed out that 'conventional neurological assessment' will likely reflect normality when applied to such children.

However, during the past twenty years several pediatric neurologists have formulated neurological evaluations likely to detect symptoms reflecting below-average motor coordination. For example, twenty years ago Touwne and Prechtl (1970) two Dutch neurologists, and more recently others (Tupper 1987), have incorporated measures of motor awkwardness and neuromotor immaturity into well designed evaluations for children with 'minor nervous dysfunctions'. Several contemporary neurological-evaluation schedules have been designed to be used following conventional neurological assessments. Thus it appears that using contemporary assessment tools and sophisticated strategies, signs of motor awkwardness are medically identifiable and diagnosable with reference to the presence of associated neurological dysfunctions.

The definition by Gubbay also did not seem to consider that motor ineptitude is sometimes found among groups of youngsters who are otherwise considered normal. Gubbay seems to suggest that poor motor is invariably accompanied by other problems including mental retardation, learning disabilities, the presence of either acquired or congenital brain tumors, and/or within various other medically identifiable atypicalities. In it becoming increasingly apparent, however, that some awkward children present symptoms exclusive of other obvious medical, educational or psychiatric disorders.

Recently, clumsiness in children has been defined by Hall (1988) as 'a deficit in the acquisition of skills requiring fluent coordinated movement, not explicable by general retardation or demonstrable neurological disease. This more enlightened definition seems based upon contemporary evidence making it increasing clear that a child may evidence motor awkwardness independent of, and without the presence of, other medical conditions and problems. Furthermore, research data appearing in the 1990's is beginning to identify the existence of various sub-syndromes within what was once viewed as a rather global and undifferentiated type of movement problem. (Hoare & Larkin 1991) (Miyahara 1992).

These modern views of motor awkwardness also make it increasing clear that youngsters may evidence clumsiness independent of other possible medical problems that may or may not be present. Furthermore, each youngster should be accorded a precise evaluation focusing upon his or her unique set of symptoms. The current literature also strongly suggests that follow-up remediation should be applied with precision, be accompanied by reasonable goals, and be symptom and syndrome specific. The nature of motor awkwardness within, and independent of, other syndromes is discussed in Chapter 3. Descriptions of various sub-syndromes are found throughout the text, particularly in Chapters 5 and 7. Guidelines for remediation are located in Chapters 7 & 12.

Awkward children and youth, however, continue to reside in a diagnostically 'grey area'. They are youngsters who make their peers tense and resistive during play, and who also present management and educational problems to parents, teachers and to professionals who deal with them. Similar to what is said about learning disabled children, awkward children possess hidden disabilities, problems that may only become apparent when complicated motor tasks are expected of them.

INCIDENCE

Poorly coordinated children are present in significant numbers in groups of youngsters from which the obviously physically, mentally and sensorially handicapped have been identified and removed for special help. The incidence of children evidencing poor coordination, according to various estimates, ranges from 5% (Bremmer & Gillman 1966) (Gubbay 1975) (Henderson & Hall 1982) (Iloeje 1987), to 15% (Hoare & Larkin 1990, and even to 20% of school populations, from which the obviously handicapped have been removed (Paine 1968) (Clements 1966). Their presence has been documented in Europe (Gubbay 1976) Asia, Africa, (Iloeje 1987), Australia (Hoare & Larkin 1991), and in North American. Thus throughout the world it appears as though there is at least one awkward child within most classroom settings containing at least 20 youngsters. Thus motor awkwardness appears to be a pervasive problem among contemporary children and youth.

Gender differences

It has been assumed for several decades that clumsiness is more prevalent among boys than among girls (Henderson & Stott 1977) (Lazlo et al 1988). However recent evidence suggests that this problem may be as common among young females as among males

(Short & Crawford 1984) (Hoare & Larkin 1991). In the past a preponderance of awkward boys, have been usually found among both experimental and clinical populations studied. However, this sex bias may have been due to the tendency to refer boys, more often than girls, to remedial programs. In many societies there also may be more social pressure applied to boys at younger ages to excel physically, than is placed upon their female classmates. Thus, in numerous sub-cultures, physical awkwardness in boys may be noticed more by peers, and teachers, than is true than when girls are observed. Further research should be conducted to determine the incidence of awkwardness among both sexes, and the possible reasons for possible imbalances discovered.

New Populations

Throughout the world, in the late 1980s and early 1990's, the numbers of awkward children seem to be increasing. Additional sub-populations of motorically delayed youngsters are emerging as the result of numerous conditions, infants and children who are likely to evidence both mild and severe problems in physical coordination. These new groups include infants born to an increasing number of mothers who use "abusive substances" during pregnancy. Infants before and after birth have been exposed to other noxious substances ranging from abrasive chemicals in polluted air, to lead and asbestos in the environment. Fetus damaging chemicals have even included poorly formulated baby food. Pervasive malnutrition in many parts of the world is likely to produce developmentally deficient children whose symptoms include motor delays. Thus, numerous youngsters in these emerging and expanding populations of the developmentally delayed, thus pose continuing and challenging problems to a army of professional workers, both in the United States and elsewhere. Reference to some of these 'new' populations is found in Chapters 3 and 4, and in other sections of the text. (Cratty 1990).

HISTORICAL BACKGROUND

Scientific interest in what has sometimes been termed the 'clumsy child syndrome' has been varied over the past sixty years. Whether or not these youngsters are noticed by behavioral, educational and medical specialists has seemed to depend partly upon the affluence of the culture. Understandably the subtle problems of motor coordination have often not been of great concern of those in developing countries. Among educational and medical communities in "third-world" nations one usually finds an emphasis placed upon children and adults with obvious and profound medical problems.

There are several historical trends, beginning from the pioneering efforts of Nicholas Oseretsky in Russia during the 1920's. The qualities of clumsiness evaluated subsequently were often dependent upon performance demands and upon values attached to physical prowess in various sub-cultures, and upon the orientation of the professionals assessing motor ineptitude in children.

Historically the assessment of motor coordination by professionals has taken numerous forms. The outcomes of such measurements have thus been varied. The identification of these youngsters has depended upon the validity of the instruments, the orientation and interpretations of professionals giving the tests, as well as upon how conservatively or liberally test-givers were willing to bestow the labels "awkward" or "clumsy" upon an individual child, or upon a population of such youngsters.

Since the first decades of this century professionals from a variety of disciplines, ranging from medicine to physical education, have researched, written about, and interpreted the problems accompanying poor coordination in children. Articles focusing upon the awkward child may be found in journals of pediatrics, neurology, education and learning disabilities. In 1975 three books focusing upon awkward children were published. Two had similar titles 'The Clumsy Child." (Gubbay 1975) (Arnheim 1975). A third book titled "Remedial Motor Activity for Children" (Cratty 1975) also dealt with the identification and remediation of clumsiness children. More recently a text by Laszlo and Bairstow (1985) has covered selected aspects of the evaluation and remediation of perceptual-motor behavior in awkward children. Still other contemporary work has illuminated the nature of neurological soft-signs, included both sensory and academic symptoms prevalent among children with poor coordination (Tupper 1987)

Numerous writers have promised that the identification and remediation of poor coordination in youngsters will dramatically improve both school readiness and academic success. The titles of their books and articles often reflected these cheery speculations, and included "How to Develop Your Child's Intelligence". (Getman 1952) and others (Kephart 1955). As a result some unsuspecting teachers, parents, and other professionals eagerly exposed children to structured regimens of motor activity in attempts to improve reading and other academic, perceptual and cognitive skills. Most of the time, however, the expectations and hopes these theories generated were not realized. Additional discussion about possible links between motor ineptitude and learning is found in Chapter 9.

Contemporary Viewpoints

Recent research should encourage professional workers to view physical awkwardness with more precision, than was true in the past. (Miyahara 1992) (Hoare & Larkin 1991). These data are also beginning to encourage the formulation of symptom-specific remedial procedures. Some of the pertinent literature appearing during the past two decades, has begun also to focus upon both poor physical coordination as a problem separate and independent of academic learning disabilities. Lastly newly developed imaging techniques have begin to result in the identification of some of the neural substrates underlying subtle coordination difficulties (Knucley et al 1983).

THE PRESENT FOCUS

This book is an effort to illuminate the causes, characteristics and educational ramifications of below average physical coordination in children. It has been attempted to write in terms that are clear to parents who are interested in understanding the problems of their awkward offspring. The effort has also been made to satisfy the needs of professionals in education, medicine, para-medical specialities, and also workers within other areas who may profit from an orientation to problems symptoms and causes related to motor incoordination.

The book is based partly upon available research data containing information about how the nervous system develops and how malfunctions may produce motor incoordiation. The clinical experiences of the author and his colleagues have also been drawn upon to illustrate the nature of the condition and to describe the various symptoms and syndromes discussed. Several thousand awkward youngsters we have dealt with within a clinic program over the past three decades have provided numerous personal experiences and observations that continue to expand our interest and knowledge.

The text thus contains information reflecting a wedding of both clinical observations with data from the available research literature.

Readers may thus select chapters for review corresponding to their unique interests and backgrounds. For example, those with some knowledge of the nervous system may be more interested in exploring Chapter 4 and surveying other sections dealing with neurological underpinnings. Educators, parents and others interested more in the behavioral, social and educational dimensions of motor awkwardness may be drawn more to chapters 5 through 10.

The Audience

There are several groups of professionals. It is hoped to reach with this material. In addition to parents who may wish to understanding the physical efforts of their children, it was desired that the book's contents would interest more pediatricians in the identification and social-educational implications of subtle 'soft' neurological signs reflecting motor development problems. In this way it is hoped to improve the sensitivity of some who may not be aware of the presence of numerous poorly coordinated youngsters they are encountering in their practices. The available literature makes it clear that some of their medical peers have evidenced increasing interest in the neural and behavioral ramifications of motor ineptitude (Tupper 1987).

It was also intended to stimulate paramedical personnel, including both physical therapists and occupational therapists, to consider the developmental ramifications of what they might offer to younger clients. Children do not only require the services of therapists when they have cerebral palsy, incur serious burns, or when they are obviously damaged in accidents, but also when moderate motor problems may be making their young lives extremely difficult. There is a large number of awkward youngsters who may benefit from the expansion of therapists' goals and programs (Goodman-Edwards S.A. & Cermak 1989).

It is also desired that more teachers may, after reading the text, become more aware of the presence of and problems among, poorly coordinated children in their classrooms. Furthermore after awkward youngsters are identified, it is hoped that this material will encourage classroom teachers to extend, or seek, special help to improve physical skills needed at play to assist efforts expended when printing and writing. Awkward children are looked upon by some teachers as unwanted children whose slowness when attempting to complete assignments present vexing classroom management problems. It is hoped reading the material in this text will help some teachers to engage in more sophisticated observations of developmentally delayed youngsters they are likely to encounter, than is presently the case.

It is believed also that physical educators, special educators, and adapted physical educators have important moral, professional and legal obligations to assess and to attempt to rectify motor coordination problems present both in pre-school as well as in school-age populations. It is hoped that the following material will assist them to reach these goals. Moreover the following discussions may prove to be the impetus for new courses in curricula for both regular and adapted physical educators.

Unique Biases

There are several bias that the author harbors, and has carefully nurtured, over the years. It is felt important to state these initially so that readers may be forewarned, as these prejudices are undoubtedly reflected in the forthcoming pages.

(1) While it is apparent that physical awkwardness is often associated with other kinds of problems, it is also true that incoordination may exist as a syndrome, or as set of symptoms, in relative isolation, among populations of youngsters who are adequate or above-average in other respects. The problem of incoordination in children, it is believed, thus needs addressing as a viable subject of scientific research, as well as from educational and remedial viewpoints.

(2) There is often a need to "neurologize" (to speculate about the neurological underpinnings of a behavior), particularly about a condition that is mediated by the central nervous system. However, independent of what some conclude are the 'neurological underpinnings' of physical incoordination, is the need of clinicians to determine what kinds of remedial activities may be useful and then to apply these in precise ways to each youngster.

(3) Poor physical coordination is a condition worthy of study, of assessment, and of attempts at remediation in and of itself, and not necessarily as a means to correct other academic, intellectual and/or sensory deficiencies. For example, the inability to write

and to print well (dysgraphia) has been identified as a specific learning disability, and thus is in need of improvement when encountered, independent of other academic strengths and weaknesses a dysgraphic youngster may display.

Contemporary Classifications

In the United States, during the 1980s, poorly coordinated children have become increasingly recognized as an important sub-division of youngsters requiring special testing and services. This recognition is reflected in legal-educational descriptions which guide the diagnosis of all atypical children. The 1987 revision of the Assessment Code, contained in the Diagnostic and Statistical Manual employed by psychologists and psychiatrists in the United States, contains detailed descriptions of what are labeled. "Specific Developmental Disorders" (Axis III). One is termed a "Developmental Expressive Writing Disorder" (315.80), and a second a "Developmental Coordination Disorder" (315.40) reflecting poor integration of the larger muscle groups.

An emphasis upon early recognition of physical awkwardness in children as a medical problem has also been evidenced by the inclusion of this condition in standard neurological texts in the 1960's (Walton 1966) (Brain and Walton 1969) (Ford 1966). Often this problem has been categorized as a type of minimal cerebral dysfunction, or as a type of neurological soft-sign (Deuel & Robinson 1987).

Prognosis for Change

As is true of other remedial programs, including physical therapy, speech-language enrichment and occupational therapy, the outcomes of attempts at improving motor coordination are often difficult to predict. Prognosis is particularly difficult when trying to determine what effects a program may have whose efforts are directed a given child. Moreover the nature of the possible neural adjustments, underling modifications of physical skills, are also not well known at this time.

Gaps in knowledge of possible outcomes, however, should not preclude the institution of intelligent efforts directed at attempting to improve the coordination of a child with motor problems. These attempts may include also strategies to circumvent a problem (learn typing to avoid manuscript writing), adjusting the demands placed upon an awkward child (reducing the quantity of written work required in a school setting). Discussions of the possible effects of motor training are found in Chapter 13 and elsewhere.

Finally it is believed important to consider the constant, and often serious, social-emotional hurdles encountered by poorly coordinated children. They often suffer more social punishment, at the hands of both peers and adults, than do those with more obvious handicaps. An understanding of, and acommodation to these social pressures is essential when working in positive ways with such youngsters. This aspect of the problem is dealt with in Chapter 10.

Readers, with various backgrounds and orientations, may select various chapters and sections for consideration. For example, Chapter 11 dealing with assessment, may be of minimal interest to a parent. Chapter 10 covering social emotional factors may be more important to both parents and teachers who attempt to cope with awkward youngsters on a daily basis. While readers with a background in clinical neurology may also find parts of the text useful, while those neurologically naive may not wish to survey various sections. It is thus hoped that different groups of readers will use the text in the variety of ways intended by the author.

QUESTIONS FOR DISCUSSION

1. Why might be said that an awkward child possesses hidden problems?
2. What variables might cause the incidence of motor ineptitude to vary from population throughout the world, and between sub-culture within your country?
3. What kinds of family and social perceptions are likely to result in a child being referred for an assessment of motor awkwardness?
4. What variables are likely to influence the percentage of girls versus boys referred to remedial programs designed to improve motor coordination?
5. What problems are excluded by current definitions of physical clumsiness in children? Can you formulate a definition of your own?
6. Discuss current historical trends reviewed in the chapter. What trends to you see reflected in your community programs, and/or in the literature you may have reviewed on the subject?
7. What labels have been applied to clumsy youngsters? How to various labels reflect either a neurological-medical or behavioral-psychological approach to the problem? How might the kind of labels applied by various members of society result in lowering the self-esteem of an awkward youngster?
8. Discuss whether or not a child may be physically awkward, independent of, or in addition to, learning disabled or hyperactive. What kind of motor problem is likely to bunt the academic efforts of a child in a classroom?
9. How might different measures of motor abilities be used and be interpreted by various medical, para-medical and educational professionals?

10. In what ways might parents react to a poorly coordinated child in the family? Might reactions of various family members differ, in what ways? How might the parents first become aware of, and/or be informed of their child's coordination problems? What social and family variables might influence the intensity and type of parental reactions to the clumsy child's efforts?

Chapter 2
Historical Background

EARLY HISTORY

For centuries dramatic and obvious movement anomalies, observed in both the brain damaged and among the emotionally disturbed, attracted the attention of medical doctors and of scholars within other emerging scientific disciplines. Aurelous von Hohenheim, who lived from 1493 to 1541, was among the first within the Western World to describe the signs and symptoms of a number of movement disorders. Included among his writings are descriptions of actions he labeled 'choreas' (from the Latin "to dance") consisting involuntary spasms seen in the face, trunk, and limbs (Barbeau 1982).

For the next four centuries other medical pioneers, with increasing sophistication, explored the causes, symptoms and potential cures of other movement disorders. The problems they illuminated ranged from subtle twitchings and tics, to vigorous pathological actions of the entire body. For example during the 1600s Thomas Sydenham, referred to as the 'English Hippocrates', laid the ground work for understanding seizure disorders, and began to illuminate various types of cerebral palsy. In the 1700s James Parkinson identified both the neural structures and symptoms of a condition he termed 'the shaking palsy'. In the next century Gilles de la Tourette and others began to classify movement disorders marked by verbal and motor tics.

The scientific awakening of the 1800s was reflected in writings forming the bases for numerous disciplines ranging from genetics and biology to archeology and anthropology. During this same century parallel progress was made by neurologically oriented physicians, as they continued to explore the nature of various movement disorders. During the latter part of the 1800s William Hammond, a surgeon-general of the United States, wrote a landmark text, titled 'Treatise of the Diseases of the Nervous System.' It contained vivid and useful descriptions of both progressive and non-progressive types of movement anomalies. Hammon's book, first published in 1871, was reprinted in nine editions, the last of which appeared during the beginning of this century (Hammond 1871).

THE 20TH CENTURY

As the 20th century dawned, advances continued to result in clearer understandings of the causes and effects of other movement abnormalities. In addition the literature continued to provide increasingly useful treatment strategies. In 1910 J. M. Charcot, for example, advanced the first effective treatment of some forms of Parkinsonism. An epidemic of encephalitis in Europe in 1915, stimulated work by Kinnier Wilson and Wagner von Jauregg, resulting in clearer descriptions of this infection's symptoms.

Coordination Problems

During the first decade of the 20th century coordination problems in children were first mentioned in the literature. Prior to this time poor coordination was primarily studied as a collection of symptoms appearing in older stroke patients. In 1911 Dupre described what he termed a 'motor deficiency syndrome' seems among children (Ford 1966). He wrote that this syndrome was characterized by signs that included awkwardness of voluntary actions, excessive tendon reflexes, mild hypertonicity, and neurological overflow. Dupre believed this disorder to be different from other previously identified motor disorders, due partly to the fact that the neurological underpinnings of signs moderate awkwardness were not easily identifiable. During this same decade Collier also identified a group of children, whom he labeled 'congenitally maladroit' (Ford 1966).

Thus the medical literature reflects a long history of interest in the obvious movement disorders. During the previous centuries the focus had been upon describing and explaining dramatic movement problems often appearing involuntarily, and usually at times when an individual wishes to remain at rest. By the early 1900s, however, some scholars began to focus upon coordination problems in children that were often hidden, and appeared only when reasonably complex tasks were attempted. Therefore it has only been within this century that attention has been paid to subtle motor dysfunctions including physical awkwardness among maturing children.

AWKWARDNESS IN CHILDREN

By the 1920s and 1930s symptoms of poor motor coordination were viewed in several different ways. At first awkwardness was considered as a symptom in combination with other behavioral and medical problems. Later motor awkwardness was noted to exist as an independent neuro-behavioral entity, worthy of measurement and study. The Russian researcher-clinician, Nicholas Oseretsky was among the first to express this viewpoint (1931).

During the 1920s Oseretsky, working in the Moscow Neurological Institute, developed a assessment instrument to measure what he called 'motor idiocy'. This test spawned numerous descendants over the years (*see Chapter 11*). His test established tasks within different skill categories, reflecting various levels of difficulty, for children in different age groups. Thus the make-up of his test resembled the 'mental levels' concept appearing fifty years before within the make up of the first intelligence tests developed by Alfred Binet.

In the United States, at about this same time, Samuel Orton wrote about the presence of awkward children within groups of learning disabled subjects whom he was studying. Orton described a 'mild incoordinate type . . . (of dyslexic child) . . . in whom many exact motor acts are acquired slowly and with difficulty' (Orton 1925).

By the 1930s neural pathological conditions began to be viewed by some as valid ways to explain the presence of poor coordination in children. In 1937, for example, one writer concluded that incoordination was as an aftermath of encephalitis and thus was tied to a traditional neurological disturbance (Schain 1972).

In the 1930s Samuel Orton, continuing his interest in poor coordination among dyslexic children, apparently viewed the problem through bi-focal glasses. He wrote that physical awkwardness could be either rooted in behaviors associated with nervous system dysfunction, or was not aligned with neurological damage. He thus seemed to decide that motor incoordination could reflect both a neurological disorder of praxis (motor planning problem) and also a difficulty caused by poor visual spatial recognition, independent of neural pathologies. (Orton 1937).

Orton thus apparently believed that the signs of awkwardness tied to these behavioral-visual conditions were somehow separate from clumsiness associated with neurological damage to the main neural pathways mediating movement, lesions in the extra-pyramidal pathways, or to cerebellar dysfunction. Orton was also among of the first to recognize that motor dysfunctions were often multi-dimensional. He concluded that symptoms of poor coordination were evident when youngsters attempted to perform a variety of tasks including walking and running, and also when they labored to execute manual skills, including printing and writing.

Orton was also among the first to notice that awkward children were likely to evidence emotional problems. Several observers, during the years that followed also postulated that that motor coordination problems in children could often led to feelings of social inferiority and to low-self esteem. (Orton 1937) (Gubbay 1975) (Cratty 1975). Orton's early contributions to information about awkward children, were thus significant.

During the next two decades several issues arose, producing conundrums that continue to plague those attempting to understand awkwardness in children and in adults (Gordon and MacKinlay 1980). One issue was whether or not clumsiness may best be described with regard to the resemblance of its symptoms to mild forms of the traditional types of cerebral palsy, or whether other frames of reference are appropriate with describing awkwardness.

Soft Signs

One approach to diagnosis emerging in the 1970s, was to place motor awkwardness within a broader classification system that included a variety of 'soft signs' or "neurological soft signs". These 'signs' were defined as the obvious . . . "evidence of manifestation of an illness or dysfunction of the body." (Taber 1973). These have been thought by most to reflect subtle neurological disturbances, that are difficult to detect using traditional diagnostic strategies. (Tupper 1987).

Lists of soft signs reflecting movement abnormalities, have come to include general motor awkwardness, together with other qualities such as choreas (sight jerky movements), tremors, synkinesia (involuntary spreading of tensions and movements) and several types of motor planning problems (dyspraxia) (Duele & Robinson 1987). Soft signs also include symptoms that reflect reading problems, attentional difficulties, and sensory-perceptual deficits. Motor awkwardness, however, is believed by some studying these subtle neurological problems, to be the most 'handicapping' of these soft-signs (Ford 1960) (Walton et al 1965) (Orton 1925).

Soft signs, it was noted, were unlikely to be accompanied by easily detectable pathological symptoms and causes. In contrast, more obvious 'hard signs' of neurological dysfunction were, and are, considered to be accompanied by clear-cut evidence of organic neuropathologies, including tumors and obvious lesions. List of soft signs, thus included global symptoms of motor incoordination as well as more subtle movement symptoms that are sometimes difficult to assess.

Soft signs thus are usually considered less severe than hard signs. Hard signs can include, for example, dramatic and obvious symptoms of various types cerebral palsy. Additionally soft-signs, were sometimes found to appear inconsistently in evaluations conducted during several sessions. Thus these subtle behavioral anomalies began to present two types of diagnostic problems. One conundrum encountered was the aforementioned, reliable detection and assessment. The second problem involved attaching significance to their appearance, or/and to their persistence over time, in the life of a child (Towbin 1987).

Classification

Various classification systems have been formulated with which to 'organize these 'soft-signs'. These systems have included groups of as many as ninety-nine different symptoms of this nature. Most of time the presence of soft signs have been identified using neurological evaluations designed specifically for their detection (Clements 1966) (Small 1982).

In the 1970s an assessment battery, focusing upon soft signs, was formulated by the Early Clinic Drug Evaluation Unit of the National Institutes of Health, located in the United States (1973). This instrument, was labeled The Physical and Neurological Examination for Soft Signs (PANESS) (Rie 1987). Its presence stimulated the formulation of other measuring tools with similar purposes. These additional devices have included a pediatric evaluation schedule for use with children of from seven to nine years (Levine et al 1983).

The meanings of the presence of soft signs usually have been divided into categories: These include

(a) Indices of subtle manifestations of traditional pathological motor symptoms including modifications of muscle tone, distorted reflexes and the like, and

(b) Soft signs that suggest developmental processes are not proceeding in the expected ways and at the hoped-for speed.

This latter cause suggests that some 'lags' are being evidenced in the unfolding behaviors and capacities of the child (Tupper 1986).

Several persistent and frequently encountered movement qualities accompanying general awkwardness, include dyspraxia, apraxia and synkinesia. These and other types of soft-signs and symptoms are discussed further in Chapter 6, dealing with various qualitative aspects of motor abilities.

The Search for Definitions and Causes

Some scholars have focused upon formulating definitions of physical awkwardness. Others have seemed more preoccupied with determining causality. At times the formulation of a definition reflected a parallel effort to determine cause. Edgar Doll (1951), for example, was one of the first to employ the term 'minimal cerebral palsy' to describe clumsy youngsters. In truth, however, various forms of motor awkwardness may stem from a number of sources including lack of experience in, and exposure to, movement demands, and subtle endocrine problems. Other causes of awkwardness are likely central nervous system deficits, causing symptoms resembling mild forms of cerebral palsy.

Some scholars, including Birch (1975) expressed the opinion that neurological explanations for motor awkwardness are often not accurate, and when used may unduly alarm parents. Thus Birch argued that clinicians and educators should replace vague, neurologically oriented terms, when discussing awkward children with their parents, with other word-labels less likely to induce parental concern. Birch recommended using 'developmentally delayed' or 'irregular motor maturation' when referring to awkward children. (Birch 1975). Currently the search continues for descriptive labels that are both accurate and acceptable to professionals, and at the same time non-abrasive when heard by parents.

Awkwardness and Intelligence

The issue of whether awkwardness is associated with scores on standard tests of intelligence often has often arisen. This complex relationship currently continues to interest both parents, and professionals (Annell 1949) (Rie 1987). Some writers have referred to the lack of correspondence between academic intelligence and motor skills. For example, Annell in 1949, after explaining that awkward youngsters have problems in various self-care skills including dressing, noted that clumsy children often evidence good intelligence.

Other writers, however, adopted a contrasting viewpoint, and have closely aligned motor incoordination with other unwanted developmental symptoms, including academic problems and poor attention. Strauss and Lehtinen in their book titled *Psychopathology and Education of the Brain Injured Child,* (1947) were among the first to describe a syndrome that, in addition to signs of motor incoordination, also was comprised of academic learning deficits, perceptual problems, and attentional deficiencies.

Thus throughout the final five decades of the 20th century, some scholar-observers, and educators have grouped minor to moderate motor dysfunctions with learning disabilities. These speculations have influenced an army of clinicians, both amateur and professional, to encourage educators to attack academic-learning disabilities by attempting to remediate motor incoordination.

Ellen Rie, recently exploring data illuminating these relationships, concluded that no consistent relationships are found between various soft-signs including motor awkwardness and learning disabilities. However, she tempers her conclusions by the admission that available studies often contain poorly conceived tests, applied to diverse and often loosely identified populations (1987). These subtle relationships are explored further in Chapters 8 and 9.

In contrast to those advocating that learning disabilities and movement problems are both closely associated, and thus mutually influential, are others whose research data strongly suggests the independence of movement capacities and academic performance. For example, information from research by Walton (196l, 1963, Walton et al 1962), conducted in the 1960s, indicated that motor clumsiness may exist separate and apart from learning disabilities and/or hyperactivity. His work resulted in the identification of children with severe clumsiness. Walton was also one of the first to employ the term "The Clumsy Child Syndrome". The data from a recent study by Miyahara also supports this supposition (1992). Walton also included dysgraphia as a symptom within the syndrome he first named.

Walton, and later others, including Gubbay (1975), Henderson and Hall (1982), Hoare and Larkin (1991) (Miyahara 1992) and Laszlo (1988) in Australia, have continued to study the make-up of youngsters evidencing "The Clumsy Child Syndrome". They have included under this broad classification, several sub-groups of children whose motor symptoms are not easily aligned with traditional measures of neurological dysfunction.

As more data was obtained, researchers began to view awkward youngsters as consisting of at least two major sub-types, including

(a) whose academic-learning characteristics are deficient, and

(b) a second group of clumsy children whose academic capacities and potentials range from average to superior (Henderson and Hall 1982) (Miyahara 1992).

Contemporary research evidence about the characteristics of poorly coordinated youngsters has revealed other ways to classify this condition. For example, one group of clumsy youngsters may consist of some whose motor problems appear within a variety of tasks including graphic behaviors, gross motor behaviors and in the finite action-sequences needed when forming articulate speech. In contrast, there are awkward youngsters whose motor dysfunctions lie within a single and specific competency area that may include a problem *only* when writing, *or* when executing gross motor tasks involving ball skills, locomotion and balance and the like. (Henderson 1987).

Another two-way classification rests upon a developmental perspective. On one hand, it has been postulated, are children of pre-school age who may mature out of, or be quickly educated out of, their motor problems. In contrast another group, it has been hypothesized, consist of youngsters whose persisting signs of motor dysfunction will require continual exposure to remedial efforts applied throughout their school careers.

A promising trend is the appearance of recent cluster analyses by Hoare and Larkin (1991) and by Miyahara (1992). Data from these studies have begun to describe, and identify, sub-types of children within what was previously referred to globally and imprecisely as 'The Clumsy Child Syndrome'. The increasing precision with which various sub-types are being identified is reflected in the content of Chapters 5, 6, and 7. These data together with clinical-observations, prompted the plural title of this text reflecting the multi-dimensional perspective taken by the author when surveying symptoms and causes of motor awkwardness.

HISTORICAL TRENDS: AN OVERVIEW

Several historical trends may be identified within the literature. Initially there was a period of about four hundred years during which subtle neurological-behavioral dysfunctions were largely overlooked. This period of time was marked by the first explorations by neurologists-anatomists of relationships between obvious brain damage and dramatic aberrations and alterations in motor behavior. This first period lasted up until the end of the last century.

Next the decades from 1910 to 1960 were marked by the appearance of writings by both medical and psychological-educational specialists reflecting an interest in the a number of awkward children that appeared in their clinics. These scholars then either related the condition to mild but traditional neurological-medical problems such as cerebral palsy, or suggested that the problem was primarily educational in nature.

During the latter portion of this period, from about 1940–1960, motor incoordination came to be viewed by many as inseparable from learning disabilities, perceptual dysfunctions and hyperactivity in school children. During this time period a number of terms were employed to describe the syndrome, and also to label the youngsters evidencing motor incoordination. These name-tags included minimal brain damage, minimal brain dysfunction, delayed or irregular maturation, and minimal cerebral palsy (Ford 1966).

The third period, beginning from about 1960 and lasting until the present, has been marked by a more sophisticated consideration of clumsy children. Evaluations of awkward children by some during these decades thus included a thorough dissection of a variety of aspects of their total personalities, including their intellectual-academic potentials. Further this contemporary work has illuminated the sensory-perceptual bases of their difficulties, various symptoms of motor dysfunction they display, and also the social and emotional problems that are likely accompaniments to poor motor coordination.

Data from this third 'modern' period has thus resulted in the realization by some that the clumsy child syndrome is made-up of several sub-classifications of children. These sub-groups includes several dichotomies, including those with and without associated academic problems; and youngsters whose problems appear within several motor-tasks areas, versus those whose dysfunctions are rather specific.

Still another way of classifying clumsy children has consisted of postulating the existence of a group whose problems appear to be the result of immaturity, and secondly a sub-group of youngsters whose problems appear to be more lasting. (Silva and Ross 1980).

This latter period is also marked by the appearance of measurement tools of increasing sophistication. (Laszlo et al 1988) (Henderson 1987). A graphic look at these trends is seen below.

CONTEMPORARY ISSUES

A Neurological and/or Behavioral Problem

Several problems appear important to consider within the historical context of the 1990s. One persistent issue revolves around whether to view awkwardness as a neurological or as a behavioral phenomenon. For example, Gubbay (1975) and others (Pond 1960) have described clumsy children solely in behavioral terms, sometimes directly, and sometimes indirectly, suggesting that minor or moderate motor dysfunctions have no neurological etiology. Some have coined the term minimal brain damage, to describe children who are clumsy, thus suggesting that motor incoordination is a direct and visible sign of neurological disturbance.

Chart 2-1. Major Historical Trends

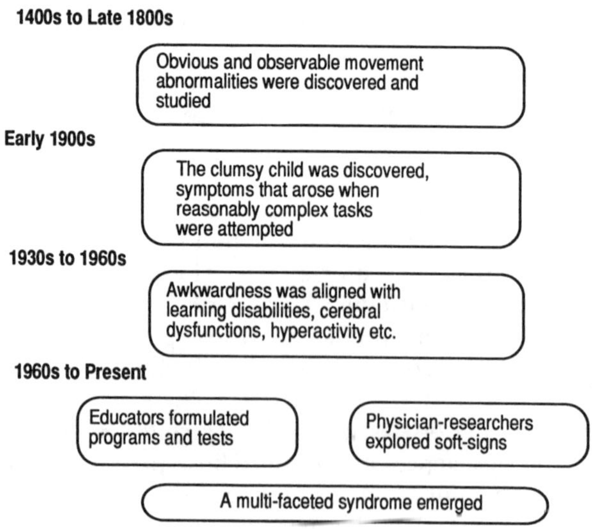

The scientifically and medically murky area of 'neurological soft-signs' also provides numerous pits of quicksand into which some may fall when attempting to sort-out the meanings, definitions, and significance of motor incoordination. (Tupper 1987) (Small 1982). However, ignoring the neurological underpinnings of motor incoordination, just because they are difficult to locate, appears to be short-sighted. Simply because signs of motor awkwardness do not always correlate to traditional signs of obvious brain damage, does not mean that moderate motor dysfunctions appearing developmentally in children, in common with all other behaviors, are not mediated by the central nervous system.

A recent longitudinal study has demonstrated the persistence of motor soft signs in a group of thirty-two awkward children over period of ten years. Thus instead of ignoring the neurological ramifications of motor awkwardness, perhaps because of the effort one should obtain and employ appropriate measurement devices. Neurological schedules, containing motor items, specifically designed for children with moderate coordination problems are appearing in the literature with increased frequency. Included in this list are assessment devices designed by Touwne and Prechtl (1970) (Henderson 1989) (Stott et al 1984) and others (Milani-Comparetti-Gidioni 1968) (Henderson 1987). A brief overview of these contemporary instruments is found in the Appendix of the text by Tupper (1987).

Additionally new methods of scanning the brain have begun to prove useful as diagnostic strategies, and are providing avenues of promising research. In the 1980s, for example, computerized scanning techniques have delineated marked structural differences in the brains of some clumsy youngsters. (Knuckey et al 1983).

Social-Emotional Symptoms

A second issues involves the illumination of the social emotional accompaniments of motor incoordination. Numerous statements may be found in the literature, pointing out that clumsy children characteristically evidence several types of psycho-social problems including low self-esteem, the tendency to display abrasive and inappropriate attention getting behavior, as well as other social mal-adaptations. (Cratty 1975) (Gubbay 1975). However it is difficult to locate studies in which the appearance of these less-than-useful compensations, and psycho-social problems, are clearly documented. Twenty years ago my colleagues and I found that self-esteem problems were prevalent within a population of clumsy children (Cratty et al 1970). This and contemporary evidence illuminating this problems is surveyed in Chapter 10.

Academic Learning and Poor Coordination

A third issue involves the vexing job of sorting out relationships between academic learning and motor ineptitude. To state that a child may be generally clumsy and thus does not evidence academic problems is simplistic. The inability to write-well (dysgraphia) has been labeled a specific learning disability in and of itself. A clearer definitions of what sub-types are found within learning disabled populations should further clarify the symptoms seen in motor sub-types within the same group of academically deficient youngsters.

Awkwardness and Visual Perception

A fourth issue is whether visual perceptual problems cause, are correlated to, or are independent of movement problems. Data on this topic continues to be researched (Hulme 1982, 1984). Finding low positive correlations between tests of kinesthetic and visual perception, and motor competencies does not infer causality. Children with minimal or moderate neurological dysfunction may evidence a variety of problems. These problems that may be contributed to by a similar deficits in the central nervous system. For example, a lack of maturity of certain structures in the brain stem may cause attentional deficits that can lower performance in similar ways as a group of children perform a number of tests including those reflecting intellectual, perceptual and/or motor functions. Relationships, both causal and statistical, between perceptual, academic and motor problems are explored further in Chapters 7 and 8.

Sub-Syndromes

A fifth issue that requires additional illumination is the nature of, and description of various sub-syndromes found within large groups of clumsy children. Current research strongly suggests that symptoms of clumsiness appear as a multi-dimensional condition. As more information of this nature is forthcoming, additional work should result in the formulation of more productive syndrome-specific remedial strategies

Finally the suggestion that some children with coordination problem may simply grow out of their ineptitude requires examination. This kind of assertion is what some parents may like to hear, in order to exclude troublesome, and often expensive, early remedial help.

The fact that signs of motor clumsiness may be designated as developmental abnormalities *does not necessarily mean* that an poorly coordinated child will inevitably grow out of his or her awkwardness. The adjective 'developmental' applied to various symptoms of motor incompetence indicates that in the course of normal motor development some children are not progressing in the expected ways and at reasonable rates (Duele & Robinson 1987, pp 96).

There are indications in the literature that:

(1) Early remedial help of a number of kinds is more likely to succeed, than if such assistance is rendered in late childhood, that

(2) Mild problems are more correctable than are moderate or marked problems and that

(3) It is difficult to be certain, given the present knowledge of neural-behavioral relationships, just what early problems may evidence positive changes through maturation.

Information covering the prediction of change due to interventions is found in Chapter 13.

It has been my observation that awkward children of five years, when tested, evidence few accompanying social-emotional compensations. However when six year olds suspected of motor delays are evaluated there is often a marked emotional accompaniment to their physical awkwardness. This more distinct emotional overlay is apparently caused because six year olds have had an additional year to ponder the extend of their awkwardness, a period during which they have also received negative social feedback from their parents, peers and teachers. By middle childhood problems of several types are likely to multiply if remedial help has not been extended to poorly coordinated youngsters during their early childhood years. Data in Chapter 12 strongly suggests that leaving an awkward child alone to simply "mature out" of his or her problem will likely result in further delays in motor performance accompanied by an increase in symptoms reflecting a negative emotional "overlay" to the coordination difficulties present.

OVERVIEW

Since the 15th century observable movement abnormalities began to be classified by medical pioneers, and by the 1700s and 1800s their neurological significance probed. These included ataxias, athetoid movements, Parkinsonian signs and other extraneous and often dramatic atypical movements of the body and its parts, usually displayed when individuals were attempting to remain at rest, or immobile.

Not until the 20th century, however, did motor signs of clumsiness attract scientific attention. Motor incoordination in children began to be studied when it was noted that when a complex task was attempted by some youngsters they experienced frustration and failure. Thus signs of incoordination that have been explored only recently. These symptoms consist of disruptions of actions that occur when youngsters attempt to engage in useful motor tasks in which most children, of a similar age, are expected to be successful.

Motor awkwardness in children was first written about in 1911. By the 1920s evaluation devices began to appear. Among the most influential early tests was that devised by Nicholas Oseretsky in 1922 at the Moscow Neurological Institute, to identify what he termed 'motor idiocy'. Oseretsky' test has been translated into numerous languages and has undergone many modifications. It has formed the basis for the numerous contemporary evaluation instruments that have followed. (Oseretsky 1948) (Bruinink 1978) (Stott and Henderson 1976). The condition Oseretsky began to study in the 1920s was not labeled the "clumsy child syndrome" until the 1930s. This label was first formulated by observers of coordination difficulties in children evidencing post-encephalitic complications. (Schain 1972).

After the World War II, interest in awkward children expanded, as motor ineptitude appeared as a symptom in several syndromes. Included in these syndromes were symptoms reflecting learning disabilities, perceptual problems, and hyperactivity. From the late 1940s, to the present, programs to remediate learning disabilities through movement activities proliferated While coordination as a treatment area was popularized, however, improving motor skills, was often viewed a strategy useful in the correction and improvement of academic learning.

By the 1960s, symptoms evidenced by clumsy children began to be studied by many as a separate syndrome independent of other problems encountered in maturing youngsters. In the 1970s books and research literature dealing with the problem began to appear. These writings dealt with both practical and theoretical-medical issues including the association of motor awkwardness with other "soft" neurological dysfunctions and minimal brain damage. In the 1980's. and early 1990's. several scholars began to arch for and to identify, various sub-syndromes reflecting motor awkwardness. (Miyahara 1992) (Hoare and Larkin 1991). Productive work in the 1980's has also included the exploration of the sensory-perceptual processes that underlie motor awkwardness, the development of more useful assessment instruments, and studies exploring improved strategies for change.

QUESTIONS FOR DISCUSSION

1. How was the history of the scientific pursuit of a better understanding of motor problems differ before, and after 1950?
2. Historically in what ways have scholars viewed the neurological underpinnings of motor awkwardness?
3. How did an interest in remediating learning disabilities influence that amount of attention devoted to coordination problems within this century?
4. What names are important to consider as main contributors to understanding the nature of physical incoordination during this century? What were the contributions of each persson you named?
5. Explain the interest displayed in evaluating and explaining neurological soft-signs? What problem areas, and questions, within this literature require further illumination.
6. How do hard-signs differ from soft-signs? How conceptually and definitionally do soft-signs differ from symptoms of motor incoordination?
7. How might a neurological examination uncover signs of motor incoordination? Was it suggested in the chapter that standard neurological examinations (schedules) are likely to assess motor soft-signs?
8. What are useful contemporary trends in the literature, cited in the chapter, that deal with awkward children? Has your reading uncovered any other types of research that may be viewed as important?
9. What types of neurological problems were first, viewed and considered by doctors and neuroscientists between 1500 and 1900?
10. Historically what definitions of motor ineptitude appeared? How did the various definitions reflect different viewpoints about relationships between motor clumsiness and neurological functioning.
11. Before the turn of the century who were some of the early contributors to knowledge about motor dysfunctions ? What were the contributions of each one you name?
12. During the decades ahead what research seems needed to further an understanding of awkward children, and to formulate more effective remedial strategies?

Chapter 3
Selected Movement Disorders in Childhood: Causes and Descriptions

INTRODUCTION AND OVERVIEW

The question most asked by parents after their child has been evaluated in our clinic, is why? Some parents apparently hope that if the reason for poor coordination is discovered the 'cure' will be more quickly forthcoming. This kind of reasoning has perhaps been conditioned by the usual relationships between causes and cures which the medical fraternity and sorority traditionally depend upon when dealing with the sick and injured. Unfortunately however, the reasons for the presence of symptoms reflecting mild to moderate physical awkwardness are usually obscure, and often impossible to delineate precisely. Furthermore, forming reasonable hypotheses as to why youngsters may evidence coordination problems do not always facilitate the formulation of more effective remedial strategies than if no reason for the incoordination is arrived at.

Numerous conditions may cause a child to be unskilled at play and in the classroom. These problems range from those emanating from the family or from the sub-culture in which the youngster is raised, to inborn genetic anomalies. An uncoordinated younger may be one who has been deprived of adequate exercise and physical experiences by parents, who may be following the norms of a sub-culture which dictates that caretakers should act in overly protective ways toward their young.

It has been found, for example, that infants raised within families who tend to 'smother' their efforts to explore and to move, displayed delays in motor development (Levy 1942, Beller 1959). In contrast, motor precocity is likely to occur within cultures encouraging unrestricted, and that also sanction early motor training, (Werner 1972). Thus within such diverse environments, as would be expected, a cause-and-effect chain of mutually influential variables begins to form. Positive attitudes coupled with parent encouragement and training inevitably lead toward superior motor performance capacities and skills. Even in highly stimulating settings, however, awkward children may be present, and withdraw from play, even though they may evidence a desire to participate fully. (Clifford & Bundy 1989).

It is difficult, however, to separate the possible effects of various influences upon physical skills. Some factors reflect family norms and values, other variables are biological and/or genetic. It has been found that there more delays in motor development occur among children from older mothers, than are present among infants and children from younger birth givers. (Gillberg et al 1982). In addition, firstborns are often subjected to more motor training by parents. Those later in the birth order, in contrast, are more likely to have play skills stimulated by their older siblings. (Schabel-Dickey 1978, Alberts and Landers 1978). However, these and similar conditions could result in motor capacities attributable to either genetic or cultural variables, or to some subtle a combination of both.

Personal-social causes may combine with various biological and genetic variables to blunt motor development. For example, older parents may discourage vigorous physical activity exhibited by their offspring, tolerating less 'confusion' than may younger parents. Thus youngster's motor-exploratory behaviors may be suppressed among these older and hypothetically more sedate parents. However older parents may also differ biologically from younger parents, resulting in differences in the vigor of their offsprings.

Birth order may also constitute both a societal, as well as a biological variable. Children born first in the family are delivered by mothers whose bodies may be less adapted to giving birth easily, and thus may be more likely incur peri-natal problems. Children born later are often less difficult the mother to deliver; and thus are less likely to experience less peri-natal trauma. At the same time firstborns may more likely assume dominant leadership positions in games, than are those appearing later in the birth order, resulting in increased physical competencies.

Both experiental and inborn conditions may combine to blunt the motor abilities and performance capacities of children. If youngsters are born with less than adequate coordination, the result is usually a withdrawal from vigorous playground games, because of the social abuse they may receive from their peers. With withdrawal results in what has been termed a 'disuse syndrome' reflecting a diminution of physical capacities experienced, because the child fails to exercise and to play vigorously on a daily.

Parental neglect is another potential contributor to poor coordination. Lack of practice in early and middle childhood may thus combine with innate qualities to further reduce the awkward child's capacities to display adequate force and to correctly time skilled actions. Similarly when children who may have inherited various types of dysgraphia are forced to try to print in a classroom withdrawal from and refusal to try academic work is often encountered. This results in a lack of practice which then is likely to blunt further their abilities to execute accurate letters and words.

Some symptoms of motor ineptitude are found within rare syndromes. These conditions, consisting of infrequently encountered, progressive problems, are often inherited. Within such syndromes motor ineptitude is usually only one of several early symptoms of trouble. The early and accurate diagnosis of these conditions is sometimes made difficult because their motor may be masked and covered up by normal maturational processes during the early months and years of life. Thus within some progressive syndromes motor and/or muscular difficulties may not become apparent until the third or fourth year, or may even remain hidden until the child is ready to enter school at the age of five or six.

Within the past several years new and vexing problems, contributing to motor development delays, have surfaced. For example, during the middle 1980s the increased availability of inexpensive street-drugs to young mothers, such as 'crack' cocaine, contributed to births of large numbers infants evidencing several kinds of developmental anomalies. Many of these motor development problems, along with other atypical behaviors are now found to extend into childhood and adolescence. (Cratty 1990). Many of these infants are now entering school, displaying either overly passive withdrawn behaviors, or agitated and aggressive tendencies. Both types of symptoms are presenting significant challenges to primary school educators.

For the most part however, the vast majority of uncoordinated children evidence symptoms that are non-progressive, and whose precise whose etiologies are obscure. When some cause is apparent (or hypothesized), the reasons given are sometimes similar to those believed to cause various forms of cerebral palsy. However, the incidents or traumas that have caused minor to moderate coordination problems are less severe manifestations of the variable(s) to which some of the traditional types of cerebral palsy are attributed.

For example, minor birth anoxia (deprivation of oxygen at birth) may cause minor coordination problems that do not appear until the school years are reached, and the necessity to print and opportunities to play ball are encountered. In contrast a more prolonged period of oxygen deprivation at birth is likely to cause obvious abnormalities including pronounced alterations in muscle tension and in abnormal movement characteristics appearing during the pre-school years as well as in early in early infancy. It should be noted, however, that the parents of many moderately clumsy children report no unusual events occurring within the birth histories of their children.

This chapter contains a brief survey of several of the most common conditions seen among children, problems accompanied by motor and muscular dysfunctions. The discussion has been divided into three sections. Reviewed first are several of the more commonly encountered syndromes that are accompanied by progressive motor delays. These conditions are often inherited and may involve the deterioration of peripheral neuromotor processes and/or the diminution of structures and mechanisms within the central nervous system. These problems include various forms of progressive ataxias.

The two progressive syndromes described are relatively rare. However, those whose professions bring them into contact with large numbers of pre-school youngsters, including nursery school teachers and the like, should become familiar with the nature of the motor symptoms occurring among younger children that may signal the onset of these serious problems. If these symptoms appear, the child should be quickly referred to appropriate medical specialists. Non-medical educators and developmentalists who assess and attempt to improve the movement characteristics of children, including adapted physical educators, should be aware of the limitations that a one-time evaluation may have when applied to a child whose motor difficulties may part of a be progressive syndrome.

A second section contains a brief overview of two types of inherited conditions that contain movement abnormalities, Down Syndrome, and Tourette Syndrome. These two syndromes by no means represent all of the possible genetically transmitted problems that are accompanied by motor difficulties. However, these two syndromes contain symptoms that represent marked and often dramatic aberrations of movement behaviors. Moreover they are among the most encountered inherited conditions accompanied by motor development lags.

The final part of the chapter deals with possible causes of the stable, non-progressive, symptoms exhibited by the majority of uncoordinated children and youth. These problems may be caused by various insults to the fetus occurring before birth, traumas experienced during the time of birth as well as various post-birth accidents and encounters. In this last group are children labeled as evidencing one of several types of cerebral palsy. In this final group also are some children whose prenatal environments were not biochemically poisonous, but who somehow experienced more subtle insults that resulted in clumsy, uncoordinated behaviors. The motor involvement among 'cocaine children' at times also may resemble mild to moderate forms of cerebral palsy.

PROGRESSIVE CONDITIONS

Many conditions, often inherited, involve gradual deterioration of motor functions controlled by the cerebellum, brain stem, the spinal cord and/or the peripheral portions of the nervous system. The aberrant motor symptoms that appear may be due to atrophy of nerve cells in central structures and within peripheral neural pathways. Some of these conditions are due to defects in biochemical processes which influence the use of blood sugar by the muscles, and by other process essential to normal muscle metabolism.

Friedreich's Ataxia

Friedreich's ataxia has been described as the most common type of progressive cerebellar deterioration occurring in childhood (Menkes 1974). The condition was first identified during the middle of the last century. In common with other medical problems that involve cerebellar degeneration, there is a demyelination (breakdown of the nerve sheaths) in both the long ascending and descending sensory-motor pathways, together with a degeneration of the axons in the cerebellum, and brain stem.

There are a wide variety of symptoms connected with this condition, ranging from diabetes, to skeletal-postural problems. These latter difficulties include abnormalities of the structure of the foot, including a high and rigid longitudinal arch (Pes Cavas), kyphosis (round shoulders with protruding scapulas), and spinal mal-alignments including scoliosis. (*See Plate 3-1*) Although the symptoms characteristically appear during the third decade of life, the onset of one type of this inherited condition may begin in childhood.

The signs of motor incoordination appearing, include unsteadiness coupled with balance problems, tremors in the hands, Thus difficulty in writing and to printing legibly is experienced. The symptoms appear gradually and may progress slowly. At times symptoms reflecting neuro-motor deterioration may stabilize for various periods of time. Speech problems occur, involving both difficulties in articulation and difficulties when attempting to maintain the control of the respiratory processes underlying speech.

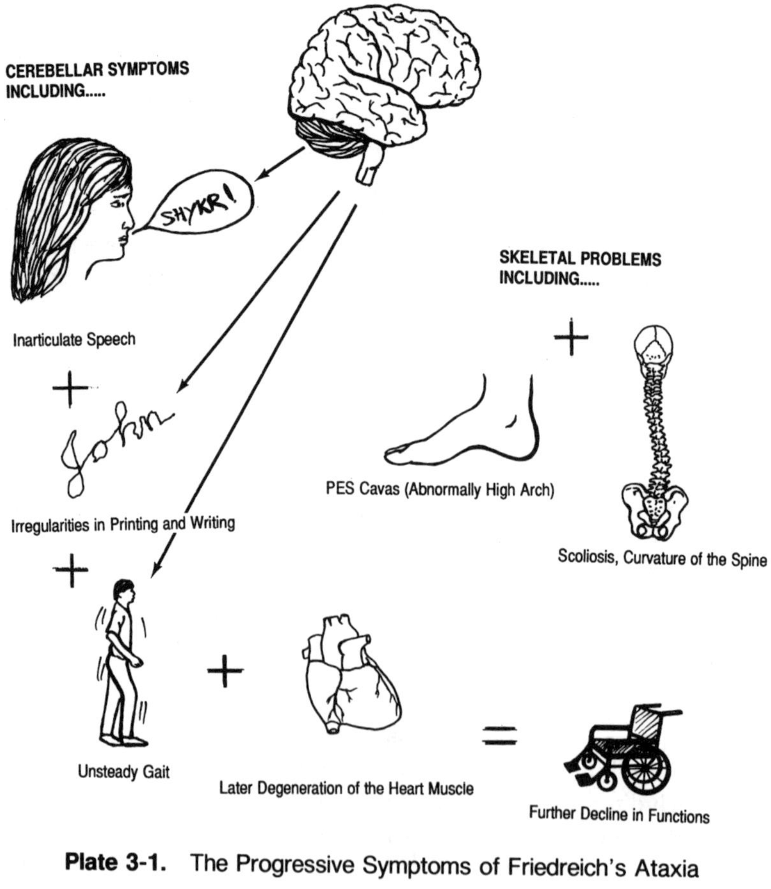

Plate 3-1. The Progressive Symptoms of Friedreich's Ataxia

Other symptoms include retinal degeneration, as well as problems with bladder control. Menkes (1974) and others recommend effective movement therapy, involving carefully taught motor tasks, for children exhibiting this condition. Moreover most experts suggest that these youngsters should remain active as long as possible, and should be encouraged to acquire appropriate recreational skills of reasonable difficulty.

Ataxia-telangiectasia

The second most prevalent type of progressive ataxia seen in children is termed Ataxia-Telangiectasia (also labeled *Louis–Bar's Syndrome*). This condition was first identified in the 1970s. Many early signs of motor incoordination exhibited by these children appear similar to those seen in other types of progressive ataxias, involving the atrophy of cells in the cerebellum. The condition, however, is not accompanied by skeletal mal-formations as is seen in Friedreich's Ataxia. The motor symptoms of Ataxia Telangiectasia may be masked by normal development until the third to sixth year of life, as is sometimes true of similar progressive problems.

When the symptoms begin to appear they can include athetoid-like movements, instability of the trunk, tremors in the hands, abnormal eye movements include nystagmus, and general muscular weakness. Other problems that may be present include diabetes, the appearance of tumors, problems in the immune system as well as mental retardation. The condition first may first present motor symptoms resembling Friedreich's Ataxia. A clear and differentiated diagnosis, however, is relatively easy when various signs emerge including ocular and cutaneous lesions are considered. (Jerusalem & Bischoff 1972).

Like children with other progressive ataxias, those manifesting Ataxia-Telangiectasia, should be exposed to motor development therapy of moderate intensity. Easily acquired recreational skills should also be taught. However stemming the ultimate course of this condition, and of similar problems, is not possible at the present time.

Other Progressive Conditions

Other syndromes partially involve the progressive deterioration of parts nervous system regulating motor functions. These motor symptoms may include pathological conditions that are the result of the growth of tumors in the spinal cord, the frontal areas, in the cerebellum and in other parts of the central nervous system, including the visual pathways, and the mid-brain. In addition to adequate medical diagnoses and treatment, these problems are at least initially blunted by help in the form of developmentally oriented therapy intended to slow the deterioration of motor qualities in the involved youngster.

MUSCULAR DYSTROPHIES

Muscular dystrophy is a categorical term that includes several conditions involving deterioration of the muscles and of their neural connections (motor units). These conditions include diseases of the motor neuron including poliomyelitis, and spinal muscular atrophy (Werdnig Hoffmann disease); diseases involving the deterioration of the axon, aberrations of the neuromuscular junction including myasthenia gravis; and pathologies of the muscle itself including myotonic dystrophy (or atrophy), and muscular dystrophy.

Muscular dystrophy is inherited, and the muscle itself is the site of the disease process. It is marked by a gradual appearance in early childhood marked by symptoms that include a loss of muscle tone, diminished deep tendon reflexes, and an apparent enlargement of the muscles, particularly in the lower legs (pseudo-hypertrophy). An accumulation of fat cells between diseased and atrophied muscle cells is partly responsible for this false enlargement of muscles seen in children with this condition.

Muscular dystrophy is accompanied by degeneration in cardiac muscle, and also a breakdown of imperative muscles in the pulmonary system, including the diaphragm. This deterioration eventually leads to death. Accompanying inactivity can also produce obesity in the children afflicted with the muscular dystrophies. Additionally muscular dystrophy may be accompanied by mental retardation in some youngsters, a diminution of mental functioning t believed to be caused by modifications of nerve cells within the cortex.

Although a great deal of investigative work has been conducted, the precise causes of the various types of muscular dystrophies is not entirely clear. Among the hypotheses vigorously pursued is the supposition that the condition is caused by various anomalies within in muscle protein. Although there are three types of muscular dystrophy, the general symptoms are similar.

The two kinds of muscular dystrophy that appear in childhood include Duchenne's type, appearing earlier; and the less prevalent Facioscapulahumeral type, usually not seen until later in childhood. The fascioscapulahumeral type affects the face, the shoulder and upper arm, and deterioration is not as rapid as in Duchenne's. A third type, Limb-girdle muscular dystrophy, does not occur until the teens, and is not as likely to occur as are the other two kinds.

The symptoms of the Duchenne's type are often subtle and appear early in childhood simply as signs of muscular weakness. Duchenne's type of muscular dystrophy is the most prevalent, and appears in one child in about 25,000. The condition is transmitted through sex-linked recessive manner.

During the pre-school years young children afflicted with Duchenne's type of muscular dystrophy may be seen having problems arising from the floor. They may need to first lock their legs, and then use their hands to 'walk' up their legs until an upright position is attained. This 'Gower's sign' is one of the first indicators of the presence of the condition, and may be accompanied by the enlargement of the lower legs as was described above, accompanied by a tightness of the hamstrings.

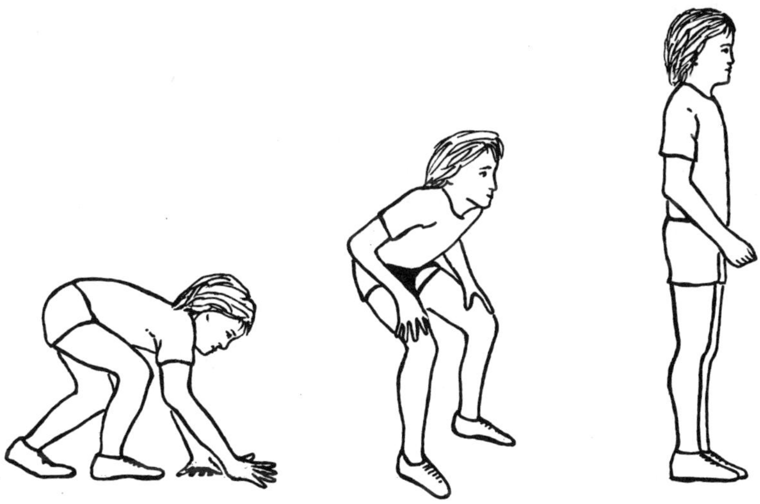

Plate 3-2. Gower's sign of the early onset of muscular dystrophy "Gower's Sign" is seen as a child attempts to arise by first 'walking with the hands up toward the legs, next straightening the knees, and then attaining an upright position by alternately pushing and moving the hands up the legs until an upright position is attained.

Muscle deterioration is accompanied by degeneration of the heart muscle, due to the same infiltration of fatty cells. The cells in the heart muscle also become more fibrous. Mental retardation seen in some children with Duchenne's muscular dystrophy was earlier believed to be due to the presence of the physical handicap. Recently, however, retardation has been attributed to modifications within the cortical cells.

Motor development therapy seems most effective, in lessening the rate of deterioration, if the program is initiated early in the life of the child and contains tasks of moderate intensity. Various hormonal and steroid therapies are currently being researched with some success. Day-care workers, and others dealing with pre-school age children should be aware of the subtle early signs that children afflicted with the dystrophies may evidence, so that early and appropriate medical referral and diagnosis takes place.

INHERITED NON-PROGRESSIVE CONDITIONS

Tourette's Syndrome

Tourette's syndrome was first identified in the last century as a group of symptoms that include various types of involuntary motor tics, single-cycle spasms, together with vocal tics consisting of both meaningful and nonsensical utterances. It is the most prevalent of a group of tic disorders, and is typically first seen in childhood. In recent years Tourette's syndrome has attracted the attention of the general public, partly because of an increased number of children diagnosed with the problem, and also because of the tendency of some to utter obscene vocal tics (Cohen 1988). The problem appears to be inherited, through the mother, based upon data from twin and family studies (Shapiro & Shapiro 1986). Tourettes occurs among boys about four times more often than among girls.

Thorough surveys focusing upon the prevalence of motor awkwardness within this population are not available. These youngsters have been found to exhibit attentional deficits, learning disabilities, and several kinds of obsessive behaviors. Thus thorough studies of their coordination and movement capacities also should be useful. The tic episodes they display, involving both unusual verbal and motor outbursts, typically disrupt normal classroom functioning and their efforts at play.

It is thus believed essential that youngsters with this condition receive help in learning and executing essential motor tasks. Several children, evidencing this disorder, seen recently in our clinic, evidenced problems in carrying out play skills at expected levels for prolonged periods of time, as well as difficulties when printing and writing.

The tic episodes that result in a diagnosis of Tourettes may appear as early as one year. Typically, however, by five or six years of age the majority of youngsters with various forms of this syndrome are diagnosed (Shapiro 1986). The tic symptoms seen in various youngsters differ widely. They range from spasmatic movements of the head and face, and may also include the less frequently seen movements of the trunk and lower limbs. Vocal episodes (tics) are also heard in about 30% of all youngsters diagnosed with Tourettes. These vocalizations can include noises made by the tongue and throat, repeating phrases spoken by others (echolalia), socially unacceptable words and phrases (corprolalia) and may even include expressing obscene gestures.

Sensory tics may also be present, in addition to the over 300 vocal and movement tics that have been classified among this population of youngsters. These unusual sensory-perceptual experiences are reflected in reports by youngsters that they experience recurrent feelings of sensations in the joints, bones, and muscles. (Shapiro & Shapiro 1988). Some of these youngsters have reported that they need to move around to relieve these annoying sensations. Sensory-perceptual tics may also include unexplained feelings of lightness, of heat , and/or of cold.

The treatment that seems most promising includes biochemical interventions, in the form of neuroleptic drugs that alter dopamine transmission. These have sometimes altered tic severity (Shapiro 1988). These drugs, including Haloperidol and Primozide, have been found to reduce tics by from 50-60%. However, their use has reportedly produced unwanted side effects in from 40-60% of the youngsters to whom they have been administered. These side effects include those of which a teacher-therapist should be aware, and may include increased hyperactivity and distractibility, social problems, and school phobias, as well as loss of memory.

Other physiological side effects reported include constipation and weight gain. Thus the administration of the drugs appear appropriate only for youngsters displaying the most marked and frequent symptoms of Tourettes. (Jankovic 1986). Non-neuroleptic drugs have also been used including Chlonidine, which seems to "down-regulate" neurons in the brain, although it is reportedly less effective than the other agents discussed. (Cohen 1988).

Some have suggested that psychological-psychogenic factors trigger the appearance of Tourette's symptoms. For example it has been found that the tics represent an outpouring of suppressed sexual or aggressive tendencies. These hypotheses have sometimes prompted some clinicians to employ psychotherapy as part of the treatment of Tourette's youngsters. (Cohen 1988).

Behavioral modification has also been used, with limited success, in efforts to diminish the symptoms evidenced. Youngsters have been rewarded either for suppressing a vocal or motor tic, and/or substituting an appropriate action or word for undesirable ones. A kind of 'flooding' technique has also been used, involving encouraging a child to "over-exercise" a tic by voluntarily expressing it intensely for prolonged periods of time. It is hypothesized that the muscular or psychic fatigue resulting will reduce the incidence and/or intensity of the unwanted mannerism. The data from this and other treatment approaches is not encouraging, relative to the production of long-term permanent changes.

Young-patients have also been encouraged to try to willfully suppress their ticks. Relaxation training has also been shown to be helpful in the short-term reduction of motor tics. Although only moderately successful, these behavioral-psychological efforts may have the advantages of offering individual emotional support, and attention to these socially and emotionally disrupted youngsters. (Cohen 1988).

In summary the results of therapy, or the self-efforts of the child-patients, when attempting to control tics, may result in changes of short durations. Often, after a short period during which they have been suppressed, the tics then will suddenly burst out in intense episodes as though their suppression has somehow resulted in additional pressures building up which need to be relieved after a period of their non-expression. However some hope may be obtained from the consistent finding that the incidence of tics tend to diminish as the youngsters get older.

Therapists attempting to improve academic, social-emotional and motor skills of children diagnosed as evidencing Tourette's syndrome should attempt to conduct or to obtain a detailed evaluation of the unique symptoms each youngster may evidence. There are currently two scales available for this type of assessment. These include The

Shapiro Tourette Syndrome Severity Scale, (Shapiro & Shapiro 1988), and the Tourettes Syndrome Global Scale (Shapiro & Shapiro 1988). These measurement instruments evaluate the frequency, type, and social impact of the tics experienced and expressed. Furthermore, while administering motor and academic therapy, the behaviors of medicated youngsters should be carefully observed in order to detect the appearance of any undesirable side-effects that may occur.

These youngsters should be dealt with patiently and with compassion, as the tic-behaviors they evidence cause them severe social trauma among their peers, and often with adults with whom they come in contact. The introduction of motor tasks including playground skills, and printing-writing activities should be done patiently and sequentially, with care taken not to further frustrate these emotionally volatile youngsters.

DOWN SYNDROME

This syndrome was first identified in the last century by an English physician, James Langdon-Down. Searches for the cause of this condition, conducted throughout the 19th century, finally terminated in the 1950s when the invention of the powerful electron microscope permitted genetic scientists to observe the chromosomal aberrations that mark this syndrome. Down Syndrome is currently the most prevalent chromosomal abnormality seen in children.

Abnormalities of the genetic-chromosomal material of which the cells are made up, appear by the third week after conception, and usually involves a breaking away of the 15th chromosome, and the formation of an additional chromosome (an extra #21). Thus the cells of most Downs youngsters contain 47 rather than 46 chromosomes. Thus in essence the Down youngster is a genetic mutation, and is likely to evidence deficiencies and abnormalities in many, if not most, bodily systems and structures. Twenty to sixty percent evidence abnormalities of cardio-vascular function including the presence of congenital heart disease, and ventricular septal deficits. Other abnormalities include gastrointestinal problems, and mal formation of the spine, particularly of the upper cervical region which may produce neurological symptoms (Dzenitis, 1966) (Cooke 1984).

Marked hypotonia, coupled with a hyperextensibility of the joints, are among the primarily muscular symptoms of children evidencing various types of Down Syndrome (Morris et al 1982). At birth, infants with Down Syndrome, are easily recognizable. Their unique almond shaped eyes, and the presence of other easily identifiable facial and bodily characteristics, enables their early diagnosis. They do not present the difficulties encountered when assessing infants with other types of developmental problems discussed in this chapter.

The Down's youngster, by the second and third years of life, characteristically evidences measurable delays in motor as well as in intellectual and linguistic development. In contrast, during these same years of early childhood, the abilities of normal infants have been described as exploding!

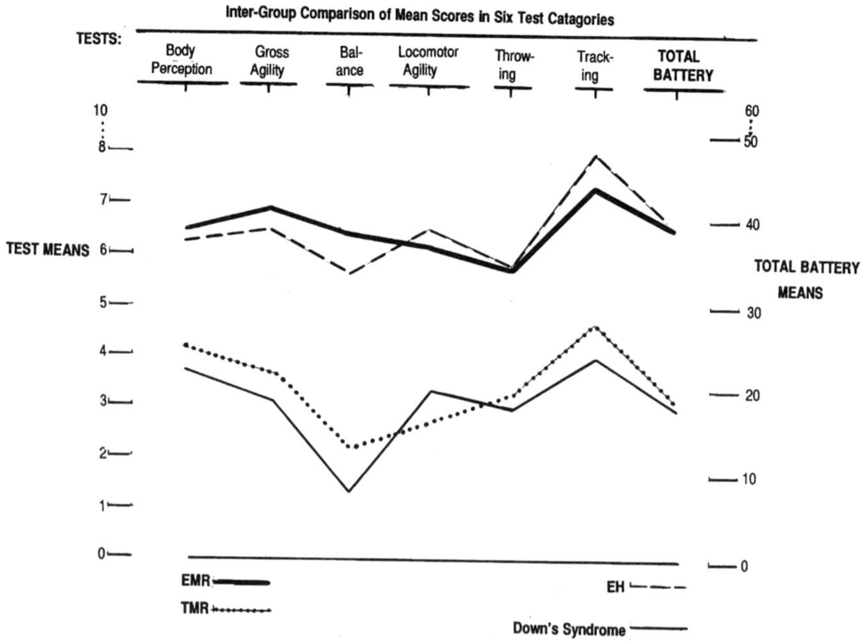

Chart 3-3. Inter-group comparisons of the motor abilities of retarded children

The data indicates that Down Syndrome youngsters scored lower on tests of motor ability than any other sub-groups, including various classifications of retarded youngsters. Moreover the EH Classification, Educationally Handicapped, scored lower on three of these sub-tests than did children classified as Educable Mentally Retarded.

The deficiencies of Down youngsters are also reflected in the late acquisition of walking, a skill that is sometimes not mastered until the third year of life. Problems are also encountered when attempting to reproduce intelligible speech. Graphic skills also are delayed. Although there are marked individual differences among Down Syndrome youngsters, the average group of Downs Youngsters are from two to four years behind normal youngsters in most motor abilities. (Cratty 1967).

They are measurable genetic differences between the two most prevalent types of Down youngsters, the trisomy and translocation groups. However behaviorally, and developmentally, members of the two groups are indistinguishable. In contrast, however, are the characteristics of a rare third category, the "moziac type," in which only a portion (about 10%) of whose cells evidence chromosomal abnormalities. Members of this third sub-group may evidence only minor motor and intellectual problems, and at times are never diagnosed.

Down youngsters evidence marked inter-individual differences in various aspects of development, including movement capacities. Some are mute, while others can carry on lengthy, socially acceptable conversations. Some are markedly retarded, while others can read at the first or second grade level. However due to a variety of neurological problems, and developmental delays virtually all require extensive practice to acquire rudimentary self-care tasks, and to engage in simple recreational and printing skills. For example the frontal lobes of the cortex, and the optic pathways remain under developed (lackcomplete mylination), and thus their ability to easily acquire visual stimuli and then to process the information are likely to be poor. Downs youngsters characteristically lack adequate balance, while the integration of input and output in tasks requiring the sequencing of a series of actions is also likely to be deficit.

Despite this seemingly gloomy picture of their potential reflected in inherent neurological problems, it has been found that motor development programs when carefully applied early in the lives of Down children may produce positive outcomes. Likewise carefully programmed educational efforts often have produced good results. (Esenther 1984) (Connolly et al 1980) (McInerney et al (1982) Contemporary efforts to control their diets, and stem the obesity that was formerly characteristic of these youngsters also has proved useful.

CEREBRAL PALSY

For several decades that been noted that signs of clumsiness in children often appear as mild to moderate forms of cerebral palsy (Gubbay 1974) (Walton et al 1962) (Dare and Gordon 1970). The problem is that there is no way to "pathologically confirm" cerebral palsy in clumsy children as is sometimes possible when a child evidences obvious forms of cerebral palsy. Electroencephalographic evidence, coupled with other traditional forms of neural assessments usually fail to confirm specific neuropathologies which may accompany moderate motor ineptitude in children. Clinicians have also reported over the years that mild clumsiness appears in the form of cerebral-palsy sub-types. Presently at our clinic are three children who evidence mild ataxias. The movement patterns of another half dozen reveal mild spastic qualities.

It thus seems that cerebral palsy, as a non-progressive central nervous system condition producing poor coordination, should be considered as a continuum. Some 'neurological intact and healthy children fall outside the diagnosis entirely. Other youngsters, however, exhibit symptoms that place them at various points on a 'motor scale: with some evidencing mild "soft" motor signs, others exhibiting more marked clumsiness. Still others possess markedly aberrant movement characteristics that place them within various cerebral palsied sub-groups as these categories are traditionally diagnosed.

Cerebral palsy, meaning brain paralysis, is a broad term which refers to non-progressive types of motor coordination problems, due to insults to the central nervous system. Most of the time cerebral palsy is present at birth, however a small percent of those with this kind of affliction have incurred damage to the neural centers controlling movement as the result of oxygen deprivation to the brain (hypoxia) occurring around the time of birth. Accidents during childhood, peri-natal and post-natal viral infections or poisoning from toxic chemicals, may also produce mild to marked symptoms of cerebral palsy.

Common Causes

Oxygen Deprivation

A main cause of cerebral palsy is some degree of oxygen deprivation occurring at birth. All structures of the body are susceptible to hypoxic injury prior to, or during, birth; however most vulnerable

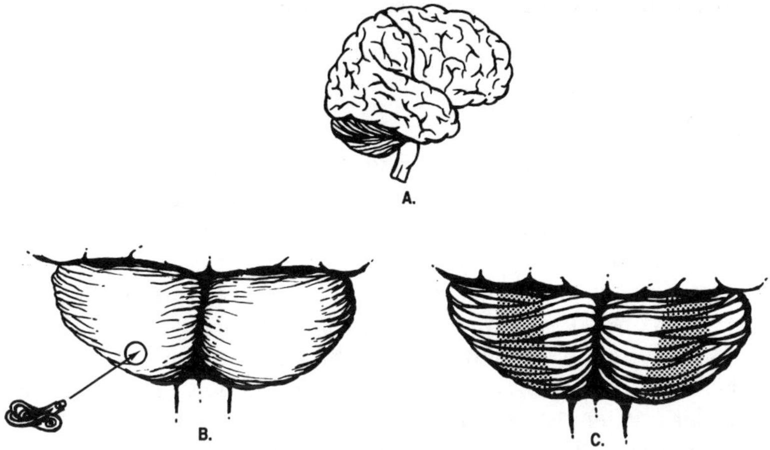

Shown from the rear in B and C, the cerebellum has numerous functions including the mediation of balance, B. and of motor programs involved in the control of rapid, skilled and well integrated movements requiring the coordination of the hands and arms, as shown in the shaded areas in C.

Plate 3-4. Functional areas of the cerebellum
Located just above the brain stem, the cerebellum has traditionally been designated as the organ that smoothes and refines motor programs. It is a neurologically primative organ appearing in evolution, when some sea animals left the sea and acquired limbs. Thus requiring a neural structure to mediate limb position.

are structures within the central nervous system. Problems encountered by the pre-mature infant, including short episodes during which breathing terminates, results in hypoxic reactions, damage to the respiratory centers themselves, and other functional problems such as a compressed or entangled umbilical cord. Severe hypoxia may cause death.

When oxygen deprivation to the brain occurs is likely to influence the type of damage incurred and also the developmental delays later encountered. For example, if oxygen deprivation occurs early during gestation the deeper layers of the brain including the several centers, controlling movement storage and programming, are likely to be influenced. If apoxia is encountered later in development, damage is likely to be seen in the cerebral cortex, and thus associational-thought processes are likely to be disrupted. However cerebral damage within each circumstance may be wide-spread and diffuse, or result in abnormalities related to a more limited area. (Towbin 1970).

Vascular incidents

Vascular accidents prior to, during or shortly after birth also cause motor difficulties ranging from the mild to the severe. These incidents can include rupturing of blood vessels early in fetal formation and thus involve the deeper layers of the central nervous system. In contrast, those occurring later during gestation or shortly after birth are likely to influence more superficial layers of the central nervous system. Near birth the cerebral cortex acquires its venous system, and thus is susceptible to damage due to one or more vascular accidents (mild infarctions).

As is true in the case of hypoxia, vascular incidents are not of an all-or none nature. Vascular accidents and incidents occur to varying degrees, as is true of oxygen deprivation. The resultant neural damage due to infarctions may thus vary markedly. Marked and obvious disruption of the motor systems occurs when these two problems occur in severe proportions, while minor to moderate symptoms of clumsiness are encountered when these problems occur to mild degrees. (Towbin 1987).

Acquired Brain Injuries

A sharp blow to the head is one cause of behavioral abnormalities which reflects trauma to the central nervous system. If no penetration of an object occurs these are sometimes collectively labeled "closed brain injuries." Delineating The precise manner in which behavior will be disturbed is not always possible upon knowing the location of the cranium which has received the blow. Striking the head may thus have unpredictable outcomes. This occurs because the blow can cause a shearing effect, in which surface neurons are scraped in ways that may cause problems difficult to predict. Often swelling produced by a blow in one portion of the brain may cause pressures in other parts, also producing unpredictable outcomes.

We have evaluated children in our clinic who have experienced trauma of this nature either at the hands of abusive caretakers, or as the result of traffic accidents. Other problems in youngsters and adolescents with closed brain injuries due to trauma, can include depression and boredom, and a reluctance to attempt motor tasks that have previously been learned. (Mercer & Bloch 1983). This stems partially from the fact that they have lost abilities they were accustomed to expressing. Their depressing is the mourning of these losses.

The movement symptoms among trauma cases often resemble those in children diagnosed as cerebral palsied. For example one-sided involvement is seen if the child has been struck on one side of the brain. Movement problems in this case appear on the side, opposite to that receiving the blow. Usually the younger the child or youngster incurring head trauma the more likely post-trauma motor functions may be positively modified with remedial efforts. Data indicate that after the middle twenties, recovery from head injuries through therapy becomes significantly more difficult. (Heiden et al 1983) (Talmadge & Collins 1983). A relatively small percent of all children with minor to moderate coordination problems have suffered some kind of head trauma. Children suffering severe head trauma may become comatose with complete recovery unpredictable.

Types of Cerebral Palsy

The various sub-types of cerebral palsy are classified relative to their location on the body and within combinations of limbs, and also by the type of movement qualities that are seen. The types, based upon movement qualities include the random writhings of the athetoid, the tremors of the cerebellar ataxic, and the hypertonicity of the spastic. Each of these types are often assigned a precise cause, which in turn has purportedly caused trauma to as specific part of the central nervous system. In reality, however, determining precise neurological sites influencing each of the several types of movement aberrations collectively termed 'cerebral palsy' is difficult, due to the interdependency of various centers controlling movement within the central nervous system.

In general, however, it is assumed by some that Rh incompatibility which is not rectified at birth is productive of athetosis. Damage to the centers which store motor programs in the central nervous system is often assumed, trauma which then results in disturbed patterns of coordination and movement. However today most potential cases of cerebral palsy are preventable, in developed countries, with the immunization of the mother and with the early exchange transfusion of the newborn infant. Thus remaining as one of the main causes of cerebral palsy, including both athetosis and spasticity.

In the United States prematurity, and its associated medical disorders including hypoxias and vascular incidents, is a pre-condition associated closely with cerebral palsy. Literature reviewed in Chapter 6 in the section dealing with developmental apraxia also strongly suggests that mild forms of motor incoordination are also common among children born pre-maturely. It has been estimated that prematurity accounts for from 33-60% of all cases of cerebral palsy in the United States. (Wright et al 1972). Other causes named for athetoid-like symptoms are prenatal infections in the mother including Rubella during the first three months of pregnancy, as well as others including toxoplasmosis, and other viral infections. The athetoid often constantly expresses random motions, engaging in meaningless and fatiguing writhings that often resemble primitive birth reflexes.

Spastics evidence movement strained and tense movement patterns. There is an absence of relaxed and controlled lengthening of muscle groups, for example, as the arm reaches for an object. The child appears bound by flexion responses on the upper limbs, while the lower limbs often appear to be in constant extension. The causes traditionally assigned to this type of cerebral palsy range from birth anoxia, and trauma, to prematurity and post natal encephalitis. Birth anoxia may occur due to mal-development of the placenta, shock due to blood loss in the mother due to injuries, as well as to a knotting of the umbilical cord.

Likewise birth anoxias may result when labor is prolonged and the birth is difficult. Most of the time it is assumed that the damage has been done to the extrapyraminal pathways (those out side the main motor pathways containing pyramid shaped cells), and to portions of the brain stem (the reticular formation). These portions of the nervous system, in a spastic, seem to have lost their ability to precisely control and to modify the tension of muscles and of movements, and to regulate reciprocal innervation, involving the interplay of flexor and extensor muscles. A rare form of spasticity is also inherited, and usually only involves the lower limbs.

Ataxias may involve damage to the cerebellum from causes not always apparent. It has been speculated also that tremors and unsteadiness seen in some infants stressed prenatally with maternal drug use have incurred cerebellar damage, due to insults to the neural transmitters, as well as to the cerebellum itself. (Cratty 1990) The behavioral manifestations of the ataxic may include an unsteady shaky gait, together with a regular mild to moderate tremor of the upper limbs. The lower limb unsteadiness results in balance problems reflected in an inability to perform various locomotor activities well. Thus the ataxic child has difficulties skipping and hopping and moving laterally in games. If there is unsteadiness in the upper limbs, accurate printing becomes difficult, and the child must learn to "anchor" the arm and wrist to the table when attempting to replicate letters.

Various portions of the cerebellum are assigned the job of refining movements either to the upper or lower limbs, as is true of the sensory-motor cortex itself. Thus damage to a restricted part of the cerebellum may result in symptoms that evidence either a lower or an upper limb ataxia. However, in most cases unsteadiness in both the upper and lower portions of the body, is seen among children who are obviously ataxic, or in clumsy children with mild signs of this condition. An ataxic syndrome seen among groups of clumsy children is described in Chapters 5, and 7.

At the behavioral level mild forms of cerebral palsy pose constant problems to awkward youngsters. The tense child, evidencing minor spasticity, struggles to relax while attempting to learn to print letters. The youngster with mild athetosis draws letters with an unevenness that may puzzle observant teachers and parents. Another youngster with a mild problem managing one side of his or her body (a hemiplegic) has trouble moving laterally with equal skill in both directions, and thus cannot retrieve balls in the outfield. The youngster evidencing mild ataxic symptoms weaves unsteadily in games, and draws figures with troubling oscillations.

The problems encountered by moderately clumsy children when attempting to master motor skills are magnified among cerebral palsied youngsters. In some ways, however, the obviously cerebral palsied child paradoxically may not subjected to as much social censure as may occur when a clumsy child spills a glass of water on a classmate. In this second case the awkward child may be believed by his classmates to have committed an intentional act; whereas the poor coordination among the cerebral palsied is well known by observers to be the result of medical conditions beyond the youngsters' control.

OTHER TYPES AND CAUSES OF MOTOR PROBLEMS IN CHILDREN

Biochemical Insults

Numerous types of biochemical insults may cause neural damage reflected in motor incoordination. One type of problem encountered in large numbers of infants in the 1980's were the influences of drug ingestion by pregnant mothers. These noxious substances include crack cocaine, discussed in the section which follows. Other abusive substances ingested by pregnant mothers including alcohol, and nicotine can cause developmental problems including motor incoordination.(Deren 1986). Lead poisoning, as well as exposure to asbestos may cause problems that are reflected partly in motor incoordination and mental confusions in executing recreational skills and self-care tasks.

Familial Clumsiness

There is relatively little data delineating possible familial influences upon motor awkwardness. It is difficult to separate 'real" inherited factors from the more general familial variables. Poor nutrition, for example, may influence more than one family member and be seen in several generations. Negative attitudes about exposure to vigorous effort that may also prevail in families.

The limited information that is available, however, indicates that familial influences may be influence awkwardness in some children. In a study, involving more than 53,000 women, sponsored by the National Institute of Neurological Diseases and Communicative Disorders, conducted between 1959 and 1965, developmental parameters including motor coordination were contrasted to variables that including family membership. It was found that the probability of a child evidencing signs of neurological dysfunctions, including motor incoordination, were 30% greater when other peers also were delayed motorically. The familial relationships extended also to linkages of moderate neurological dysfunctions among cousins.

In the same study when the presence of motor soft-signs in forty twin pairs were contrasted, the degree of predictability rose even higher (Nichols 1987). Regehr and Kaplan (1988) also have found that motor ineptitude when coupled with learning disabilities are apparently is traceable through families.

Other Insults, and Overview

Numerous other types of insults to, and problems within, the central nervous system may cause motor incoordination of either an obvious and subtle nature. These include tumors of various types that are often the result of little-understood inherited qualities. Tumors within the central nervous system are of numerous kinds. Their type, size and location will influence development in unpredictable ways. A tumor may cause an organ to mal-function, and/or crowd neural structures thus causing problems by their bulky presence. Sometimes surgical and chemical efforts to reduce tumor's effects results in unwanted symptoms including sensory, cognitive and/or motor deficits.

Other problems likely to produce either major or minor motor coordination problems, depending upon their severity, include problems in organ formation, physical injuries, as well as infections resulting in cell death prior to, or at, the time of birth. The results of the delayed or defective formation of structures (organogenosis) within the central nervous system are dealt with in Chapter 5 that follows. Other chapters also contain data from studies using animal models in which lesions induced early in organogenosis have resulted in subsequent anomalies of central nervous system structures.

SUMMARY AND OVERVIEW

In this chapter some of the possible variables and conditions that result in youngsters being labeled as clumsy are discussed. Several of the more common childhood problems that include motor ineptitude as a symptom were also briefly surveyed. Among the conditions covered were two of the most common progressive ataxias, Friedreich's Ataxia and Ataxia-telangiectasia. These problems, although rare, should be considered when observing an awkward and unsteady pre-school child.

It is thus emphasized in this section, and throughout the text, that those conversant only with the behavioral, and not with the medical aspects of neuromotor functions, should *not* assume that an awkward child whom they observe, or assess, is evidencing symptoms that are stable and non-progressive. When working with youngsters evidencing these types of syndromes the treatment-guidelines should be formulated by medical personnel, the work should be started early in life, and the intensity of the motor development program should be mild to moderate in nature.

The nature of muscular dystrophy was also surveyed, including a brief look at early symptoms that children with this progressive condition usually display. Like the progressive ataxias, normal development early in life may mask important signs of the dystrophies that may begin to be seen during the pre-school years. Well planned programs of exercise, and of motor development, instituted early in the life of such children are usually recommended by their medical supervisors.

Two relatively common non-progressive syndromes were also described. These included discussions of the unusual symptoms seen in youngsters afflicted with Tourette's Syndrome, and the movement characteristics encountered among children diagnosed as evidencing Down Syndrome. The genetic mechanisms undergirding Down Syndrome are well known. However the manner in which Tourette's is inherited is not as clear cut. The symptoms displayed by a Down infant are apparent at birth. Tourette's symptoms do not begin to emerge until the second to fifth or sixth years of life.

Youngsters evidencing both syndromes should be exposed to carefully planned programs of physical activity. These efforts if well designed, should make positive contributions to the education and emotional health of these populations. More is known about the motor developmental characteristics of Down children, than is known about children with the tic disorder covered in this section. The presence of random and seemingly meaningless spasms and jerks among Tourette's children make their social integration difficult, and thus make the job of the motor therapist a difficult one. Promising data, appeared in the 1980s, suggested that when early intervention strategies and programs are applied to Down youngsters positive developmental gains are likely to result.

The final part of the chapter contained information about the probable causes of numerous children labeled clumsy. The primary causes discussed included hypoxia and vascular accidents occurring before birth Descriptions of various classic types of cerebral palsy, together with the causes for this kind of problem, were meant to assist in the better understanding of both the sub-types of youngsters classifiable within the highly diverse group known as clumsy children.

It should be emphasized that the brief list of causes and syndromes reviewed here, does not explain the etiology of all clumsy children. Changes in what society does, and what pregnant mothers ingest, are producing new and complex difficulties, some of which are just emerging. Within this context are the thousands of infants born to mothers who are using abusive substances during pregnancy. Although most of their offspring are now within the first year or two or life, it is apparent that these infants are likely to display symptoms later in life, that include distractibility, delays in motor as well as other social and academic problems. (Cratty 1990).

Numerous other conditions and variables may cause physical awkwardness, including inherited-genetic factors, familial life-styles. A significant percent of parents whose children we evaluate in our clinic report that they also experienced problems related to physical awkwardness when they were children. There are some indications in the literature that motor awkwardness, particularly when coupled with learning disabilities, have familial origins (Nichols 1987) (Regehr & Kalpan 1988). However, more research appears needed to clarify just how general awkwardness may persist in families.

QUESTIONS FOR DISCUSSION

1. Discuss why some kinds of progressive conditions may not be seen immediately after birth, and are not evidenced until during the later pre-school years?
2. What is Gower's Sign? What presence of what condition does this behavior reflect?
3. What types of muscular dystrophy might a child evidence? What early and later symptoms may be seen in children with various types of muscular dystrophy?
4. What are the symptoms of the two progressive ataxias described in the chapter? What are remedial principles that should be followed, relative to recreational skills and fitness training?
5. Why might a motor development specialist refer a child with coordination problems to a more thorough medical evaluation when motor problems are diagnosed?
6. What are various types of Down Syndrome? What movement qualities are likely to be seen among children evidencing each type?
7. What are the various types of cerebral palsy seen in children? What are the symptoms seen in each type? In what major way does cerebral palsy differ from the progressive ataxias described in the chapter?
8. Explain the concept that symptoms reflecting cerebral palsy should be considered on a continuum?
9. Discuss familial clumsiness? What are the social and emotional implications of awkwardness among more than one family member?
10. What other variables, surveyed in this chapter, may cause delays in motor development. Can you think of other factors not covered in this chapter that could lead to awkwardness?

Chapter 4
Organogenesis and Development Deficits

INTRODUCTION

In the previous chapter some of the more prevalent syndromes, containing movement deficits were described. With these descriptions etiologies were also discussed, reflecting anomalies of neural structures and biochemical-muscular processes. In this chapter selected cellular level causes for developmental deficits in the central nervous system are surveyed. These microscopic problems may result in incoordination, because of faulty formation of neural organs and networks early in the development of the fetus and neonate.

Two processes are covered in this chapter. The first of these, *cell migration,* occurs during the time the nervous system and its structures are formed. Cell migration is the name give to the manner in which the cells are transported along carrier (glial) cells to form parts of the central and peripheral nervous system.

The second mechanism, *neural regression,* begins later in development, overlaps cell migration in time, and continues into adulthood. Neural regression refers to the manner in which the nervous system apparently rids itself of unneeded cells and connections. Neural regression is a "pruning-away process" that eventually eliminates from forty to fifty percent of the neurons initially generated.

Initially most models of human maturation postulated during the first decades of this century were behaviorally-based (Piaget 1954) (Cratty 1969) (Erickson 1950). During the 1970's, however, some researchers began to explore several, potentially important, neurobiological accompaniments to maturation. These experimentalists, employing both animal and human models, focused upon several ways that the maturing nervous system changes and is formed, during the pre-natal and post-natal periods.

The prolific developmental psychologist T.G.R. Bowers emphasized the need to delve into neural mechanisms in his text written in the middle 1970's. Bowers explained that the imperative theoretical question, 'how development takes place', could be best responded to by exploring finite neurological mechanisms underlying observable behavioral changes occurring during maturation. (Bowers 1975: page 425). Biophysiologists, some of whose work is reviewed below, responded to Bower's challenge.

Among the important maturational processes explored are the ways in which neural cells migrate and attach themselves to sensory end organs and to muscles. The manner in which neurons migrate to form neural structures is another sub-process involving neural migration that also has been investigated. (Rakic, 1977). Still other mechanisms researched have included the ways in which a normally maturing nervous system seems to "prune away" apparently excess cells, dendritic processes, and networks during maturation (Carlson, Earls, and Todd, 1988). This second process has been labeled neural regression.

The findings from the laboratories of these experimental neurobiologists are affording potentially useful insights into the nature of maturation. These data also are also assisting to explain the occurrence of developmental problems, including delays in motor coordination.

Some of this emerging information has begun to illuminate more clearly, and to substantiate some of the concepts proposed in earlier behavioral models of maturation by Piaget, and others. Comparing these newer neurological insights to speculations about how both normal and atypical behaviors emerge is beginning to offer new directions for additional research. Merging knowledge about neural mechanisms and of cellular level neurological changes to behavioral indices of maturation, should also result in application of new and useful neurobiological and medical interventions. This information, furthermore, should produce more effective educational-enrichment strategies intended to blunt or to reverse developmental delays, than are currently available.

The first sections contain descriptions of two neurological mechanisms; cell migration and neural regression. Second reference is made to the nature of various insults that may occur as the nervous system is developing. Third, various types of motor developmental problems will be considered as possible reflections of abnormal cell migration and neural regression.

In the final parts of the chapter, the nature of developmental problems within two atypical populations is examined. One of these groups is composed of awkward children, the second consists of infants subjected to maternal drug use. In this latter group motor problems present themselves at birth. Developmental abnormalities, including poor motor coordination, appear to plague many throughout childhood. The chapter concludes with a brief discussion of implications for more effective programs of infant stimulation and remedial interventions.

NEURAL MECHANISMS

Cell Migration

During the third week after conception, the nervous system emerges as a groove, along the back of the embryo. This groove then folds, forming the neural tube. By the end of the fourth week the neural tube also begins to fold, and due to an unequal amount of cell division along its length, gives rise to several bulges. These swellings later form the major components of the central nervous system including the cerebral hemispheres, the mid-brain, the cerebellum, and brain stem.

In primates, cell division along the ventral lining of this groove provides neurons, some of which then migrate toward the outermost layers of the cortex. Migration proceeds at different rates in various components of the central nervous system. For example, within the cortex, cell migration is completed normally between the 24th and 32nd weeks of gestation. Cell migration in other central structures, including the cerebellum, continue to take place after birth.

The general way which this migration takes place has researched for several decades. It is known that neurons move along the lengths of special support cells, or glial cells. These transport-glial cells carry the neurons to their final resting places to the several layers of the cortex, the cerebellum and to other parts of the central nervous system. The neurons that are generated first are laid down at levels deeper within the organs involved. Neurons formed later travel along pre-programmed routes to layers that are closer to the surface of the cortex and to other structures formed. This process reflects the principle of neural maturation termed, "inside to outside" .

Still unclear, however, are nature of the precise biochemical-neurological mechanisms causing these millions of neurons to find their proper places, initially to specific glial transport cells, and then to "assigned" layers in structures such as the cortex, mid-brain, and cerebellum. The general way in which transport occurs has been confirmed by staining techniques including the injection and tracking of radioactive thymidine, which is incorporated into the DNA

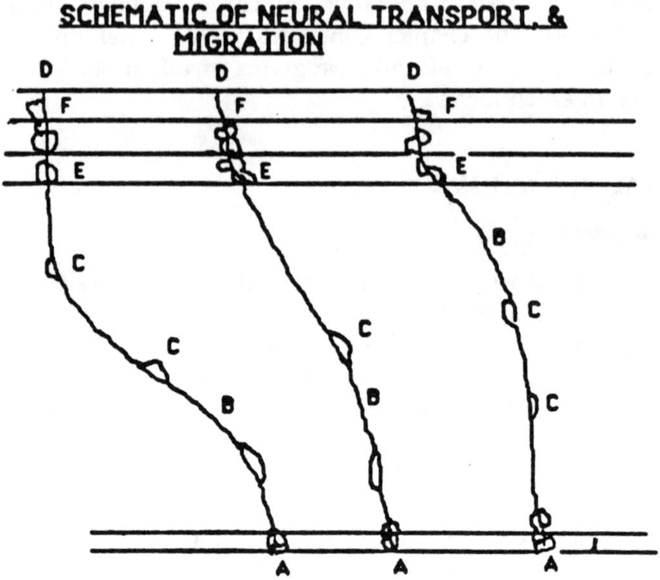

Plate 4-1. Schematic neural transport and migration cells (C) move from initial zones (A), along transport glial cells (B) to developing cortical plates (D) newly arrived cells move to superficial layers (F) by passing cells (E) which have been laid down earlier

shortly before cell division (Purvis & Lichtman 1985). However, the delineation of the precise bio-neurological processes which cause certain neurons to travel to pre-designated glial-transport cells, and then along their lengths, to specific locations within the central nervous system, is not clearly understood.

Contemporary speculations about the complex mechanisms mediating how neurons travel and arrive at their "intended" locations, include references to the formation of biochemical affinities that cause specific neuron-glial pairings. These combinations of cells it has been hypothesized, are triggered by enzymes. However, the precise nature of mechanisms governing these attractions continue to be investigated. (Levitt & Rakic, 1980)

Problems occurring during cellular level processes undergirding maturation of neural structures, and thus of behavioral functions these structures mediate, may be manifested in numerous ways among various developmentally atypical populations. These problems include movement aberrations seen in drug-stressed neonates and infants, and in various symptoms reflecting incoordination and hyperactivity in physically awkward children.

Neural Regression

A number of complex micromechanisms take place within the developing nervous system. These include the aforementioned cell migration, as well as cell division and proliferation, cell adhesion, dendritic branching, and other processes reflected in the formation of structures that assume essential supportive functions. One of these processes attracting the attention of experimental neurologists and of embryologists with increased frequency is termed neural regression.

Neural regression refers to the tendencies of a normally developing nervous system to evidence selective cell death. This mechanism is reflected in the elimination of extraneous and apparently unneeded dendritic connections. The presence of too few cells and networks, is labeled *dedifferentiation*. The overabundance of nerve cells and neuronal networks is termed hyperdifferentiation. The material in this section thus deals with the problem of hyperdifferentiation.

Pioneer work by Hamberger and Levi-Montalcini (1949) began to illuminate this processes over fifty years age. Their germinal research has led to more contemporary investigations further clarifying how this 'pruning' of the nerve cells, and of neural connections, takes place. (Hamberger, 1980). Initially investigators, using chick embryos, found that cells within the sensory ganglia normally atrophy as maturation takes place (Hamberger & Levi, 1949).

Subsequent studies, explored the formation of several neural structures, using other animal models. The emerging data indicated that about fifty percent of all cells initially produced within the central nervous systems of primates, and in other animals, eventually die. It thus began to appear that an initial overproduction of nerve cells taking place during the fetal period, is followed by a second phase during which the elimination of apparently unneeded neurons takes place.

In vertebrates these regressive processes usually occur prenatally, within various neural structures reflecting this process at different times in development. In humans, however, neural regressive processes apparently continue into at least the fourth decade of life. Evidence exists that, for example, in the frontal cortex of humans, normal neuronal death continues to occur during adolescence and into adulthood. (Huttenlocher, 1979).

In the 1980's researchers employing invertebrate models concluded that neural regression is programmed by the cell itself. (Horvitz et al, 1982). One of the two sister cell dies as soon as cell division occurs. Among vertebrates, however, programmed cell death has not been similarly documented, perhaps because cell lineages and linkages are more difficult to study, as they are more numerous than is usually true within simpler nervous systems.

In vertebrates cell death has been attributed also to a second mechanism involving neural interactions with "targets" that include other neurons, and also muscles and glands. This second process first involves first the production of too many neurons for a given target, and then later the elimination of excess neural connections when the target structure begins to function.

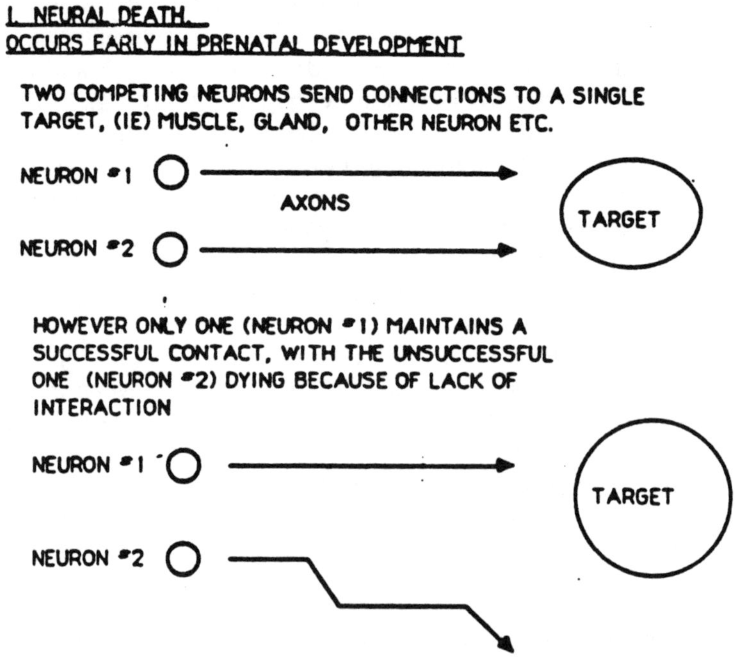

Plate 4-2. Neural regression; neuronal death

Experimentally this phenomenon has been replicated in two types of investigations. For example, in ablation studies, after a given "target cell" has been eliminated, the neurons and their dendrites that were attached to the target-structure then die. Illustrating this are the results of an early study by Hamberger and Levi (1949). They found that the removal of a of chick's limb bud resulted in death to connecting neurons. In contrast when a target is increased in size then more neurons are apparently produced. In a 1980 study by Hamberger, for example, the implantation of an extra limb bud seemed to 'salvage' neurons that would normally have died.

A second mechanism resulting in neural death, occurring during neural maturation, involves the elimination of one, of two, connections to a given neuron, when only a single connection is eventually required. Most studies of cell death have employed organisms possessing relatively simple nervous systems. However, researchers studying the elimination of dendritic processes have also employed primate species, including humans. In humans, cell elimination has been found to occurs primarily before birth; however, the elimination of dendritic connections apparently continues into the post natal period.

Nerve reduction processes have been found to occur in the auditory, visual and somato-sensory cortexes of both primates and humans. For example, in the human visual cortex synaptic density is highest at eight to twelve months of age, and then decreases by about 40% in adulthood (Huttenlocher et al, 1982). Some of the most elegant work of this nature has been conducted by Weisel, 1982), and by Hubel (1977) and his colleagues. In addition Rakic (1977) has investigated neural regressive processes within the visual cortex of primates.

Several hypotheses have been advanced in efforts to explain the reasons for the normal death of neurons and the elimination of dendritic connections during maturation. The process is believed by some, for example, to represent a 'fine tuning' of the nervous system, resulting in the precise matching of neurons to target tissues of various sizes (Hamberger and Oppenheimer, 1982). Other scholars have proposed that neural regressive processes produce 'healthy' nervous systems that are better nourished by available nutrients. In contrast is normal cell-network elimination does not take place, and the nervous system retains an overabundance of nerve cells and of neural networks less efficient use will be made of available biochemical nourishment.

Researchers have also begun to speculate that aberrations or interruptions of normal cell death and/or of useful dendritic elimination result in various types of unwanted behavioral con-

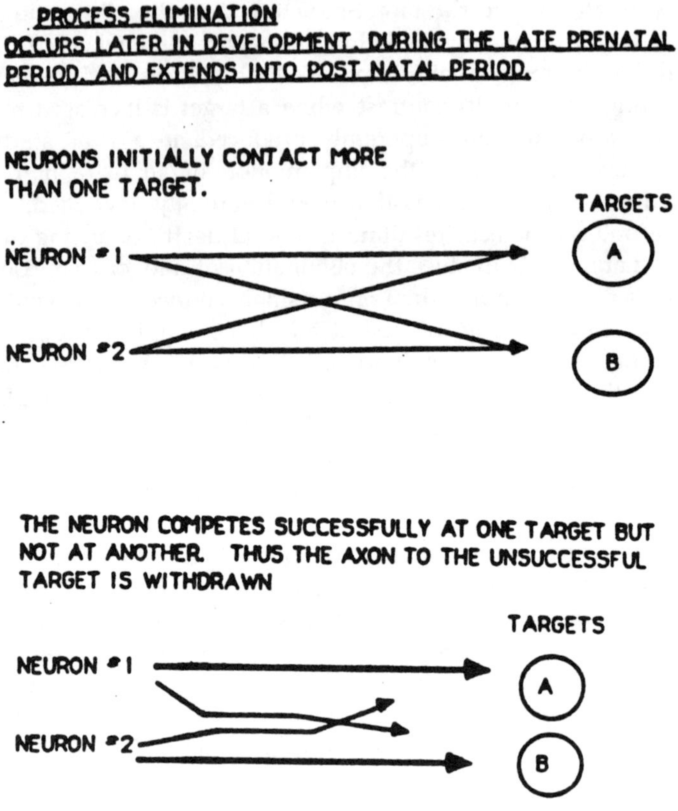

Plate 4-3. Neural regression: process elimination

sequences (Carlson, Earls and Todd, 1987). Among the problems explored have included the disruption of perceptual-motor processes, speech difficulties, and the appearance of negative personality traits, including distractibility (Carlson, Earls, and Todd, 1987).

Among the hypotheses that have been proposed is that various symptoms, including marked by hyper-reactivity of the sensory or/and of the motor systems, are caused by defective nervous systems in which normal cell regression has not occurred. In the following sections the symptoms reviewed include, hyperactivity, developmental anomalies seen among drug-stressed neonates, and selected characteristics of youngsters with coordination problems.

DEVELOPMENTAL DEFICITS, BEHAVIORAL OUTCOMES

Introduction

Numerous developmental deficits may be attributable to anomalies in cell migration, the presence of insults or of lesions in the central nervous system. Other problems can be traced to anomalies in the manner in which layers of cells are laid down within various structures including the cerebral cortex. Aberrant clusters of misplaced cells, termed plaques, are also cited as disruptions in neural development, leading to both academic and to sensory-motor problems. (Duane 1991).

Still other difficulties may be caused by defects in neural regression, and hypothetically may consist of various symptoms reflecting hyper-sensitive to different types of environmental stimuli. The appearance of these symptoms thus may suggest that the individual is '"over-wired". These symptoms may be reflected in several types of aberrant behaviors, that may include hyper-reactivity, and the presence of excess motor activity.

Hyperactivity

Hyperactivity and/or deficits in attention have been given numerous labels since scholars began to become interested in distractible children during the 1930's. One of the more recent labels applied to distractible children is *attentional deficit disorder* (ADD). This label continues to be expanded due to the observation that attention deficits are often coupled with hyperactivity. Thus recently the observation that an attention deficit coupled with hyperactivity is seen displayed by many dysfunctional youngsters has resulted in an elaboration of the term.(ADHA).

This collection of symptoms may be expressed, and observed, in a variety of ways. Some children may be seen to move too often around a classroom, leaving their seats at inappropriate times. Other children bearing these labels may remain relatively immobile, but display constant and inappropriate manipulative behaviors. Still a third type of youngster may not evidence distractibility physically, but display cognitive inattention. This latter symptom is seen as youngsters allow their thoughts and/or eyes to stray to subjects irrelevant to the lesson, or situation. It is common, however, to find a child expressing this type of upset in a variety of ways, by evidencing distractible, hyperactive, as well as impulsive behaviors when confronted with various situations throughout the day.

The causes for these symptoms may be classified into two main groups. One group includes including behaviors having social-emotional roots. This would include hyperactive and avoidance behaviors caused by too permissive, or overly abusive, parenting. The avoidance of difficult school work because of a perceived threat to the self-esteem, constitutes can still another emotional-social cause for hyperactivity.

A second group of causes is labeled, with little precision, as 'neurological.' The neurological underpinnings of inappropriate attention, however, might include defects in numerous structures and systems within the central nervous system. Among those neural centers blamed for undue distractibility are portions of the brain stem. The reticular formation, for example, has sometimes been named as a mediator of attention. However other structures also cited as causing hyperactivity, including portions of the mid-brain controlling, or failing to control, feelings and emotional behavior. Problems within the visual centers located in the frontal cortex, controlling 'gaze' characteristics, also may make it difficult for a children to to rest their eyes for prolonged periods of time upon appropriate targets and tasks.

Another set of structures whose malfunctions may contribute to hyperactivity are portions of the basal ganglia. The basal ganglia, when functioning well, collect and store motor programs prior to their expression in conjunction with other parts of the central nervous system. Problems within these have been hypothesized by some to contribute to the faulty storage of motor programs, resulting in the failure to delay the output of important motor programs, when delays are appropriate.

The failure to delay and store perceptual-motor programs, after they have been formulated, likely results in what is termed impulsive behavior. This includes actions that are seemingly engaged in without thought, and includes a collection of undesirable behaviors that often serve an impulsive youngster poorly within social situations, among family members, and at school. In contrast effectively delaying behaviors by first thinking through possible courses of appropriate actions, is apparently the product of a sound and intact "neural storage system."

Subtle problems within the frontal areas of the brain are also possible contributors to hyperactivity, resulting in or "executive functions" and organizational skills by a clumsy child. The frontal lobes have, during the past decade, been studied with increased sophistication. A main function of this evolutionary newer structure, unique to man in its proportions, is to focus attention and formulate useful and reasonable programs of action and thought. (Benson 1991). Hyperactive, impulsive youngsters thus seem to lack adequate 'executive functions' mediated by areas within the front of the neurocortex.

In addition to neural mechanisms mediating motor output, a hyperactive child is often unable to select and screen out unwanted input. Thus defects in sensory receptors, and in the neural mediators of sensory information, may cause various forms of hyperactive and/or distractible behavior. In this context one could postulate, for example, that the occipital area at the rear of the brain, mediating visual information, may contain too rich a network of dendrites within the nervous systems of some overactive children. Thus habitual and continual over-reactivity of these youngsters may reflect a failure of this important structure to select and to reduce visual input effectively. Therefore one could postulate that processes involving normal neural regression have not taken place within the visual-receptive area.

Indirect evidence suggesting the validity of these assumptions comes from several sources. For example, stimulant drugs that are often employed to control hyperactivity, constrict the openings of the eyes' lenses. Therefore this family of medications may help to arrest over-activity, at least in part by reducing excess visual input. Thus Ritalin and other stimulants may serve to control the excess visual input that apparently bombards and disturbs distractible children who have not been medicated (Ross et al, 1982).

Examples of environmental accommodations to apparent hyper-reactivity of the visual-sensory system may be found by examining strategies traditionally employed by special educators. For decades many teachers attempting to assist the efforts of distractible students, have limited visual and auditory information to which they must attend. One strategy employed has been to provide distractible youngsters with office-like cubicles in which they are able to work and study, during a portion their school day. This methodology often has met with success. Distractible youngsters have been reported to chose to retire from their chaotic classroom settings, and go to their 'office-cubicles' when they find themselves unable to exert control over unwanted impulses. (Cruickshank, 1961).

Both educational interventions and biochemical strategies, therefore, have been employed to reduce levels of stimulation among youngsters evidencing attentional deficits. These successful attempts at stimulus reduction may reflect the possibility that both visual-sensory end organs and also neural structures mediating vision may by over-reactive, due to defects in normal neural regression. This same hyperdiffereniation may be present within the auditory systems of youngsters who habitually over-react to auditory stimulation including autistic children. Further research using both animal and human subjects should help to further illuminate these speculations.

Physical Awkwardness

Physically awkward children evidence a variety of abnormal movement characteristics. Many, for example, display associated movements (termed synkinesia) consisting of extraneous posturings in body parts, not directly involved in the task(s) at hand. (Cratty, 1989). Research data and clinical observations have led to the conclusion that the persistence of these unusual actions into middle childhood and beyond suggest the presence of both specific and of general maturational delays. (Cohen et al, 1967) (Touwen and Prechtl, 1970) (Fog and Fog, 1963).

Within current research, neuromotor overflow of this type has been found to correlate with the presence of attentional deficits (Waber et al., 1985), to motor awkwardness (Hsu et al., 1989) and to disruptive classroom behaviors (Szatmari & Taylor 1984). Wolff and his colleagues also suggest that the failure to inhibit these extraneous movement is valid indicator of general neuromotor immaturity (Wolff et al., (1983)).

The appearance and persistence of neuromotor overflow, or synkinesia, pose problems for a maturing youngster. For example, if these unusual posturings are noted by a clumsy youngster's classmates, derisive comments may be forthcoming. Additionally skill may be disrupted because of the faulty biomechanics that often accompany the appearance of such movements. For example, if the arms consistently flex at elbows, when the legs are activated, smooth and powerful jumping patterns may be disrupted.

Faulty neural regression may be at least partially responsible for the appearance of some of these unusual actions among some youngsters. After an idea requiring action is formulated in the associational areas of the brain, muscle combinations are somehow selected from the motor cortex. The motor program must then be synthesized and formalized as a pattern in the appropriate motor centers. The motor program, after being refined by portions of the cerebellum and brain stem. may then be stored, or acted upon immediately. Deficits or delays in neural regression may cause selection processes within the motor cortex to occur in inefficient ways. In contrast, precise functioning and interaction of these complex processes can occur, it could be hypothesized, only if an optimum number of neuronal connections and dendritic networks are present.

Motor overflow is typically observed in normally developing neonates, and among infants. When a one-month old infant becomes overstimulated, general excitability spreads quickly to most muscle groups. The normal thrashings of infants have been described as reflecting a stage of "normal athetosis" (Cratty 1989b). Thus when young infants become agitated, arms and legs move wildly and in concert, thus reflecting that neural regressive processes within the neuromotor system still are not complete.

It might be hypothesized, that as normal neural regression takes place, the process is accompanied by a parallel increase in the precision of muscular tension and of effort, marked by decreases in extraneous movements occurring when normally maturing youngsters become excited. Thus it seems possible that when normal cell regression occurs within the sensory-motor cortex, excitatory processes begin to influence the selection of increasingly specific and appropriate muscle combinations, producing actions more likely to correspond to the precise tension and accuracy demands required by specific motor tasks. In contrast, youngsters whose nervous systems do not exhibit appropriate neural regressive processes, may continue to exhibit neuromotor overflow when they are confronted with motor tasks requiring both precision and effort.

Emerging technology might be used in order to clarify relationships between various behavioral signs of immaturity, and faulty maturation at the cellular level. For example, through the use of some of the newer imaging techniques subtle defects within the nervous systems of awkward children may be found to accompany faulty efforts at ordering sub-movements of skills into their proper sequences. (Villafana 1988) (Filipek & Kennedy (1991)).

Problems in the formation of various parts of the nervous system may result in different types of apraxia, or dyspraxia. For example, defects or delays in the formation of portions of the basal ganglia, and both the primary and secondary motor cortexes, may cause ideomotor apraxia.. Ideomotor apraxia denotes confusions in the manner in which sub-sequences of a skill are ordered. In contrast faculty neural development, marked by incomplete or defective cell migration, of the frontal, associational centers in the neurocortex might be found among those who exhibit what is called ideational apraxia..

This second general type of apraxia is marked by an initial inability to formulate the idea underlying a movement. Thus youngster afflicted with this problem may pause several minutes to think through an action before even attempting a moderately complex motor task. Likewise hesitations in the formation of words, phrases, and sentences by children evidencing language-speech problems ("formulation aphasia") may also be due to problems in the normal maturation of programming sections of the brain. Various forms of apraxia, and neural models attempting to explain these conditions, are discussed more thoroughly in chapters 5 and 6.

THE DEVELOPMENT OF DRUG-STRESSED INFANTS

Infants evidencing developmental delays, due to the use of noxious substances by their mothers during pregnancy, have concerned observers for over a century. Abnormal structural and behavioral symptoms, reflecting what is now labeled the "fetal alcohol syndrome", were first noted during the final part of the last century among neonates born to women English prisons (Rossett & Sander 1979).

Throughout the 20th century, the use of a wide variety of noxious substances, including heroin, PCP, marihuana, cocaine, and specially concocted "designer drugs," has been the cause of a great deal of concern (Deren 1988). It was the easy availability of a cheap form of rock cocaine (or crack) in the 1980's, however, that resulted in a plethora of infants born with this kind of potential poison in their circulatory systems (Kumer et al 1989). One author has described the epidemic as producing a disadvantaged 'bio-underclass" of children. (Greer 1990). Currently in the United States it has been estimated that almost a half million infants are born each year who have been damaged by maternal drug use (Miller 1989).

Biochemically the processes that may occur within the systems of these infants are just beginning to be understood. Pharmacological actions of adult cocaine use are believed to consist of (a) the blockage of sodium channels to membranes of excitable cells within the body, this results in an inability of the cell to propagate action potentials to neighboring cells. (Commassaris 1989).

A second action taking place is the blockage of the uptake of the catecholamines, dopamine and norepinephrine into presynaptic nerve terminals. This latter mechanism results in an increase of both norepinephrine, and of dopamine-mediated effects, both in the brain and in the peripheral structures. (Commassaris 1989). It is possible that disruptions in these important bio-neurological processes, during the maturation of the nervous system, have injurious consequences to several imperative developmental processes, including normal cell multiplication, dendritic proliferation, transport of neurons, structure formation, and neural regression.

It is probable that the influences of cocaine upon adults are be not precisely the same as, the chemical the effects exerted upon the nervous systems and behaviors of infants. For example, the presence of cocaine in the circulatory and nervous systems of babies may be particularly dangerous because of the continued persistence of benzoylecgonine (a primary metabolite of cocaine) for up to four days after birth. Babies cannot metabolize cocaine quickly as adults, because of the lack of necessary enzymes (cholinesterases) and thus probably do not as quickly rid their systems of this chemical poison. (Rodriquez 1989).

Gaining a clear understanding of the biochemical parameters of the problem is complicated for several reasons:

(1) When drugs pass back and-forth between the mother to the fetus several times, they appear to alter their chemical forms, in ways not fully understood. The infant is not simply a chemical 'sink' passively accepting a drug, but is an active modifier of substances, that probably pass in altered form to the mother, and then undergo further chemical modifications as they re-enter the fetus' blood. (Szeto H. (1988)).

(2) The kinetics (effects of the drug overtime) of the various abusive substances are not easily studied in the fetus, and are thus not known. There is some evidence illuminating how continuous drug exposure acts upon an adult's nervous system. Addiction is usually followed by varying degrees of accommodation (Ambre 1989). However the subtle biochemical and neurological modifications that might occur over time during the nine-month exposure to drugs that the fetus endures, are not easy to research and thus little understood.

(3) Mothers of drug-stressed neonates, both before and after their infant's birth, typically falsify the duration time they have used drugs, and lie about the types they have ingested. In addition, it is commonly found that these mothers have taken more than one drug in various combinations during vaguely defined times during pregnancy. Thus determining precise cause (drugs-used and when) and effects (developmental delays of infants) with these poorly delineated variables present is at best an extremely difficult undertaking.

(4) Finally it is possible, that abusive substance use by fathers detracts from the development of infants evidencing the presence of drugs in their systems at birth. Thus to thoroughly 'get at' the problem, both the nature and influence of paternal drug use upon infant development needs to be investigated. At this point little evidence is available reflecting the possible paternal participation in producing developmentally delayed infants.

Several types of distortions in development, often observed in drug-stressed infants, suggest damage has occurred to selected and specific neural structures and mechanisms. The exotic motor behaviors seen include both rapid tremors and intermittent spasms (choreas). The locations on the body at which both kind of atypical actions occur, and the time in the life of the infant that they make their appearance and disappearance, may also have useful diagnostic significance. The unique and unusual motor behaviors exhibited by these infants have required the development of contemporary assessment tools, as the traditional measures of infant development have not proved adequate in the task. (Cratty 1990). (*See Appendix*).

From a neurological standpoint the tremors reported in cocaine-stressed infants both by caretakers (De Oliveira 1990), and by researchers (Chasnoff 1986) may be partly attributed to damage to important maturational processes critical to the healthy development of the cerebellum. The appearance of these tremors, often not starting until the second or third week of life, (Cratty, 1989) coincides with the time the cerebellum becomes normally becomes neurologically stratified (Rakic, 1971; 1981). The cerebellum, after birth continues to generate and to relocate neurons, in contrast to other organs within the central nervous system in which neurogenesis has been completed at birth. It is possible, therefore, that cerebellar damage may result when drugs have been ingested later in pregnancy during the time of cell migration is taking place, and the cerebellum becomes stratified.

Cerebellar damage to the drug-stressed fetus may initially result in the 'restive tremors' reported. These actions consists of vibratory activities, by the neonate, while the hands are clenched, and the elbow joints flexed (DeOliveira, 1990). The sudden termination of these tremors, observed at about the third to fourth month, may occur when the higher centers become mature, and thus mask these cerebellar dysfunctions (Cratty, 1990). The termination of these tremors may also result because the transport of neurons within the cerebellum has been completed. (Rakic, 1981) (Rodier, 1980)

It has also been reported that cocaine-stressed infants continue to show inaccuracies in reaching behaviors (dysmetria) later during their first years of life, and into the second year. This finding thus suggests that earlier damage to the cerebellar cortex may have resulted in what are termed 'terminal tremors", oscillating and inaccurate motor activity occurring at the termination of movements. (in this case at the end of reaching responses) (Cratty, 1990) (De Oliveira, 1990).

Other caretaker reports have indicated that children of eight to ten years whose histories include maternal cocaine use, continue to evidence unusual movement qualities. For example one foster mother informed me that she sometimes had observed older children, stressed prenatally with maternal drug use, twisting out of their clothes when they became agitated (Cratty, 1989)! Thus early cerebellar damage may, among some, have long-term negative effects.

Cocaine seems to absent itself from the blood stream of infants about 72 hours after birth. However these early noxious effects may result in neural damage during the latter stages of gestation and during the first three days of life, that exert lasting trauma to precise motor functions that continue to be seen during early and middle childhood. This early chemical damage that cocaine may exert may thus include not only the blunting of neural transport functions as outlined above, but also the disruption of normal cell regression.

Another type of abnormal motor activity reported by caretakers of drug-stressed neonates are single-cycle jerking actions (choreas). These spasms seem to persist longer during infancy, than do the tremors discussed above. Some caretakers have suggested, when interviewed during periodic developmental examinations accorded their charges, that this type of abnormality are more useful predictors of the appearance of later problems, than are the tremors that appear earlier during the neonatal period (Cratty, 1990).

These irregular jerking actions may stem from damage to portions of several motor control centers whose functions include the formulation and storage of motor programs. Damage to portions of the basal ganglia has been traditionally hypothesized to underlie irregular athetoid movements common to some kinds of cerebral palsy. Exploration of fruitful hypotheses, as well as the formulation of useful neural models, are likely to come about when newer imaging techniques are used to explore to the nervous systems of drug-stressed infants (Vallifana, 1988).

Other developmental anomalies seen in drug-stressed infants, including those exposed to cocaine, include hyper-reactivity to stimulation, as well as tonus abnormalities. Among the two types of muscular-tone problems, consistently reported, include extreme hypertonicity as well as "floppy" behavioral patterns that signal hypotonicity (or dystonia). Some children, influenced earlier by maternal cocaine use, are now entering school. Observers report that these youngsters continue to evidence either hypotonic-sleepy reactions, or hypertensive, distractible, overly aggressive and restive behaviors. (Deren 1986).

Caretakers report that successful mothering techniques for calming hypertonic, and restive cocaine-stressed infants include reducing stimulation. Thoughtful foster parents state that they are careful not to move the infants too rapidly, or expose them to lights and sounds that are too intense. Further, caretakers inform investigators that making sure stimulation of various kinds is present in moderate amounts, is critical if one is to avoid triggering behavioral disruptions by their young charges. They say, for example, that sudden movements of the infants are disruptive to the infant's emotional state, while gentle rocking movements are calming. Soft lighting and soothing music reportedly proves calming, whereas sounds that are too loud, or lights that are too bright are likely to be highly disruptive. (De Oliveira & Cratty 1991).

This hyper-reactivity of cocaine-stressed infants to various kinds of stimulation encourages the speculation that processes involving normal cell regression have not occurred in a normal, both within sensory end organs, and in areas of the brain that receive and mediate sensory information. Thus it could be hypothesized that abnormally high numbers of neurons, and/or an overabundance of dendritic connections, are present in such structures as the auditory receptive areas of the parietal region, in the visual-receptive (occipital) areas, as well as in the somato-sensory cortex that mediates movement sensations. Contemporary scanning techniques are presently being applied to objectify the nature of normal and abnormal brain development occurring in youngsters afflicted with perceptual-motor problems. (Knuckey et al 1983). The further use of these newer and exotic strategies should further clarify aberrations in mediating sensation among these drug stressed infants and children.

Longitudinal studies are needed to determine whether higher-associational centers have been negatively influenced by maternal cocaine use, and by the ingestion of other drugs and abusive substances. It has found in some primate species that the neocortex evidences signs of neural maturity before the basal ganglia, and cerebellum are complete (Rodier, 1980). Therefore it is possible that heavy drug use early in pregnancy may negatively influence the placement of cortical cells, and thus the associational processes usually assigned to the higher centers, including the frontal lobes.

IMPLICATIONS AND OVERVIEW

Consideration of the hypotheses raised in this chapter lead to numerous implications and speculations. These hypotheses include suppositions of interest and importance to scholars researching bio-neurological concomitants of maturation, to physicians concerned with the health of special populations, and to educators and developmentalists assigned to carry out the difficult and jobs of modifying development and aberrant behaviors. Thus useful conclusions may be drawn, from the research evidence discussed, both by those interested in the medical bio-neurological aspects of developmental problems, as well as individuals focusing upon modifications of aberrant behaviors in adults and in children.

Biochemical interventions may be useful in reducing neural damage in neonates during pregnancies marked by maternal substance abuse. Politicians might consider mandating hospitalization and treatment for neonate-mother combinations in which types of noxious chemical interchanges are obviously taking place. Laws might be passed based upon the supposition that a felony is taking place, chemical child abuse, when this type of apparent poisoning is apparently going on among pregnant mothers. However the precise nature of medical interventions that may prove useful are not clearly apparent, given the scarcity of presently available evidence, and the difficulty of monitoring the chemical environment of the drug-exposed fetus.

Medications may also be further refined to more precisely assist youngsters evidencing various forms of stimulus over-reactivity. Children with various classifications, including the autistic, the hyperactive, as well as the emotionally disturbed, may be assisted in this way.

Youngsters within a variety of exceptional groups may thus be aided with the development of increasingly sophisticated medical-chemical interventions intended to inhibit and/or control neuronal growth and to enhance the formation of healthy and intact neural structures both during gestation, and also during the early months of life. These potential clients range from drug-stressed neonates, to hyperactive and/or awkward school children.

Biochemical interventions appear needed to stimulate processes of normal cell regression, within neural structures and to control systems and structures that appear to be oversensitive to various kinds of stimulation. Biochemical interventions may also eventually appear which will trigger useful 'pruning' processes (neural regression) within structures whose mal-functionings may result in excesses of unwanted motor output, or produce hyper-reactivity among various populations.

At the behavioral level the contemporary literature describing the development of important neuronal processes surveyed in this chapter, suggests several implications. For example, it is increasingly clear that one should apply programs of infant stimulation with precision, rather simply expose young clients indiscriminately to a large quantity of experiences. Too much stimulation will likely prove counter-productive. Remedial efforts should result in programs that contain experiences which calm, as well as those which enhance productive cognitive and motor explorations. Failure to heed this principle of optimum stimulation, will likely result in programs containing components that are less-than-useful behaviorally, and that may even result in youngster's behaviors regressing. Unless such programs are carefully constructed, a neonate, child or adult client may be exposed to experiences that, at the neural level, could contribute to the proliferation and maintenance of an undesirable number of neurons and neural networks, and which will thus sustain unwanted behavioral and perceptual outcomes. The caretakers of drug-stressed infants and some educators of hyperactive awkward and/or learning-disabled youngsters) seemed to have already accepted this principle intuitively. (Cruickshank (1956) (DeOliveira 1990).

Much of the material in this chapter related to dysfunctional human development is admittedly speculative. However studies with animal models have indicated that (1) lesions inserted into the central nervous systems of rats early in development lead to anomalous cell migration (Dvorak et al 1978), and (2) early cortical lesions can alter connectivity and the ultimate location of axons in hamsters (Frost 1988). Future research should result in the further illumination of how early insults to the human nervous system are later manifested both neurologically and behaviorally.

QUESTIONS FOR DISCUSSION

1. Differentiation between the terms *dedifferentiation.* and *hyperdifferentiation.*
2. What are some of the writer's main hypothesizes relating neural development to behavioral abnormalities? What evidence is needed to substantiate the speculations found in the chapter?
3. What kinds of neural dysfunctions were listed in the chapter as occurring during neurogenesis (development of the nervous system pre and post-natally) that purportedly can lead to behavioral and developmental lags in infants and children?
4. What two mechanism were given as illustrating the nature of neural regression.
5. What movement characteristics of infants stressed prenatally with maternal cocaine use were discussed in the chapter?
6. What symptoms seen in clumsy and hyperactive children were attributable to faculty neural regression? What were the mechanisms that were hypothesized as causing these behavioral-neural relationships?
7. What mechanism and processes were described as mediating cell transport?
8. What animal studies were cited in the chapter as illuminating both cell transport and neural regression?
9. Discuss neural regression within a developmental framework, from conception to adulthood.
10. What kinds of additional neuro-behavioral studies are needed to support the various hypotheses advanced in this chapter?

Chapter 5
Sub-syndromes

INTRODUCTION

Upon reviewing available contemporary research it is strongly suggested that several sub-syndromes occur within the groups of youngsters evidencing various symptoms which mark them as having poor coordination. It is purposed within this chapter to identify and to describe the characteristics of the more prevalent sub-syndromes presently emerging in current research obtained among populations of awkward youngsters. This exercise in identification is believed important for several reasons. The description of viable sub-syndromes should result in more useful diagnostic and remedial guidelines being formulated, than are presently available. Secondly, this analytical undertaking might serve to stimulate needed research focusing upon awkward children.

The following sub-syndromes were formulated by consulting two types of information. The first source consisted of research studies. In these investigators employed factor and cluster analyses of performance attributes, obtained from groups of awkward children.. (Miyahara 1992) (Hoare and Larkin 1991). Groupings of neurological soft signs have also been explored using factor analytic methods, and have provided another source of objective data. (Tupper 1987)

Information was also derived from our own clinical observations. Clinical descriptions, available in the literature, were also consulted. These have based upon the experiences of numerous professionals working with neurologically suspect infants, children and adolescents within remedial-educational settings. These two sources of information, one scientific-statistical and the second observational, suggest strongly that various sub-groups of awkward children are likely to exhibit predictable groups of atypical behavioral symptoms.

ATAXIC SYNDROME

The cerebellum was one of the first parts of the central nervous system to evolve. A rudimentary cerebellum began appearing as a bulge at the top of the brain stems of the first amphibians when emerging from the sea. One of the main functions the cerebellum performs is to provide information about the positions and locations of limbs. The amphibians thus apparently required this neural center when they began to evidence appendages suitable to locomotion, and which enabled them to move around land for the first time.

Cerebellar functions in humans have been studied for decades. For example, symptoms reflecting a moderately dysfunctional cerebellum have been measured in late childhood have been associated with low birth weight by Lesny and others (1980). Cerebellar problems are thus likely among numerous populations of developmentally delayed youngsters.

The cerebellum has several imperative motor functions, making it an important neural center to fathom, when attempting to understand the nature of various kinds of poor coordination. One of the main jobs of the cerebellum is to refine and smooth motor programs, as they emerge from the central nervous system, and journey to the muscle-collections that combine to produce smooth and purposeful action patterns.

The cerebellum also is believed by some as responsible for controlling and pre-programming various rapid automatic patterns in which some muscle groups engage. These automated movements may include the rapid throws (saccades) made by the eyes when reading. Other times the eye jumps in this rapid manner is when tracking fast moving objects (moving more than about 50 angular degrees per second).

These repetitive actions made by the eyes, occur too rapidly for conscious control, from 3-8 a second. Thus their precision and direction may partly mediated by the cerebellum, rather than by higher control centers.

The groups cerebellar-motor symptoms seen in a child also may include tremors and inaccuracies of the larger muscle groups, as well as hand hand-eye coordination difficulties. taken together they represent a mild form of cerebral ataxia. Problems controlling precise eye movements important when engaging in sports containing rapidly moving objects and people may also be caused by cerebellar dysfunctions.

Various components of the cerebellum control precision of movements within different parts of the body. The amount of cerebellar tissue devoted to the control of various body parts corresponds to the complexity of the actions of which each part is capable. Thus larger parts of the cerebellum are devoted to controlling the precise movements of the mouth, lips, and hands, as is true of the main sensory-motor cortex. In contrast, smaller portions of the cerebellum, mediate the less precise movements of which the trunk, and lower limbs are capable. This is an important principle to keep in mind, when considering the specific nature of various cerebellar 'soft-signs' that awkward child manifest.

Among the main behavioral signs of some kind of mild form of cerebellar 'involvement' are unsteadiness and mild tremors. As only a portion of the cerebellum may be involved, in some youngsters the tremors may be seen as regular low amplitude fluctuations only in the hands, or of the pencil when drawing, and may not be apparent in the lower limbs. In other children unsteadiness is only evidenced in gait, or when attempting to balance. The presence of unsteadiness and tremors in both the upper and lower parts of the body is most likely, however. Unsteadiness in the upper limbs may be seen as the child produces lines in which there are marked by tremors, and unsteadiness. The total figure or letter may be recognizable, however the quality of the lines making up the figures may be poor.

Further problems in hand-eye coordination can also surface, including dysmetrias, difficulties in making accurate lines, and making reaching movements of exact lengths. (Chapter 7) Additional problems can include a decomposition of rhythmic and fluid movements, into disjointed and disconnected ones.

An awkward child, within this syndrome classification, may exhibit a mild lower-limb ataxia. This symptom involves an unsteady gait, and other locomotor problems including the inability to hop consecutively at the expected age. The support phase within the walking cycle is not likely to be followed by a relaxed flexion of the leg at the knee, but by an unwanted spasm-like kick-out or extension (a clonic reaction). This type of problem will also negatively influence both static and moving balance. Keeping a stable position, required in tests of balance, is dependent upon maintaining precise tension in the lower limbs, including the ankles and feet.

Infants and children, suffering moderate to mild cerebellar damage, may evidence different types of tremors at various stages in maturation. The negative effects of pre-natal cocaine exposure has been found to result in rapid, low-amplitude tremors shortly after birth. These are 'restive tremors' and occur with the arms flexed, and the hands placed near the shoulders. These restive tremors may suddenly cease, to be replaced by terminal tremors. The latter are inaccuracies that occur as the cocaine-stressed child attempts to engage in accurate reaching behaviors.

It has been proposed that the initial 'restive tremors' are evidence of initial cerebellar damage caused by a failure of the formation of the organ during the latter stages of gestation and during the first days of life. It has further been hypothesized that 'restive' tremors signalling this initial damage may become less apparent, and are replaced later by other 'cerebellar-signs' consisting of terminal tremors occurring as these children attempt to accurately reach for objects. (Cratty 1990).

Other types of cerebellar symptoms include poor kinesthetic awareness of limb location. This child, for example, may need to watch his or her arm as it is drawn back in an overhand throwing motion, or it may simply 'disappear' from the thrower's consciousness. Difficulties in alternating rotary movements of the arms and hands, as when moving quickly from supination to pronation, also are considered 'cerebellar signs'

Thus damage to children's self-esteems may be marked as they struggle with a constellation of these symptoms. These can include an inaccurate and stumbling gait, poor balance, less than adequate ball skills, plus inaccuracies in printing. Damage to the child's body may also occur, as they may often trip and fall due to balance and gait inaccuracies. Over the years my colleagues I have frequently encountered awkward children evidencing this type of 'sub-syndrome' in both our clinical and experimental programs.

Experimental verification of the existence of a sub-syndrome of 'cerebellar types' among groups of awkward youngsters may be found within the data emerging from several studies of the motor behaviors of neurologically 'suspect children.' For example an investigation by Ritter and his colleagues (1970) it was found that hopping tests frequently identified children with other neurological soft signs present, including problems when walking and turning.

Further validation of relationships between measures balance and unsteadiness is found in a ambitious study by Nichols (1987). Several useful findings emerge from Nichols' comprehensive factor analysis, conducted from 1959-1965, using data obtained from several thousand children. For example it was found that the inability to hop consecutively at the age of 4 years, together with imprecise drawing efforts were both predictive of the appearance of other symptoms later in life including hyperactivity in school settings. More directly to the point, associated signs of clumsiness including measures of poor coordination and abnormal gait. At the same time these two measures 'loaded' in the same factor as signs of synkinesia (mirror movements) and other abnormal movements (Nichols 1987).

Two recent cluster analyses conducted with populations of awkward children further confirm the existence of this sub-syndrome. Miyahara (1992) identified a sub-group within his data, that included children with poor dynamic and static balance, coupled with deficits in ball aiming skills. The linkages described earlier in this section between visual accuracy and balance, both attributes hypothetically mediated by the cerebellum, would account for this association between deficits in ball skills and balance within Miyahara data. Hoare and Larkin (1991) also identified a sub-group of awkward children evidencing specific deficiencies in balance, and the absence of other other pronounced motor coordination problems. This group constituted over 28% of the awkward children assessed in their cluster analysis (Hoare and Larkin 1991).

HYPOTONIC SYNDROME

Children beset with the hypotonic syndrome, display levels of resting muscle tone that are below average. This flaccid state may also occur in the facial region, and in other parts of the body. For example a hypotonic youngster may display a 'sleepy look' as overly relaxed muscles lifting eye lids, result in the eyes remaining half-closed even during waking hours. Among children with this condition the stomach muscles may appear flaccid (Ptosis) resulting in a 'pot-bellied' look. The term benign hypotonia has been used to describe this type of syndrome, indicating that the condition is not progressive (Eng et al 1979).

One of the five sub-types identified by Miyahara's cluster (1992) evidenced hypotonicity and poor fitness, coupled by "fair coordination." This was the fifth most prevalent sub-type within the population of learning disabled awkward children measured by Miyahara, and accounted for almost 4% of the youngsters surveyed.

This condition is usually encountered first in infancy, as delays in the assumption of various important stable and static positions are attempted. During the past two years I have assessed and devised developmental programs for three hypotonic infants ranging in age from 18-22 months who could not sit up unassisted. An additional two youngsters, whom we have evaluated, were almost three years of age, and yet had not pulled themselves to a standing position and thus had not begun to walk. The overall physical health of these youngsters was adequate and normal, nor did the condition seem to be progressive in nature. They appeared similar to floppy rag dolls when attempting to sit unaided, to assume a creeping position, or when trying to stand. Home-based programs of infant stimulation were formulated, in which their parents could participate.

Hypotonia observed by nursery school teachers in children from the 3rd to 5th years can also be important signs of more serious problems. For example several years ago, I worked with a four year old boy who evidenced muscle tone at levels below normal. He displayed the previously described, 'sleepy look' due to flaccid muscles in the eye lids. In his case, however the symptoms were precursors of athetoid cerebral palsy. Irregular athetoid movement were later seen when he began to hold a pencil and tried to draw figures and letters.

In other rare cases a pre-school child may evidence muscular weakness that paradoxically may be accompanied by an apparent enlargement of the muscles. This kind of observation may constitute early signs of muscular dystrophy. The apparent muscle enlargement (termed pseudo-hypertrophy) is due to a replacement of muscle cells with fat cells (*See chapter* 3). However, The status of most young children evidencing below-average levels of residual muscle tone, remains constant and benign, and they do not develop more serious and progressive neuromotor problems later in life.

Currently in our program we are working several hypotonic youngsters including a boy of six years. His hypotonic symptoms are accompanied by a slow reaction time, as if often the case. We have worked over one and a half years, for example, to enable him to catch a large ball after first dropping it at his feet. He was first unable to accomplish this task, due to a slow reaction time. His hand-eye reaction time was slower, than the time taken for the ball to descend, and bounce up again.

He and other hypotonic youngsters with whom we have worked (and are now working) also often evidence the inability to exert sufficient pressure when trying to make marks on paper, during attempts to draw and to print letters. Hypotonia as a sub-symptom of dysgraphia is discussed further in Chapter 7.

Hypotonic youngsters may at times display average motor abilities, if a moderate amount of force is not required for the task (Miyahara 1992). However the general impression they make upon others is one of laziness, despite the fact that their problems is neurologically based, rather than due primarily to a disinclination to exercise.

A comprehensive factor analysis by Nichols (1987) a delineates both the motor symptoms and personality characteristics hypotonic youngsters. In Nichols' investigation a measure of hypoactivity loaded in the same factor as did tests denoting 'withdrawal' and "social-emotional immaturity". (Nichols 1987). Nichols' data confirms a compensation frequently seen among hypotonic children, 'learned helplessness'. This emotional quality is discussed further in Chapters and 7 and 10.

The hypotonic youngster often evidences attention deficits, but does not frequently engage in hyperactive behaviors. This type 'dreamy' youngster often seems out of contact with teachers parents and peers. He or she may display periodical lapses of both visual and cognitive inattention.

As reflected in the data by Nichols (1987), the hypotonic child is likely to withdraw both cognitively and socially from both interaction in play and in academic environments. Thus a hypotonic child was once described to me by a teacher as a 'bell jar' youngster. While seated quietly at their classroom desks these children seem often to be cut-off from what is going on, as though separated from others by a glass encasement placed over them, like a bell jar! Hypotonic youngsters usually do not wander around classrooms, or excessively and inappropriately manipulative available objects. To the contrary they are often still and passive, sometimes within an inner world of their own making.

Various neural structures, including components of the brain stem are usually hypothesized to control and maintain levels of resting muscle tone. A steady stream of impulses mediated by the gamma efferent system, for example, is believed by some to sub-serve resting tonus levels. Thus deficits in these structures and systems are blamed for the presence of hypotonicity.

The reasons for low levels of resting muscle tone also may be include deficiencies in muscle metabolism, or be caused by other subtle problems that require the diagnostic skills of an endocrinologist. Logical interventions in a remedial program for such youngsters include exercises of various kinds. However, it may useful in some cases to supplement exercise programs with biochemical-nutritional supplements prescribed by a physician. The reticular formation and associated structures hypothesized by some responsible for the maintenance of normal residual muscle tone are depicted next page.

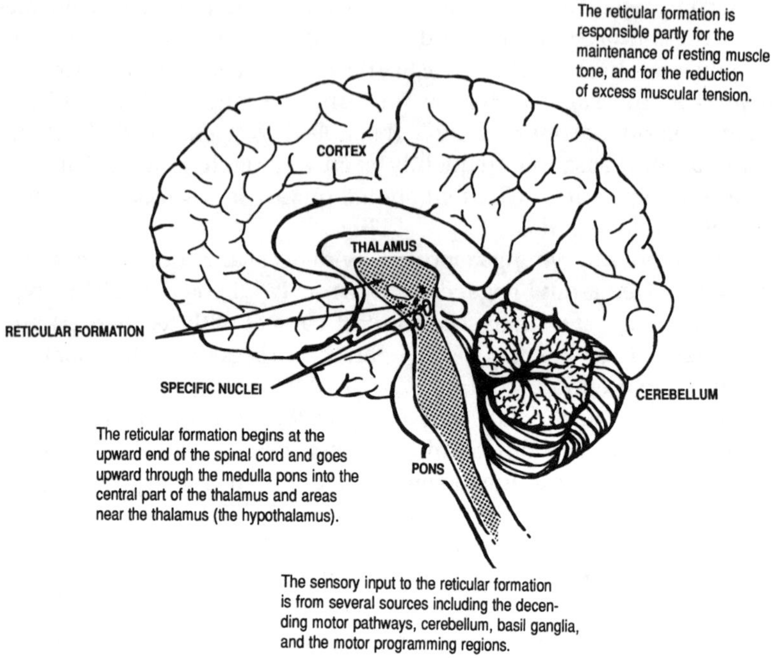

Plate 5-1. The reticular (net-like) formation

Usually a child evidencing hypotonic symptoms remains consistently hypotonic. However it has been observed recently by some of those who take care of drug-stressed infants, that while most evidence consistent signs of hypertension or hypotonia, some alternate between hypertonic and hypotonic states evidencing of frequent changes between abnormally high and unusually low levels of resting muscle tone.(Cratty 1990) . These same patterns of hypotonia and hypertension are reportedly persist among these same children upon entering kindergarten and the first grade.

TENSION SYNDROME

Some youngsters labeled 'clumsy' display constant and excessively high levels of muscle tone. In contrast to hypotonic children previously discussed, a youngster evidencing a tension syndrome displays signs of hypertonicity while attempting skills, as well as when at rest. The tension levels seem to rise when the movements become more difficult, thus compounding their struggles to execute complex skills.

This syndrome is often accompanied by excesses in overflow or associated movements (synkinesia), discussed more thoroughly in Chapter 6. When a hypertonic child is required to engage in a forceful movement with the hands, the mouth may grimace excessively; and when vigorous jumping movements are executed, the upper limbs may move and flex. Reaching movements are restrained, because as they attempt to extend their arms toward objects the smooth elongation of the flexor muscles of the arm do not occur. Instead the biceps may become tense and inhibit coordinated extension.

The tension syndrome, within groups of awkward children, may represent mild to moderate forms of spastic cerebral palsy. The neurological mechanism underlying spasticity are purportedly due to lesions in the large nerve pathways within the brain stem, that lie outside the main motor pathways. Since these main motor pathways contain pyramid shaped cells, it has been hypothesized by some that extra-pyraminal lesions contribute to muscular spasticity.

Other structures are also hypothesized to control muscle tone and thus if damaged may cause the excess tonus displayed by children evidencing symptoms reflecting this syndrome. These structures, include the net-like (reticular) formation of cells that wind their way around the brain stem, shown earlier. The manner in which associated pathways enhance motor programs emanating from the cortex is illustrated next page.

It is likely children with excess amounts of muscle tone also typically evidence hyperactivity. This includes exhibiting locomotor and manipulative behaviors that are in excess of those desirable within a school setting. Data from the study by Hertzig and Shapiro (1987) suggest the consistent presence of hypertonic signs, within populations of pre-mature children.

Similar data as resulted from an investigation by Nichols (1987). In Nichol's study one of the combinations of frequently occurring 'soft signs, included the dyad of poor coordination and abnormal reflexes. This pairing of symptoms was obtained in data from 331 of the children tested.

Unlike hypotonic children, who often seem to be in dream-like states for a good part of the school day, awkward youngsters evidencing a tension syndrome frequently leave their chairs in a classroom, grab for objects and swipe at other children who may

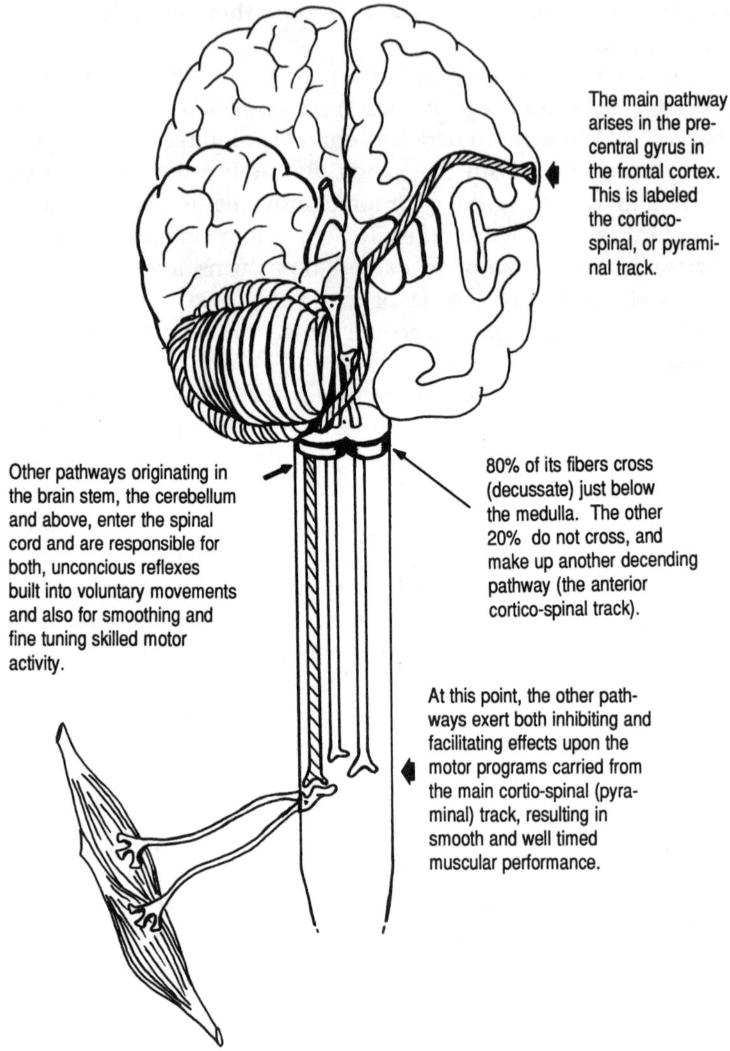

Plate 5-2. Descending motor pathways

pass in reach. The data from the factor analytic study of neurological soft signs by Nichols (1987) contains correlations between emotional fluctuations, short-attention span, and muscular tensions coupled with impulsivity. Thus there is statistical evidence that confirms the existence of the tension syndrome with accompanying attentional deficits and impulsivity.

Attempting to acquire printing and writing skills usually presents problems for this type of youngster. Learning to print letters may result in the frequent 'overshooting' of a line, or ending point. (dysmetria). This problem is sometimes 'solved' by the child by trying to both start a movement and to inhibit a movement(s) at the same time. Thus a great deal of excess tension may accompany efforts to improve graphic skills. Relaxation training is often a helpful accompaniment to writing and printing lessons, when working with this type of child. A case study of a dysgraphic child evidencing a tension syndrome may be found in Chapter 7.

Various movement sub-qualities may be blunted, when children possessing symptoms within this 'tension syndrome' attempt various motor tasks. Kinesthetic perception of limb velocity, location, and direction are frequently poor in such youngsters. Furthermore children evidencing tension symptoms also have problems in skills requiring motor planning (Chapter 6), and many appear to evidence ideomotor apraxia to varying degrees. This type of problem frequently arises when they are confronted with the necessity to learn cursive writing, particularly when attempting to replicate capital letters.

Skills needed in many team sports are often beyond the capacities of a youngster evidencing signs of a 'tension syndrome.' Additionally their motor problems may become compounded, when social derision and ridicule surface. When punishing outbursts from peers cause their tension levels to rise, they may become almost paralyzed due to embarrassment and to heightened anxiety they usually experience within such socially stressful performance situations.

Within a clinical setting children evidencing 'tension syndromes' need careful and patient attention. Frequent rests from tension producing practice may be necessary. Breaks during which relaxation training, or similar techniques may be applied, are often useful. At the termination of motor skill lessons it may be necessary to apply additional relaxation strategies to reduce their tension and to produce a positive emotional state before they proceed home, or to other parts of a school program. If we do not employ strategies intended to "deactivate" and calm these children before they leave our clinic program in the late afternoons, it then may become difficult or impossible for them to eat their dinners, or to sleep well that night.

DYSPRAXIC SYNDROME

Some awkward children cannot effectively plan and chain together series of sub-movements into smooth, well-integrated motor skills. Their levels of muscle tone may not be excessively high or lower than average, nor do they evidence the unsteadiness reflecting some kind of cerebellar involvement. Their problem may be reflected primarily in poorly sequencing sub-actions of movements into whole skills. They may be identified as dyspraxic.

Evidence for the presence of this sub-group is found in data from two recently completed cluster analyses of the abilities of awkward children. Miyahara, for example identified a sub-group who evidenced poor "dynamic coordination". This was the third most prevalent syndrome within his population, consisting of over 30% of the total group surveyed. (Miyahara 1992).

Two Australian researchers also found a group within the population they measured evidencing poor motor abilities independent of perceptually 'loaded' tasks. For example, these apparently apraxic children did poorly in tasks involving complicated assembly work. (Hoare and Larkin 1991). These youngsters constituted about 10% of the group surveyed by these researchers "down-under" (Hoare and Larkin 1991).

Neurologically it is possible that in the case of some dyspraxic youngsters the condition is due partly to problems within the integrating centers just above the ventricles of the brain, the basal ganglia. These centers are believed by some to both assist in the formulation of motor programs and also to store and delay a program's output. Damage to, or pressure upon, the basal ganglia thus may also cause these centers to be deficit in the storing of motor programs.

Corroborative evidence has been obtained in one study in the 1980's that abnormal formations of the ventricles adjacent to the basal ganglia were more likely in clumsy children evidencing dyspraxia. (Knuckey et al 1983). The enlarged ventricles found in over 20% of the dyspraxic population evaluated by Knuckey and his colleagues, conceivably could result in pressure to the two portions of the basal ganglia immediately superior to the ventricles hypothesized to formulate motor programs. Moreover 39% of the dyspraxic youngsters evaluated evidenced other identifiable brain abnormalities. Dyspraxia in children apparent in late childhood has also been associated with hyperactivity as well as with birth histories containing records of low birth weight. (Lesny 1980). A more thorough look at neural-models attempting to explain dyspraxia may be found in the following chapter.

After formulating a movement idea a child afflicted with the apraxic-dyspraxic syndrome may often act impulsively, rather than displaying the self-control typical of neurologically more intact youngsters. This portions of the frontal-associational centers may be also be deficit in these youngsters. Hypothetically portions of the central nervous system of a severely dyspraxic youngster has received an insult, either hypoxia or a vascular accident, relatively early in pre-natal development. (Towbin 1987). This kind of neural pathology thus may have influenced the adequate functioning of one, or more, of the several the neural structures believed to interact in their control of motor programming, storage and retrieval.

The poor motor planning skills typical of a youngster displaying an apraxic syndrome also may be accompanied by excessive muscular tensions. These tensions continually arise because of the emotional frustrations experienced as they attempt to execute important self-care skills, and master complex playground tasks.

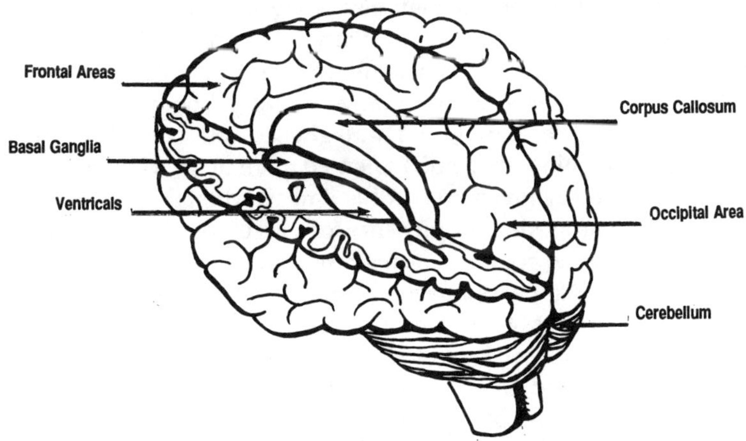

The basil ganglia, composed of four parts, lays just above the ventricles as shown. They are storage and integration stations for motor programs. Branches also go to the spinal cord, to the motor cortex, and the cerebellum. Thus, they are critical mediators of motor coordination and motor programs.

Plate 5-3. Left side of the brain, cut away to show basal ganglia

These heightened tensions may further contribute to problems of motor planning and execution. Thus awkward children who simultaneously evidence signs of the presence of both a tension and dyspraxic syndromes are common clients of clinic programs.

The dyspraxic syndrome may also involve several specific subsymptoms, including ideational apraxia, and various types of ideomotor apraxia. Ideational apraxia are delays taking place when thinking about the general idea of a task, and before acting. This kind of prolonged hesitations may signal the involvement of the higher associational areas of the brain (frontal lobes), or may simply result because these youngsters' backgrounds of failure make them cautious before even starting tasks. Delays in initiating a task may also be seen among some youngsters displaying apraxia behaviors, accompanied by varying degrees of mental retardation.

Some data has suggested by both types of apraxias (ideomotor and ideational) are inseparable in groups of children (Gubbay et al 1965) (Deuel et al 1984). However in other investigations the test batteries administered resulted in data dividing the two apraxias. (Rutter et al 1970). A more thorough look is taken at both behaviors reflecting several types of apraxias, dyspraxias, and related agnosias in Chapters 6 and 8.

Symptoms of dyspraxia may also appear more markedly within some parts of the body than within others. Deficits in motor planning skills may, in various children, lie primarily in the hands, limbs, or when they attempt to move their total body with accuracy through space. I recently tested an eight year old boy who executed drawings resembling those of a talented adult artist. However, when asked to replicate movements of his limbs and total body he proved completely confused. The presence of these specific types of limb and trunk apraxia, resulted in this boy evidencing an extremely low self-esteem. He appeared severely depressed because of the social abuse of peers consistently accompanied his efforts to participate in playground activities. However, several months of individualized instruction resulted in measurable improvement in his ability to engage in sequenced playground tasks.

Dyspraxic in these children may also be reflected in speech-articulation difficulties. Correctly sequencing the complex movements of the tongue, lips, and other parts of the mouth, when forming word sounds, may present profound problems for youngsters evidencing the 'apraxic-dyspraxic syndrome.' Numerous neurological schedules assess speech-articulation problems along with other movement-type soft signs. (Rutter 1970) (Hertiz and Shapiro 1987). Speech pathologists often remark at the unusual percent of children with gross motor problems who come to them with speech difficulties. This problem has also been labeled oro-apraxia., and buccofacial apraxia.

When working clinically with these type of children. It is important initially to expose them to various tests of motor planning. It has been found that motor planning deficits, and strengths, are task specific (Cratty 1989g). When found deficit in these types of tests these children and adolescents should be taught multi-faceted skills using progressive-part methods. For example, a complex skill should be first broken down into parts, and after a single component is introduced and mastered, it should be combined with a second, then a third part, until the entire skill is mastered. Exposure of these children to impatient teaching and to ill-prepared instructors, who demand the quick mastery of skills, are likely to result in negative emotional outcomes. Gordon and McKinlay have also written about strategies useful when working with dyspraxic youngsters (1986). The evaluation of other program intended to reduce dyspraxia are found in Chapter 13.

MANUAL-GRAPHIC SYNDROMES

It is common to evaluate children whose main symptoms only reflect difficulties with tasks requiring manual dexterity and/or who display problems when attempting to draw letters and numbers. Two separate global manual syndromes appear to exist. On one hand there are children whose fingers fumble when attempting to button their clothes and who often drop their forks and spoons while eating. Some of these, while holding their pencils in a fist-like grip, will display average or above average abilities to reproduce figures, letters and numbers.

In contrast there are other children whose dexterity is adequate, but whose graphic skills, including letter reproduction ranges from labored to nearly absent. Indeed the factor analytic literature strongly suggests that in adults there may be several more independent manual-dexterity qualities or abilities within their overall 'movement profiles.' (Cratty 1975d).

The available evidence suggests that by the age of five children evidence three separate, distinct and uncorrelated manual-graphic abilities. These sub-abilities include:

(a) Graphic skills, involving the ability to draw figures, people, places and things. These are spatial-motor tasks involving the right-hemisphere
(b) Printing-writing skills in which are may be mediated primarily by left hemisphere programs. and
(c) Dexterity and related skills which may be subjected to control by the basal ganglia, and augmented by cerebellar refinements.

For decades the independence of gross and fine motor abilities has been documented in the experimental literature dealing with motor learning (Cratty 1975d). Thus it is not unexpected that some manually and/or graphic deficient youngsters may exhibit either average or above average skills when the larger muscles are employed. These contrasts in abilities often puzzle their parents who sometimes state, . . . " But my child is really well-coordinated, he performs well in little league baseball on Saturday . . . I just can't understand why his teacher says he has a coordination problem". A youngster with these contrasting abilities is the subject of a case study in Chapter 7 dealing with dysgraphia.

Scientific verification for the independence of several manual qualities may be seen in the data from numerous factor analyses. Oseretsky (1931) intuitively seemed to realize that a separate group of dexterity tests was needed in order to sample independent qualities independent of ball skills, balance and the like. Follow-up work first by Thams (1955) and later by Bruininks (1978) and others, using factor analytic techniques verify the independence of several types of hand-eye coordination as qualities separate from groupings of scores obtained by testing the larger muscle groups.

Rarick and Dobbins (1975) conducted a factor analysis that classified children into "person-groups" for effective competition and interventions. Each group evidenced a distinctive and individual motor profile of both strengths and weaknesses in both fine and gross motor skills. They also found that a 'fine motor factor', was separate and independent of clusters of test scores obtained by evaluating strength-power, coordination of larger muscle groups, and balance.

In several neurological schedules, intended to identify groups of soft-neurological motor signs a separate group of sub-tests are typically employed to identify fine motor skill deficits. Touwen's 'schedule' contains 10 sub-groups of items, including "fine manipulative' ability. He found this skill group which to be independent of other ability groups including tasks involving gross motor functions, posture, balance of the trunk, and coordination of the extremities. Chapter 7 contains a more thorough discussion of various groups of symptoms evidenced by dysgraphic youngsters.

VISUAL-PERCEPTUAL CLUMSINESS

There are numerous visual and visual perceptual problems that may result in awkward motor behaviors. These problems may range from ocular-motor problems involving the erratic or inefficient movements of the muscles moving the eyes, to severe retinal deterioration. In addition, the camera-like eye may take a clear and accurate 'picture', but the child may not interpret, and organize visual information well and quickly. This latter type of confusion is often referred to as perceptual rather than a visual difficulty.

Hoare and Larkin (1991) recently identified a sub-type within the population of clumsy children they surveyed as evidencing problems in tasks heavily loaded with visual-perceptual components. This sub-group, consisting of 18% of the group they surveyed, had difficulty in "visually loaded" tasks while evidencing average and above-average performance in other motor skills.

Visual and visual perceptual problems interfere with accurate movement because the eyes and motor systems are neurologically and thus functionally intertwined in innumerable ways. Poor balance may occur, for example, because the eyes are unable to focus well thus de-stabilize the child's space field. This type of problem may be seen when the youngster is able to balance in a static position better with the eyes closed, than when they are open. In these cases a confusing visual field, when temporarily eliminated by closing the eyes, permits the motor system mediating balance to function better. In contrast, when some visually and/or perceptually inadequate children attempt balance tasks with their eyes open, below average scores may result.

Despite their interactions, there are measurable differences in various visual-motor functions, and other measures of motor incoordination. Thus most evidence strongly suggests the existence of a multi-faceted visual syndrome. In the extensive factor analysis previously cited by Nichols (1987), tests reflecting both nystagmus and strabismus loaded in factors separate from scores reflecting abnormal gait, and other abnormal movements.

Problems causing unclear vision may also inhibit accurate movement. We are currently working with a child of six whose vision was markedly deficient, until he received corrective lenses about a year ago. Upon 'entering the world' and becoming able to see clearly for the first time in his life, he first exhibited marked problems in ball interception and in similar skills. However after about six months of skill training, he has become able to vigorously compete in a youth soccer league. His main problem involved visual acuity, rather than motor deficiencies of the larger muscle groups.

The presence of erratic (nystagmatic) eye movements, that may reflect the presence of various visual pathologies, may also prevent a child from intercepting and extracting information well from moving objects. Serious visual-neurological problems may also result in inability to intercept moving objects well. These can include the presence of a tumor, at any one of several points within the optic pathways in the front of the brain (the optic chiasm). These types of tumors may restrict the size of childrens' visual fields, and thus prevent them from tracking balls through the same wide arc, available to youngsters whose visual fields are normal in size.

Accommodation problems, also commonly prevent children from focusing upon written work at a desk near the eyes. This problem involves the inability of the ocular muscles to draw the eyes toward each other and to focus at written work on the desk. Thus accommodation problems are likely to inhibit effective hand-eye coordinations needed when learning to print letters. Most of these difficulties, however, are modifiable with corrective lenses.

We recently worked with a boy of almost six years, whose accommodation problem was obvious. He simply could not seem to bring his eyes together and focus upon the letters he was attempting to draw. Near-point fusion was obviously deficit. He would begin trying to print each letter by first moving his head up, and then down, in apparent attempts to bring a clear picture into the retina. These tactics, however, proved unsuccessful. He then would finally try to resolve the visual-motor problem encountered by placing his arm at full length and to the side, attempting to continue printing letters with his hand, with the pencil and paper, placed about two feet to the side from where he was seated!

Children whose visual systems are intact may lack the abilities to organize and to interpret important visual information. They appear to be beset with perceptual rather than with visual difficulties. This quality also has been found to be multi-dimensional. Groups of tests evaluating visual perceptual (organizational and interpretational) skills are applied to large groups of children and factor analyzed, a number of separate and independent qualities emerge (Smith and Smith 1966). These included depth perception, the ability to fragment space (what is halfway between you and the door?) and the ability to judge movement in space. Thus it appears that deficits in innumerable visual and perceptual problems, acting alone or in combinations, are likely to effect physical skills in negative ways.

A variety of visual perceptual problems may prevent some children from accurately interpreting and copying the action patterns of their peers, including looking at, interpreting and then performing such complex skills as throwing, running, bike riding and the like. Normal children learn a great deal from watching their peers. In contrast, however, it is likely that some perceptually handicapped children do this poorly and thus to not visually-perceptually 'pick up' appropriate skill patterns present in a number of important and complex childhood activities.

Thus innumerable kinds of visual and visual perceptual problems can interfere with a large variety of motor tasks, actions ranging from those needed when printing and writing to those important in playground skills including ball interception. Movement educators dealing with motorically deficient children should familiarize themselves with behavioral symptoms that may reflect visual problems. Clinicians should also become closely associated with local visual specialists educated in the accurate diagnosis and correction of these deficiencies.

MIXED SYNDROMES

In addition to youngsters who evidence clearly definable sub-syndromes, some awkward children display symptoms that make their precise classification difficult. Similar to the 'mixed' type of cerebral palsy that may combine athetoid symptoms with spastic qualities, the symptoms some awkward children display may also cause them to be correctly labeled 'mixed' . For example, it is often difficult to separate tensions and incoordination that may because by neurological causes, from difficulties arising an 'emotional overload, the result of continual task failure caused of poor motor planning abilities.

Ocular control problems may not only cause motor incoordination, but also be part of a pervasive coordination problem arising from central nervous system dysfunctions, also resulting in imprecise movements of the larger muscle groups. Moreover as Laszlo and her colleagues have pointed out motor clumsiness is often due to a combination of motor incoordination, integration or process problems, and to deficits in monitoring kinesthetic sensory input (1985) (1988).

Such subtle variables as differences in leg length, poor foot mechanics or other postural-structural problems can also influence motor functioning in youngsters. It is likely that about 10-20% of children who are labeled as having balance problems, actually suffer from poor foot alignment. Obvious and subtle structural problems may also impede the performance of locomotor skills, including running, skipping and moving laterally. Thus the child's structure, posture, and foot mechanics should be assessed within a comprehensive evaluation of motor abilities. I have tested two children this past year, who evidenced differences in leg length that amount to over an inch. In both cases the problem caused them to appear clumsy and to have difficulty in a number of motor tasks. In both cases the parents were oblivious to a problem that was obvious upon even causal inspection.

Youngsters falling within this 'mixed classification may evidence a variety of coordination problems, reflected in virtually every motor task with which they are confronted. Both Miyahara (1992) and Hoare and Larkin (1991) identified sub-types who evidenced pervasive and consistent difficulties in all the tasks within the test batteries the employed. In Miyahara investigation this pervasive sub-group consisted of 17% of his total population. In the Australian population surveyed by Hoare and Larkin (1991) the group of youngsters who were "consistently below average in all tasks" comprised 19% of the group evaluated.

Cerebral palsied children have sometimes been described as possessing an unique patterns of poor coordination. Each youngster, it has been said, behaves differently. They have been compared to orchestras, each of whom has different groups of instruments (muscles) playing out of tune. The same may be said of the less severely involved awkward children. Many, if not most, display individual, and specific combinations of neurological soft-signs which, when combined, to cause them to be labeled clumsy.

Acceptance of the validity of the presence of various syndromes suggests that each poorly coordinated child should be considered as unique. A knowledgeable evaluator should assume that few general qualities and parameters exist, or that predictable correlations will be obtained between tasks sampling various skill groupings. A discussion of evaluation is found in Chapter 11.

SUMMARY

Various sub-syndromes, found within groups of clumsy children were labeled, and their characteristics and causes discussed. Their identification was based upon current statistical analyses, together with summaries of clinical observations. The sub-syndromes discussed include two reflecting chronic variations in muscle tone, the hypotonic and tension syndromes. The "cerebellar syndrome" described contains symptoms resembling a mild to moderate cerebellar ataxia, and includes unsteadiness in the upper as well as in the lower limbs. Other syndromes depicted included two that are multi-faceted, 'visual-perceptual clumsiness and a manual-dexterity syndrome. A 'mixed syndrome' was also listed, composed of specific combinations of symptoms. It was thus proposed in this chapter to illuminate the characteristics of various sub-groups of children labeled clumsy.

As the following chart suggests "The Clumsy Child Syndrome" may be a collection of sub-syndromes separate and independent of other childhood anomalies that also may be reflected in movement problems. Moreover within groups of clumsy children reside various sub-syndromes including the ones surveyed in this chapter. Finally there are numerous types of movement abnormalities, some obvious and some subtle, seen when a clumsy child attempts to participate in age-appropriate motor activities. These specific characteristics are discussed next in Chapter 6.

QUESTIONS FOR DISCUSSION

1. The identification of the various sub-syndromes in this chapter is based upon what kind of evidence? How do you feel about the validity of this evidence, and the veracity of the syndromes described? What might be the use of this kind of classification exercise relative to program planning?
2. What further studies seem needed, relative to the identification of various type-types among populations of clumsy children?
3. What sub-type(s) appear to require training in muscular relaxation as an important part of their therapy-remedial program?
4. What are some of the characteristics of the 'cerebellar type' listed in the chapter?
5. Why might a dyspraxic child begin to evidence heightened levels of muscular tension as he matures and is confronted with increasingly complex tasks.

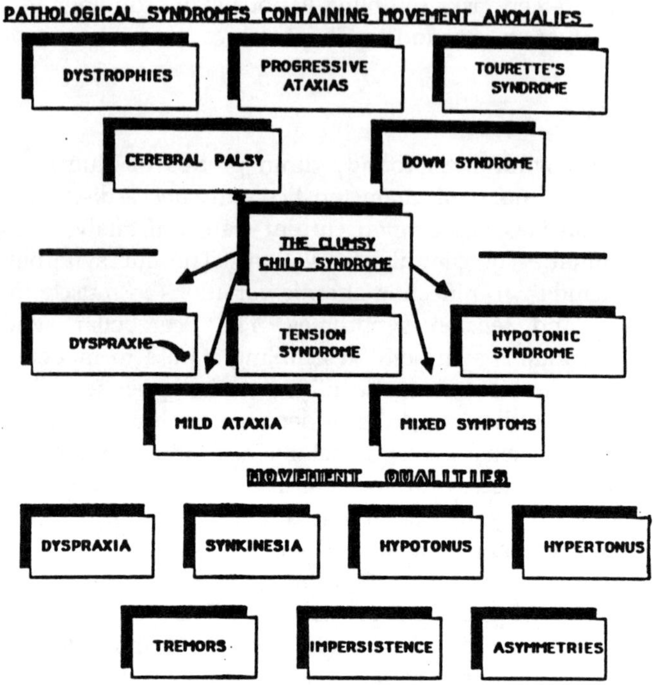

Plate 5-4. Syndromes, sub-syndromes, and movement qualities

6. Dyspraxia may be specific to the task, discuss and explain this statement, give examples.
7. What kinds of tasks might be difficult for a child evidencing visual-perceptual clumsiness? What kind of sports might be useful for such a child? What sports might best be avoided?
8. What social-emotional and physical characteristics might be observed in children labeled as evidencing benign hypotonia?
9. Why might thorough and comprehensive medical work-up be indicated in the case of a child who evidences hypotonia during the pre-school years?

Chapter 6
Movement Characteristics

INTRODUCTION

Labeling a child as simply 'clumsy', or uncoordinated, is not very scientific or precise. Youngsters suspected of coordination problems should be carefully screened and tested, to assess individual differences in obvious performance capacities. However, after this has been accomplished, even if evaluated with the most valid tests available, there remain a number of general movement qualities that are likely to be overlooked. These more subtle characteristics are likely to be seen as several kinds of tasks are attempted, skills which may involve different muscle groups.

In Chapter 5 general sub-syndromes were described. In this chapter selected movement qualities typically exhibited by poorly coordinated children are examined in more detail. Various combinations of the qualities discussed here, are found with the more global syndromes previously discussed. It is believed that the movement qualities surveyed in this chapter are important to consider for several reasons;

(1) These symptoms may have psycho-social significance. For example, the appearance of some of these qualities may make the child 'look funny' to others including friends, and family, and thus negative social responses result.

(2) Some of these qualities have important neurological significance, and reflect neuromotor immaturity.

(3) The presence of some of these behaviors have implications for the planning of program content.

(4) A thorough assessment of these qualities should help to make the problems and behaviors of awkward children more understandable and predictable.

The qualities discussed in this chapter include:

(1) Dyspraxia and apraxia

(2) Associated movements, sometimes termed 'overflow' or synkinesia,

(3) Asymmetries in actions,

(4) The contrasting qualities of motor impersistence and perseveration,

(5) Tonus abnormalities, including hypertonic qualities and hypotonia, and

(6) Unsteadiness and tremors, and

(7) The integration of body parts.

A final section is devoted to other less prevalent motor characteristics. In various combinations these movement symptoms are likely to occur within the sub-syndromes discussed in the previous chapter.

PRAXIC BEHAVIORS: APRAXIA & DYSPRAXIA

Introduction

Praxic behaviors refer to the performance of coordinated acts, that are reasonably complex, and usually consist of several parts. Underlying the production of a complex skill it is usually assumed that are several processes are important. These precursors to the 'correct' performance task include:

(1) accurately perceiving a demonstrated movement, and/or obtaining a clear understanding of verbal directions to move in some way.

(2) integrating the command or demonstration and formulating a motor plan and

(3) motorically producing the plan in a correctly ordered sequence.

Adequate praxic behaviors depend upon the adequate functioning all three of these processes.

The word "apraxia" refers to the inability to produce a correctly-sequenced, coordinated movement when demonstrated or requested. Dyspraxia, means a disruption of the abilities to produce a sequenced movement, when it is demonstrated, or requested orally. Generally the terms apraxia and dyspraxia, when applied to both to adults, and to children, reflect deficits of integrative functions within the central nervous system.

Apraxia and dyspraxia refer to motor ineptitude that excludes problems caused by structural-skeletal anomalies, peripheral muscular deficits, superficial nerve damage, and/or muscular weakness. However problems of motor sequencing may be caused by a breakdown of one, or more of the three processes including:

(a) perception of input,

(b) the central integration of input and output, and

(c) the organization of output. Thus a child scoring low on a test of motor planning may have to be evaluated further to determine which components of the three part process has gone awry.

Few youngsters may be correctly labeled 'apraxia'. A more accurate term to attach to both adults and children with moderate coordination problems is 'dyspraxia', reflecting a *disruption* of motor planning abilities, not an absence of these abilities as is indicated by the word 'apraxic'. Cermak employed the term 'dispractic' when describing dyspraxic children. (1985).

Broadly speaking the frontal lobes, portions of the motor cortex, secondary motor centers in the temporal-parietal areas, and other deeper structures, formulate and plan movements. The temporal and occipital lobes integrate sensory-perceptual information upon which to act, or information about the results of an action just-completed. This general schema is portrayed in Plate 6-2.

In the last century the term 'apraxia' was used by some of the pioneers in clinical neurology to describe the symptoms of their stroke patients in whom motor confusions were diagnosed. Over one hundred years ago Hughlings Jackson (1981), and others (Steinthal 1866), employed the word apraxia in their writings. It has also been observed for well over a hundred years that individuals acquiring various cerebral lesions disrupting coordinated movements including speech patterns, did not necessarily lose intellectual functions. Thus dyspraxia was defined in the last century, as disruption(s) of coordinated movement(s), resulting in motor ineptitude that is not accompanied by other structural, perceptual and/or intellectual problems.

During the first part of the 1900s Luria, the great Russian neurologist continued made important contributions to understanding and assessing dyspraxia in adult stroke patients (Luria 1966). Luria and others who followed have not only described apraxia and dyspraxia among those incurring neurologically damage, but also attempted to explain relationships between neural damage and these signs of poor coordination.

Currently two primarily neuro-behavioral models prevail. The "center theory" holds that specific sites in the brain are responsible for controlling motor sequencing, including the frontal Lobe (1966) and the parietal lobe (Heilman et al 1982) (Kimura 1976). Recently

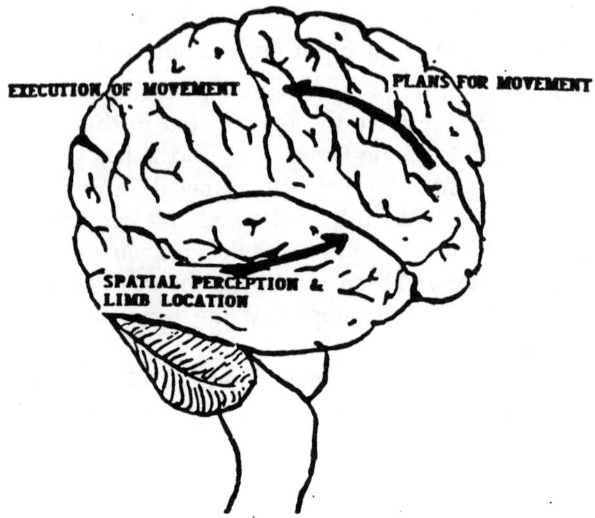

Plate 6-1. Motor planning, perception and motion
In general the front part of the brain fomulates movement plans which begin to be executed by the primary motor cortex in the parietal area just behind the associational areas. The rear of the brain engages in perceptual functions. Both of information needed to initiate movements, as well as perceptions formed after an action has taken place, both of which then feed forward to influence subsequent movement skills and effort

Watson and his colleagues postulated that the supplementary motor area is the primary center for motor programming. (Watson et al 1986).

Questions were raised by some researchers, however, who contended that specific lesion cites did not always correspond to predictable disruptions of motor behaviors, and alertness (Baso et al 1980) (Alexander & Schmidt 1980). They proposed a "disconnection theory" of apraxia. This second model, in contrast to the center theory, holds that the dyspraxic symptoms are caused by interruption in pathways linking areas involving information processing centers mediating the execution of movements. Proponents of this second model suggest that injuries within pathways connecting the two hemispheres often result in various forms of apraxia and dyspraxia. (Geschwind 1975). It is probable that insults to pathways as well as subtle lesions in various neural centers combine to cause various forms of dyspraxia and apraxia both developmentally in children and in stroke patients.

The causes of developmental dyspraxia in children have not been as clearly identified as have lesion-behavioral relationships among stroke patients. Among general causes sometimes ascribed to the condition in youngsters has been neural damage caused by low birth low birth weight (Lesny 1980) and by other perinatal stresses (Gubbay 1978). Meyer-Probst and his colleagues, for example found that high frequency of apraxia was found among those who had a history of early perinatal traumas. (Meyer-Probst et al 1980). However ascertaining specific relationships between diagnosed lesions and behavioral disruptions in children and adolescents is a difficult undertaking.

A recent study compared differences in behaviors among children evidencing two types of causes of dyspraxia. Contrasting children who had suffered organic brain damage, to those born with developmental dyspraxia, Lehmkuyhl (1984) found that the latter group exhibited a more diverse set of dyspraxic symptoms. Literature is just beginning to appear which should eventually assist in locating the mechanisms, pathways, and sites causing various forms of dyspraxia among children. However, models and theories associating various forms of developmental apraxia and dyspraxia to specific neural insults and disruptions among children, are just beginning to be formulated. A pioneer study of these associations by Knuckey and his colleagues, used modern scanning techniques. They speculated that both brain injuries and cerebral immaturity contribute in various combinations to forms of developmental apraxia, and dyspraxia seen among children (Knuckey et al 1983).

Within the past decades clinical insights and experimental data have resulted in the identification of several types of apraxia, among older populations who have incurred cerebral strokes. Similar symptoms are also seen among dyspraxic children. These sub-groups include:

Ideational apraxia

Ideational apraxia is evidenced when an individual fails to grasp the nature of a motor problem, has difficulty initially formulating an plan of action , or does not easily comprehend what is required. The motor plan may be reasonably good once decided upon, but the delay may be long-term, or result in inaction.

I recently observed the symptoms of ideational apraxia in a twenty-six year old accident case I was evaluating. When the former construction worker was asked to draw a triangle, for example, his hesitations persisted for several minutes, during which he seemed to be trying to grasp the idea of what was being requested. The triangle once drawn, however, was reasonably accurate.

Another nine-year old boy, we recently worked with in our clinic, reportedly was tied to a tree and beaten by other children at school, when his hesitations in play situations caused them consternation. He was forced into a home-tutoring program, primarily because of symptoms suggesting the presence of ideational apraxia. In other children we have encountered delays of speech-language, including *formulation aphasia* (hesitation while formulating a sentence-response in a conversation) accompanying the inability to quickly formulate appropriate plans prior to attempting reasonably complex motor tasks.

Ideomotor apraxia

A second type of apraxia, ideomotor apraxia, is reflected in behaviors that result in the several parts of motor act being executed out-of-sequence. Another client-patient we evaluated recently was afflicted with this kind of problem. His problem manifested itself in a number of contexts. This seventeen year old, high school senior, had been fired from his job in a fast-food restaurant because he could not master the sequences necessary when making hamburgers). He was dropped from the basketball team because of an inability to remember the drills. Finally, he also was a social disaster because he could not remember a series of dance steps. Despite these marked signs of ideomotor apraxia (dyspraxia), his intellect was apparently intact, as he was scheduled enter college after high school graduation.

DeRenzi and his colleagues (1968), and others (Deule et al (1984) (Poeck 1982), have studied various types of apraxia, including ideational apraxia. There are clear-cut divisions in their data differentiating damage caused within specific neural sites that separate symptoms of ideomotor apraxia from those of ideational apraxia in stroke patients. It is possible, however, that these two types may be more easily divisible neurologically in older stroke patients, than is true among in groups of children exhibiting developmental dyspraxia from birth.

Limb kinetic apraxia

This kind of subtle problem results in the sub-parts of a movement being executed improperly, while at the same time components of the movement are placed in proper sequence. An example of this behavior was described to me recently by parents of a five year old girl. She correctly reached for and attempted to use her spoon, and fork while eating, but often held them by the wrong ends! A stroke patient evidencing this condition might attempt to light a match, by striking the wrong end to the match box.

Trunkle Apraxia

This disruption in motor planning is seen when a series of movements, involving the total body, are executed improperly. In the 1960's a group of psychiatrists whom I was consulting, described their observations of what they termed 'bumping scores', recorded as they watched learning disabled, awkward children lurch around their classrooms. They were probably chronicling symptoms of trunkle dyspraxia. They further noted that the unintentional contacts made by these youngsters with trunkle dyspraxia was causing them social problems, as their classmates often responded to this contact in aggressive ways.

More recently I evaluated an intellectually bright ten-year-old girl with congenital neurological problems that had resulted in pressure to the neural structures that receive, store, and integrate motor programs. We helped her to improve her recreational skills, but it was apparent that she was also having problems simply walking accurately around the living room furniture without injuring herself. Intricate sequences of body movements essential in games, were also difficult for her to learn. The symptoms of trunkle apraxia, or dyspraxia display symptoms that resemble to maladaptive behaviors accompanying some of the general spatial agnosias discussed in Chapter 8.

Oral apraxia

This term has been attached to two types of behavioral confusions. Some writers, describing neuropathological symptoms, in the past, have used the word to denote articulation problems, the inability to correctly sequence finite actions of the tongue, soft pallet, lips, together with difficulty controlling forceful muscular actions producing air-power from the chest, as words are spoken. The terms *oro-apraxia, oromotor apraxia,* and *buccofacial apraxia,* have also been used recently to denote difficulties in the chaining of actions of the tongue, lips and mouth, when attempting to speak. (Taft & Barowsky 1989).

Yamadori (1985) has suggested that most forms of oral apraxia are similar to symptoms encountered when the diagnosis is ideomotor apraxia. According to Geschwind (1975) this type of problem is controlled by the precentral cortex and the left-arcuate faciculus, which control cranial muscles on both side of the face, and transmit information from vocal areas (Wernick's) to pre-motor areas.

A second meaning given to 'oral apraxia' has been to denote motor-task confusions occurring when an individual is given oral commands by another person, to move in various ways. Studies of children evidencing dyspraxia have contained this term, and have contrasted the abilities of young subjects when asked to respond to both visual demonstrations of motor skills, to their ability to execute physical tasks that have been requested verbally. (Kools and Tweedie 1975).

Construction Apraxia

Construction apraxia is reflected in difficulties involving the manipulation of objects, and combining parts of objects into wholes. This problem in early childhood is typically evaluated by asking a child to stack blocks on top of each other, imitating a similar stack constructed by an examiner. Difficulties when attempting to execute various self-care skills also reflect this type of dyspraxia. Shoe tying, for example, presents is very difficult to learn, for a young child who evidencing construction apraxia.

Among groups of both stroke patients and children it has been found that deficits assessed using tests of construction apraxia are often reflected in problems encountered while trying to get dressed (Bradley 1982). Attempting to manage the difficult spatial relationships needed when dressing also brings out this type of dyspraxia. Thus some observers have considered construction dyspraxias as a spatial rather than as a motor disturbance (Poeck 1986). At times the term 'dressing apraxia' is used in the literature and reflects problems both with the sensory-perceptual awareness of the body and also when attempting to formulate sequences of actions needed when putting on clothes. Recently an otherwise capable, dyspraxic seven-year-old in our clinic was unable to turn his shirt right-side out to put on, after it had been turned inside out.

I often witness this kind of dyspraxia when children in our clinic program are asked to move or adjust equipment. The other day an othewise intelligent six year old girl took almost ten minutes to figure out how to hand up a sock on a peg after the simple task was demonstrated for her several times. This task usually requires only a few seconds for most normal children her age to accomplish.

Other children in my program exhibit this type of problem when they require prolonged periods of time to put together simple jig-saw type puzzles. Another boy of seven with whom we are now working, is bright but dyspraxic. A few months ago he could not properly place his feet in foot prints adjacent to a baseball batting T, after he had been shown how. His best effort resulted in placing his back to the T, and this only occurred after numerous frustrating attempts to accomplish this spatial-motor task.

Both parents and therapists should be aware of the symptoms reflecting this kind of dyspraxia. Children afflicted with various forms of construction apraxia should patiently dealt with by their caretakers, and be given sufficient time when attempting to master and to carry out even the simplest self-care tasks. New skills, using objects, should be carefully introduced. Each new task should carefully taught, by first learning its parts. Additional information about teaching strategies taking into consideration dyspraxic tendencies among the awkward is located in Chapter 13.

Deficits in several parts of the central nervous systems of older stroke patients have been linked to various forms of apraxia. For example, in the following diagram (Plate 6-2), two lesion locations, one in the front of the corpus callosum, and the second in the parietal area within the motor cortex, have both been linked to various types of apraxia.

A lesion in the corpus callosum has been suggested as limiting the ability to plan movements that depend upon instructions passing easily from the right hemisphere to the left. This hypothesis reflects the disconnection model previously discussed. Lesions in the motor cortex has also been linked to ideomotor apraxias, that are independent of symbolic-verbal meanings. This lesion site supports the *center theory* previously reviewed. However, as been pointed out, such obvious lesions and pathway disruptions are usually not apparent when exposing dyspraxic children to neurological evaluations and to CAT scans of their central nervous systems.

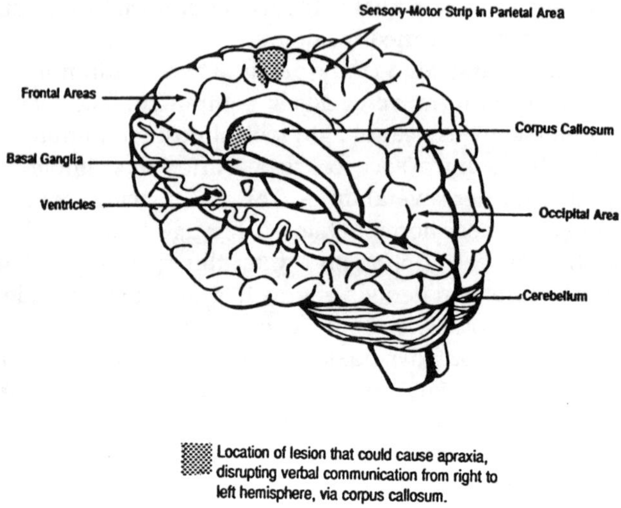

Plate 6-2. Left side of the brain cut away to show possible sites of lesions resulting in apraxia and dyspraxia

An Overview

Thus during the past several decades problems of motor disruptions seen in stroke patients have continued occupied the energies of numerous scholars (Haaland et al 1982). Data emerging from both earlier and more recent efforts afford important insights into the formulation of speech, and the development of the intellect (Kimura 1982). In addition, the available research has resulted in the formulation of theoretical models designed to explain the processes contributing to, and detracting from, accurate motor planning and sequencing behaviors (Heilman et al 1982) (Kelso and Tuller 1981).

Within the past two decades there has also been some interest shown in the nature of apraxia and dyspraxia in children. (Walton et al 1962). Currently most neurological schedules, designed to assess children with minimal problems, contain tests designed to evaluate the presence of apraxia or dysgraphia. (Tupper 1987, Appendix).

Developmental Apraxia & Dyspraxia

Dyspraxia and apraxia among children was first noted by Collier in the early 1900s who employed the term 'congenital maladroitness'.

Thereafter the terms clumsy, awkwardness, and dysgraphia in children were often used interchangeably. According to Cermak, however, there are two marked differences in the literature dealing with adult apraxics and children with developmental apraxia or dyspraxia (1985). Dyspraxia in children refers to the inability to acquire new tasks; whereas in adults the condition refers to the loss of the ability to execute tasks that have been previously acquired.

In addition the evaluation tools to which children and adults are typically exposed are often different. Adults are usually asked to engage in some self-care skill, tasks that are translatable into word formulas. These may be referred to has symbolic tasks meaning that they are able to described in words. They can include combing the hair, buttoning buttons, and the like. In contrast the assessment tools applied to children often have also contained non-symbolic and meaningless gestures. as well as self-care skills. (Ayres 1972) (Druker 1978) (Berges & Lezine 1965). However some research tests first used with stroke populations has stimulated the formulation of assessment tools later employed to investigate dyspraxia among children. For example, one of Luria's (Luria 1966) measures of apraxia, the fist-edge-palm test, was later modified to evaluate dyspraxia in children. (Cratty and Samoy 1984) and by others (Orpet 1972).

By the 1970s motor planning problems in children began to occupy the energies of several scholars. Both clinicians (Gubbay 1974) as well as experimentalists (DeRenzi et al 1980) (Kools and Tweedie 1975) focused on 'developmental apraxia'. Pediatric neurologists also began to explore the possible relationships of dyspraxia to other behaviors. Measuring neurological soft-signs, they attempted to determine possible relationships between learning disabilities, hyperactivity and to these subtle symptoms of neuromotor immaturity. (Tupper 1987) Using contemporary scanning techniques, experimental neurologists also began to obtain evidence confirming the presence of abnormalities in the brain's architecture among groups of dyspraxic-clumsy children (Knuckey et al 1983).

In the 1970s my student-colleagues and I began to study motor planning behaviors appearing in both normal and in atypical children. We also began to formulate what we believed to be much-needed evaluation instruments. (Cratty and Samoy 1984) (Cratty and Gibson 1985) (Cratty and DeOliveira 1986) (Cratty and Gong 1989). We were struck by the imprecision of the available measures. These instruments usually included only manipulation tasks, following verbal commands, or imitating a few finger postures presented by the examiner (Duel & Robinson 1987). Additionally the available tools seemed imprecise and often consisted of a check-list in which a pass or fail score was recorded. Finally many were often not suitable for obtaining data and norms among younger populations.

In contrast the testing instruments we began to develop contained relatively long series of several types of tasks. We wished to assess a broad range of praxic behaviors within various normal and atypical populations, and of both older and younger children. We also wanted to measure dyspraxia, independent of verbal symbolic behaviors that might bias the scores obtained from youngsters within various ethnic sub-cultures and from a variety of language families.

As our work progressed we found that dyspraxia in children was multi-dimensional. For example, the accuracy with which a youngster reproduced a series of hand movements, did not usually predict how well the same child could copy a series of arm-positions, or replicate locations of the total body (Cratty and Samoy 1984). In other studies scores reflecting the ability of children to replicate facial movements were found to be independent of scores from tests assessing movements of the larger muscle groups.

These conclusions, and similar findings by others, indicated that when surveying the abilities of school-age children it was necessary to develop more than one-sub test to comprehensively assess motor planning (praxic) abilities (Kools and Tweedie 1975) (Conrad et al 1983) (de Renzi 1980) (Cratty and Gong 1989). Earlier work, using stroke patients has also referred to the specificity of apraxic and dyspraxic behaviors.

As a result of our work with groups of both average and atypical youngsters, it began to appear that the list of motor planning sub-tests, in batteries designed to evaluate dyspraxia among children in a comprehensive manner should include the following:

(1) Tests to determine the accuracy of Imitation of hand and finger movements, after being given a visual demonstration.

(2) Assessment of how well a series of demonstrated limb positions may be replicated.

(3) Tests of actions that have counterparts in daily living and self-care (dressing, combing the hand, buttoning etc).

(4) Assessments of the replication of sequences of acts that involve nonsense movements, and that exclude actions appearing within a given culture, or sub-culture, actions that may be described verbally.

(5) Tests of Trunkle apraxia, measured by the attempts to replicate sequences of positions of the total body in space.

(6) Tests evaluating the ability to replicate a static positions, as well as tests assessing the qualities necessary to replicate a series of actions. (Conrad et al 1983).

The sensory information that accompanies instructions to move in various ways also appears to be influential of test results. It is usually found, for example, that responding to a visual demonstration is easier, than correctly responding after being given a verbal command. (Kools & Tweedie 1972). The following diagram reflects the various dimensions and variables that should be considered when researching and evaluating various components of praxic behaviors in both children and adults.

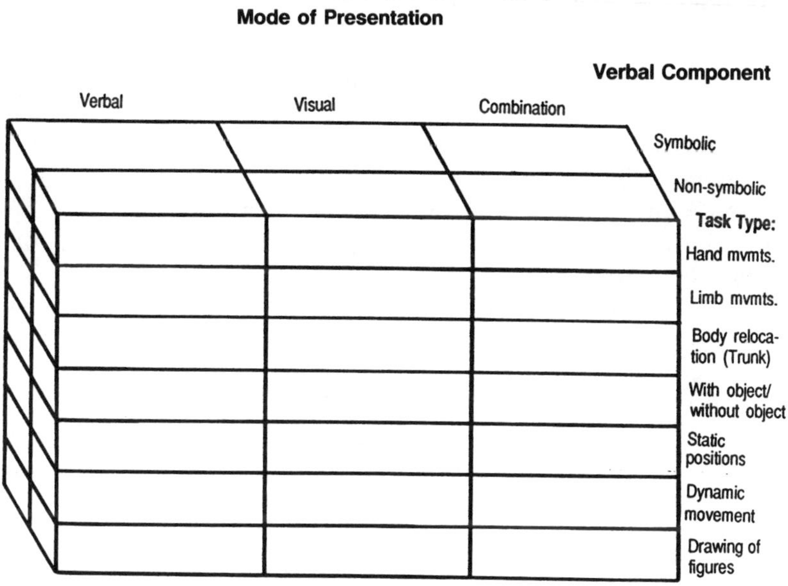

Plate 6-3. A model for the study of motor planning in children

Developmental Norms

Available findings indicate that at about six years of age most normal children respond correctly to demonstrations of typical self-care skills, and to demonstrations of moderately complex sports skills. However, motor planning abilities continue improve throughout childhood among normal populations. Currently lacking, however are well normed test batteries, based upon scores from large numbers of subjects of sexes, and from a wide range of ages, on a variety of sub-tests, including those sampling symbolic (tasks reducible to word formulas) and non-symbolic nonsense movements.

Our data began to demonstrate, however that children from about the age of 4 years to 7 and 8 years were able to replicate a series of nonsense movements (demonstrated at about one-a-second) in numbers that average about two less than their chronological ages. A four year old thus may be expected to reproduce a two-movement series, the average five year old can replicate three demonstrated movements, while a seven year old can accurately repeat five consecutive movements after they are demonstrated at the rate of one-a-second.

Dyspraxia Among Special Populations

In the 1980s my student-colleagues and I, as well as others, began to study dyspraxia in several 'special' populations. These groups included the hearing impaired (Cratty and DeOliveira 1986), the retarded (Conrad et al 1983) and the learning disabled (Miyahara, Cratty & Goldman 1990).

In the first of our studies we found that hard-of-hearing youngsters were equal or superior to children whose hearing was normal, when both were given a series of motor planning tasks. We had initially hypothesized that deaf children, perhaps deficient in internal speech, would be poorer when attempting to replicate the parts of movement series.

It was found, however, that deaf children studied were careful observers of the visually presented demonstrations. The young hard-of-hearing subjects studied apparently watched the demonstrations carefully, because they were accustomed to constantly inspecting their friends hands as they signed messages. Thus performances by the hard-of-hearing in the motor planning tasks were, in many cases, were superior to those measured among the youngsters who could hear. (Cratty et al 1986)

In a 1990 study motor planning abilities among a large population of learning disabled children were measured, using three sub-tests. The existence of several sub-groups within the group were identified among the group studied. These included sub-groups with and without dyspraxic tendencies. It was also found that the scores reflecting dyspraxia, did not correlate to traditional measures of motor ability, physical performance and fitness. Our data also suggested that dyspraxic symptoms among the learning disabled population studied, persisted from childhood into early and middle adolescence. (Miyahara, Cratty & Goldman 1990).

More details about this investigation and its implications are found in Chapter 9.

Practical Implications

A thorough knowledge of the motor planning abilities of awkward children, whom it is decided to serve, is important for several reasons. Praxic and dyspraxic qualities are important to consider when deciding teaching techniques, program content and objectives. A test battery formulated to evaluate overall motor abilities should contain at several sub-tests. Low scores in this kind of assessment should point to the need for careful teaching of an awkward child. Skills should be presented to in parts to dyspraxic youngsters, and then later the parts should be gradually synthesized into 'wholes'.

Within recent years some clinicians and researchers have suggested several types of strategies for remediating dyspraxic symptoms in children (Gschwend 1988) (Gubbay 1975). Seaman and De Pauw, for example, presented twenty-one activities purporting to remediate fifteen signs of developmental dyspraxia, they also listed. However their potentially useful suggestions were not accompanied by research data substantiating their efficacy. (Seaman & De Pauw 1982).

Gschwend (1988) also proposed a program for dealing with dyspraxia in children. The components of his program included music and art therapy, playing chess, and types of what was labeled cognitive training or will training. His suggestions seemed to constitute a more global approach to the improvement of general cognitive-motor strategies than was true within the more skill-specific program suggested by Seaman and DePauw (1982). It is obvious that research is needed focusing upon strategies that will potentially to blunt, or correct, both general and specific symptoms of dyspraxia in children. At this point the location of objective studies reflecting efforts to modify dyspraxia in direct ways, are difficult to locate. Chapter 12 also contains a survey of teaching methods applicable to the reduction of dyspraxic symptoms

SYNKINESIA: ASSOCIATED MOVEMENTS

Synkinesia refers to actions and tensions in body parts not directly involved in a task. They are thus unintentional movements that appear in the form of what might be termed muscular overflow. Several sub-types of these movements have been identified. For example, mirror movements are synkinetic actions that appear on the side of the body opposite to that of the intentional movement. Regular finger-twitching of the opposite hand when a child is asked to engage in finger opposition would be defined as a mirror movement. Thus mirror movements are synkinetic movements occurring in body parts on opposite sides of the body.

Heterotopic actions are movements which occur in muscle groups whose mediation is closely aligned within the sensory-motor cortex. Thus grimacing actions of the face, when the hands are requested to move, represent heterotopic actions. (Deuel & Robinson 1987). On Plate 6-4, various portions of the motor cortex purportedly mediating both the face and hands are shown, together with other integrative areas.

Tests potentially eliciting other types of associated movements are found in evaluation instruments directed toward awkward children. Synkinesia has also been evaluated within several populations who were labeled as 'neurologically suspect'. Low-birth weight infants, for example, have been assessed, during their early school years, using measures of synkinesia (Hertzig (1987). These measures are frequently found on neurological 'schedules' designed for application to children with suspected minimal neurological dysfunctions.

I recently was assisting two brothers, eight and nine years of age, to improve their printing and writing. Both struggled at their tasks. While attempting to form difficult letters, their heads, necks, mouths and tongues postured and moved constantly and uncontrollably. Their bodies were also in motion, as they bounced around their chairs during the lessons. I spent as much time encouraging them to relax, and attempt to diminish, these excess tensions as I did aiding them in the graphic skills they were trying to accomplish. It was obvious that the extra movements they displayed siphoned off

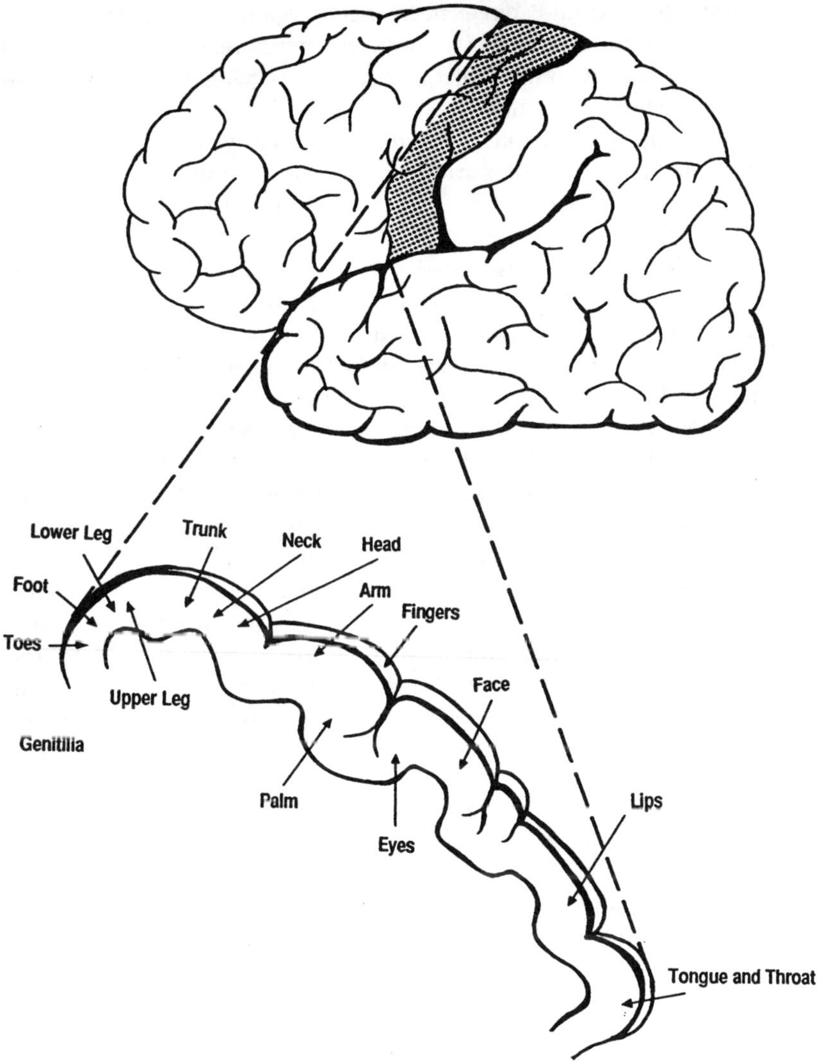

The primary motor cortex is located to the rear of the associational areas. As can be seen, more area is devoted in the motor cortex to the mediation of the more complicated motor functions, including the mouth and lip movements required in speech, as well as hand movements in manipulative behaviors. Stimulation of the various regions results in simple spasm-like movements of the corresponding parts of the body.

Plate 6-4. The motor cortex

energy that would have been better spent at the task. These extraneous jumpings and twistings, furthermore, detracted also from a calm and competent appearance, and thus created tensions in those who watched them, me!

These unusual actions were first noted early in this century and were defined as "motor irradiations that are outside the subjects' awareness and accompany but are not necessary for, the performance of an intended movement." (Noica 1912). During the decades that followed these associated movements, reflecting some kind of neuromotor overflow, have attracted the attention of neurologists, developmentalists, pediatricians, and of educators.

These extraneous posturings are frequently seen in children under the ages of seven or eight years, as a number of discrete motor skills may be attempted. After these ages, however, the neuromotor systems of normal children precise and mature. Thus with maturation the expression of associated movements is likely to diminish youngsters, and they are less frequently observed and recorded. (Cohen et al 1967) (Connolly & Stratton 1968).

The persistence of these unusual posturings into middle childhood, however, may contribute to motor awkwardness, as biomechanically correct movements may be made more difficult by their presence. The appearance of associated movement may also cause awkward youngsters to become victims of negative social evaluations by both peers and adults. Rasmussen and his colleagues, for example, found that the appearance of these overflow movements resulted in children being considered by their teachers to be both neurological suspect and behaviorally deficient (Rasmussen et al 1983).

One dramatic appearance of these actions occurs in normally developing twelve-month olds who, while taking their first steps, evidence obvious extensions in the shoulders. The hands thus are held above the head, during early attempts to walk, in what has been labeled a "high guard position".

The actions of the lower limbs as infants start to walk thus produces excess tensions in the upper limbs. However with normal maturity children's upper limbs are held lower. By three or four years of age, the arms usually swing freely in the cross-extension pattern seen in a mature adult gait.

One explanation that has been advanced for the appearance of these extraneous actions, both in groups of awkward children and among the immature, is that they are due to underdeveloped

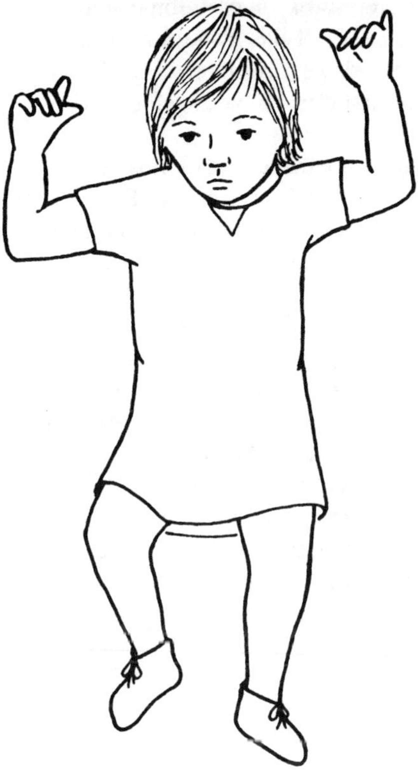

Plate 6-5. First steps taken in a high-guard position, illustrating normal developmental synkinesia

inhibitory motor pathways passing through the corpus callosum joining the two cerebral hemispheres (Fog & Fog 1963) (Wolff et al 1983). Contemporary research suggests that the manner in which these actions appear, their intensity and/or the locations on the body where they occur, have developmental significance. (Szatmari & Taylor 1984) (Waber et al 1985).

The usual hypothesis postulated is that these symptoms are signs of neuromotor immaturity and predictive of moderate behavioral dysfunctions. Substantiating this premise, data has shown that these less-than-useful actions are correlated with poor attention in children (Connolly & Stratton 1968) Wolff et al 1983), deficit school performance, with speech and language problems (Noterdaeme et al 1987) and also with other signs of emotional and behavioral immaturity (Rasmussen et al 1982). It has also found that an excess of associated movements are valid discriminators of differences between normal and atypical populations of youngsters (Abercrombie et al 1964) (Cohen et al 1967).

Evaluating the appearance, and intensity, of associated movements may prove difficult, however. For example the amount of tension induced in a given body part is likely to be influential of the overflow in another body part, thus associated movements often interact in unpredictable ways. Moreover associated movement may occur among normal subjects when they are placed, or place themselves, under high degrees of tension. Thus determining what 'normal' overflow consists of, when moderate to high levels of tension are introduced among populations of various ages, is often difficult. In one study, for example, the normal college-age subjects were asked to flex their arms, as hard as they could, against a wrist cuff mounted on a desk in front of them. Under these conditions it was found that dramatic, individualized patterns of associated movements were recorded among all of the subjects tested. (Waterland & Hellenbrandt 1964).

Evaluation

Several methods have been used to measure of these actions. One of the more popular is 'stressing the gait' by asking a client to 'walk on your heels' . . . or 'walk on your toes' . . . or perhaps to 'walk on the sides of your feet''. When extra tension is induced in the lower limbs, in this manner by encouraging distortions of gait, observations are then recorded (sometimes on a 1-3 scale) of simultaneous posturings and tensions that may occur in the arms, shoulders and hands.

The distorting-tensions, or associated movements appearing in the upper limbs, among awkward or immature youngsters, typically correspond to the types of tensions elicited in the legs and feet. Thus,

(a) if the child is asked to walk on his/her toes, the arms extend and the hands extend to the rear;
(b) when heel walking the child may evidence flexions in the elbows, and in the wrists.
(c) when walking on the outside of the feet, or when walking with the feet turned outward, the hands may also ''spoon'' and rotate outward.

(d) with the knees and feet inward the hands and elbows also rotate inward.

This "feet to hands" technique was instituted over 20 years ago (Fog & Fog 1963), and has been improved in recent years by using video-tapes to increase reliability. (Szatmari & Taylor 1984).

My students and I recently filmed arm and hand flexions, with high-speed cameras, during stressed gaits elicited among young subjects walking on a treadmill. (Hsu et al 1989). When the children were asked to walk on their heels, under this arrangement, marked flexions were filmed and recorded in at the elbow and wrists of both hands. Overflow of this nature passing between the upper and lower parts of the body has been suggested by some as due to immaturity in the ipsilateral neural pathways (Zulch 1942) Hopft et al 1974).

The functions of both bi-lateral and ipsilateral pathways, however, might be studied as functions of just how overflow may occur. For example, if more marked overflow is seen from stressing the limbs on the same side (left leg to left arm), then one set of pathways is suspect; while if the overflow moves primarily from the right leg to the left arm then the integrity of another set of pathways should be examined more thoroughly. Finally the amount of overflow seen in

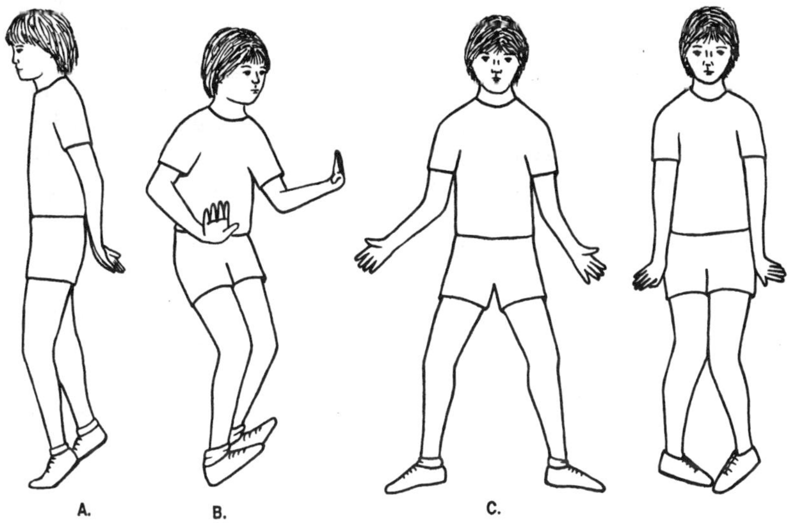

Plate 6-6. The use of stressed gaits to elicit overflow in the upper limbs

either the left or right hand and arm, when the gait is stressed in various ways, may afford clues as to whether one side or the other may be functionally more deficit.

Touwne and Prechtl (1970) and others (Tupper 1987, Appendix) formulating evaluation schedule for children with 'minor nervous dysfunctions', have included several tests for assessing associated movements. Among these were tasks producing tensions and excess posturings in the musculature of the face and mouth, applied to neurologically immature youngsters. Tensions may be seen to spread from the hands, when the child is requested to separate his/her fingers "as widely as possible", to the mouth. Synkinesia can also be recorded as flowing in the other direction, from the face to the hands, when the child is asked to smile as widely as possible. It is possible that the degree of the associated tensions produced are the result of the relative maturity of the adjacent areas of the sensory-motor cortex that mediate actions of both the hands and of the mouth. These types of associated movements are termed *heterotopic synkinesia*.

It is possible that speech-articulation problems may be reflected in an excess of muscular posturings in the mouth and adjacent musculature, when the hands and arms are placed under tension. These associated movements in the mouth and face may also provide insights into some origins of deficit language. For example, it has been a consistent observation in our clinic that articulation problems occur in children whose mouths posture excessively, while they engage in various motor tasks, including writing or when vigorously employing the larger muscle groups. Noterdaeme and his colleagues in Germany (1987) have begun to explore the possible relationships between synkinetic actions and speech-language deficiencies. The results of this kind of investigation are of potential importance to speech pathologists.

Other methods used to explore associated movement have been to induce tensions or movements in one hand then to study flexions and tensions in the opposite hand. Various methods have been used. For example, young subjects are asked to exert tension (Fog and Fog 1963) to move their (Zazzo 1960) as well as to spread their fingers (Connolly & Stratton (1960). These actions, and the tensions from one hand, to the other, that may result, have been labeled 'mirror movements'. One neurological explanation that advanced for the excessive appearance of these actions crossing the body is that pathways connecting the hemispheres are immature. (Zulch 1942) (Hopft et al 1974).

I have sometimes use these latter tasks, in lecture-demonstrations with children, to illustrate the influence of normal maturity upon the appearance of associated movements. If both five year olds and seven year olds are asked first to place their hands up and to the sides, and then to engage in finger opposition with one hand (touching each finger, in order, to the thumb of the same hand) age differences typically emerge. The more mature nervous systems of normal seven-year-old children often reflect the inhibition of similar and simultaneous actions of the opposite hand. In contrast, normal children, five years and younger, finger opposition requested in one hand will usually will be seen to spread to "mirror movements" appearing in the other.

Denckla in a 1985 study explored, with some precision, the nature of overflow due to movements initiated by intended, volitional actions of both sides of the body. She found that there were more variations in the types of overflow seen in younger subjects, when contrasted to synkinesia measured among older youngsters. She also found that there was more overflow to body parts on both the left and right sides of the body, when left-sided movements were first requested, than when right-sided movements were elicited. Denckla hypothesized that this latter finding meant that the young subjects in her investigation were likely reflected the dominant role of the left hemisphere in the planning of motor programs. Further research could be useful in illuminating the possible relationships between the type and directions of overflow to the presence of possible slight signs of hemiplegia. The location of the hemisphere(s) in which children are likely to program movement patterns, and/or verbal-motor programs might also be revealed by studying inter-limb overflow. (Denckla 1985).

Overflow in Time

Upon evaluating, and observing children in our clinic program over the past several years, it has become increasingly apparent that neuromotor overflow often occurs in *time*, as well as in the body's space. For the most part the previous discussion has centered around overflow-associated movements occurring in various parts of the body. However, associated movements may occur within a temporal framework. This second type of overflow is often marked when a neurologically 'suspect' youngster is evaluated.

This latter type of behavior usually occurs immediately after a child has executed and tried to terminate a vigorous movement. Instead of the body and limbs coming to rest, the arms legs, and sometimes the trunk, continue in motion. The most common way this is seen is in movements of the arms that resemble the flappings of birds' wings. These are likely to occur just after the youngster has released a vigorously thrown ball. At times these actions will continue for several seconds after the termination of some vigorous action.

Explanations for this temporal phenomenon are difficult to formulate. The occurrence of these after-actions may be caused by delays in the maturation of inhibitory processes within the central nervous system. Some recent work in neural regression suggests that the failure of the human nervous system to effectively eliminate unneeded synaptic connections during maturation might account for this type of phenomena. (Carlson, Earls and Todd 1988).

These continuing impulses to move often do not resemble the action just terminated. It is as if the body has neuromotor energy left over after some vigorous movement occurs, impulses that suddenly need continued expression and ventilation. Furthermore, symptoms reflecting temporal overflow may result in negative social attention directed toward the youngster evidencing them; just as is true when other types of associated movements are observed by peers and adults.

To my knowledge, temporal movement overflow has not been extensively researched. However, the observations of my staff and I suggest that (1) the form they take are relatively consistently expressed in unique ways by each youngster (2) They detract from appearance and efficiency. For example, if a youngster continues to 'flap' his or her arms after releasing a ball, he/she may then fail to be ready for appropriate actions that may quickly be required next in a game situation. Efforts to evaluate and to suppress, or to control, these the temporal aspects of motor overflow, appear worthy of further clinical and experimental attention.

Practical and Theoretical Implications

It has been suggested by Wolff and his colleagues that with further study, each type of associated movement may assume specific maturational meanings at various ages. The apparent inability of awkward and/or neurologically immature children to suppress these signs make them potentially useful diagnostic indices reflecting neuromotor maturity or immaturity. Some have suggested that inducing an excess of these movements during a neurological examination may obliterate other, important signs of neural immaturity and thus should be omitted from standard assessments (Wolff et al 1983). Most of most of the available data indicates, however, that these atypical actions are important to consider. Professionals working with youngsters whose nervous systems, and concomitant behaviors, are 'suspect' (or obviously deficit) may gain additional insights into their problems by considering this interesting and potentially important maturational sign post.

The appearance of associated movements has implications for those engaged in clinical practices intended to improve motor abilities. Tests and tasks which induce these in 'suspect' youngsters are useful, because these extraneous tensions are not easily modified by the client, and thus afford important insights into basic neuromotor maturity and immaturity.

Strategies that may reduce these unwanted movements are also important to attempt, although their blunting is often difficult for clinicians to accomplish. These interventions can include giving children visual cues revealing these unwanted actions. They may for example, be asked to perform in front of a mirror, and then to make conscious attempts to reduce associated movements. Reward systems for their suppression also may prove effective.

Reducing these extraneous posturings is not always an easy undertaking, For example, several years ago we spent time requiring a six year old girl in our program to walk a balance beam, while simultaneously attempting encourage her to extend her habitually flexed arms, by manually assisting her to do so. We had begun to feel we had achieved success after several months. However when visitors came to observe her progress one day, she first demonstrated a relaxed gait while walking the beam. Following the demonstration, however, she excitedly exclaimed to them . . . "there, how was that!!" . . . while accompanying her outburst with her habitual flexed-arm posture. With additional work, however, both remedial efforts, as well as assessment strategies are likely to improve. More research should be directed also toward illuminating the neurological significance of these unusual signs of neuromotor immaturity and dysfunction.

ASYMMETRIES

Several types of functional asymmetries take place within the 'motor personalities' of normal children. Two general categories of asymmetries include:

(1) normal hand, foot, eye and/or ear preferences, and

(2) moderate to marked motor asymmetries that may be pathological and contribute to and/or accompany motor awkwardness.

This latter type may take the form of unusual flexions, and/or muscular weakness on one side of the body, and or the limbs on one side.

Hand Preference

A normal asymmetry shared by all humans are hand and foot preferences. Preferences for using one hand (paw, or claw) are seen also throughout the animal kingdom. However humans seem unique in their tendencies to prefer to employ their right hand for difficult tasks. The causes of hand preferences in children are complex and multi-dimensional. For example inheritance seems to be an underlying factor. However hand (and foot) preferences may be disrupted by some kind of cerebral 'insult' or incident occurring prior to, during, of after birth.

Thus some youngsters have been labeled inherited right handers (or left handers) while others are 'obligate' right handers (or left handers), evidencing hand preference molded by subtle neurological traumas. The failure to establish a preferred hand, has been interpreted by some as type of atypical neurological soft-sign. (Deule & Robinson 1987).

In the past some have hypothesized that motor coordination problems may be triggered by delays in the adoption of distinct foot and/or hand preferences (Benson & Geschwind 1968). However, recent evidence strongly indicates that the incidence of both mixed handedness in groups of clumsy children is no greater than is found among groups of normally coordinated youngsters. (Armitage & Larkin 1991). This area of speculation is likely to remain somewhat 'muddy' scientifically, however, as measures of limb preference, are often highly imprecise, and unreliable.

Social factors may also influence hand usage. In some Asian countries, for example, the left hand is used to engage in essential self-care skills, and all school children are 'encouraged' (pressured into) in using their right hand when printing. This kind of social pressure results in a larger percentage of older children in the United States being labeled right handers, than is true when this same quality in younger populations is surveyed. With maturation some youngsters may be encouraged by social forces into using their right hands in the more visible tasks, such as when printing and eating.

Right sided preferences in children may be seen in infancy, when it has been observed by some that some asymmetrical reflexes are seen to persist more on the right than on the left side. (Harris 1980). In most children hand preferences emerges in a relatively consistent way in early childhood, and continues to become more ingrained throughout the years that follow (Coren 1981). However if a child seems uncertain about what hand to use in difficult one-handed tasks, such as printing, by about the time he or she enters school, various tests of hand preference might be applied. These may be constructed by a therapist or teacher, and should consist of from five to six one-handed tasks that, for that child, are reasonably difficult. This type of home-made assessment battery should be administered daily for about two weeks, in order to assess tendencies in hand use. In general leg preference is not as distinct, nor is leg preference as easy to evaluate, as is hand preference.

What is often discovered is that a child evidences a general tendency for the use of one hand, or the other, rather than a marked preference in all tasks for single hand use. In most populations of children, a group will be seen to evidence a marked left or right hand preferences in nearly all tasks. However there will be children who, while preferring to use one hand in many tasks will also prefer to use the other hand in some. Some assessment systems have employed seven categories, ranging from those who consistently use one hand, or the other, to categories reflecting mixed hand preference. Thus it is normal for some youngsters not to prefer to employ one hand in all tasks with which they are confronted.

It is usually preferable that a child is 'task consistent', that is that he or she shows consistency in hand use for important and significant tasks, such as printing. A youngster not evidencing this kind of task consistency may be assisted to do so, by affording additional cues for what hand is being used. A colored cuff, attached to one wrist, may provide such a reminder.

Hand preference is not highly correlated to the hemispheric localization of speech. Many whose speech is lateralized in the left hemisphere, are left handed, and not right handed as some might expect. The literature is also quite clear in pointing out that preferences for eye, hand, and foot use are not likely to be related. Moreover it is also quite clear that children who evidence opposite eye and hand preferences and are said to be crossed preference (or crossed dominant) are not likely to evidence more learning and/or perceptual-motor difficulties than are present among those whose eye and hand preferences occur on the same side of the body. It is clear also that left handed children, although more prevalent in atypical populations, are not more likely to evidence less effective overall motor coordination than are right-handed children. The presence of left-handers in dysgraphic populations is discussed in Chapter 9.

A knowledge of the meaning of hand use, and its evaluation is useful to all those conducting educational program for both normal and atypical children. The evaluation of various facets of the motor might also include tests of hand preference. These evaluation instruments may include measures of preference, based upon performance; children's self-reports, as well as the reports of the child's caretaker. (Benton et al 1962) (Satz et al 1967) (Tupper 1987, Appendix).

Space limitations within this chapter do not permit a thorough exploration of the complex and interesting relationships between hand use, cerebral dominance, speech localization and other asymmetries. Enterprising readers might consult the excellent texts by Bryden (1983) and Corballis (1983) for a survey of the literature, as well as review by Cratty (1989b) containing a discussion of how hand preference develops in children.

Atypical-Functional Asymmetries

Several types of subtle atypical asymmetries, may be reflected in the movement behaviors of awkward children. These asymmetries are separate and apart from normally occurring hand and foot preferences discussed in the previous section. For example, some poorly coordinated youngsters may display minor to moderate signs of a type of cerebral palsy that effects one side of the body (a mild hemiplegia). The more observable behavior signs of this condition, may involve excess flexion in the upper limb, and increased extension-tension in the lower limb on the same, involved, side of the body. Often asymmetries in an awkward child, however, will consist of subtle symptoms, signs that are not easily detected until the youngster is asked to engage in reasonably complex tasks.

Methods used to assess the presence of this type of problem can include asking the child to move laterally in a rapid manner, 'like a basketball player on defense, without crossing our feet'. If a functional asymmetry is present in the lower limbs, lateral movement may be seen to be executed more fluidly to one side than to the other. If this is the case, the child displaying a minor right-sided involvement, will move poorly to the left, as pushing off accurately and/or forcefully with the right leg proves difficult. The opposite may be also be found, that is movement to the left may be difficult because there is right sided 'involvement.' Most asymmetrical youngsters evidence right-side "involvement".

Functional asymmetries in movement may also be found among aphasic children, youngsters whose speech mechanisms are deficit, but do not lack hearing. Usually they display right-sided weakness, due to the fact that the speech deficits, accompanied by a possible motor problem, are mediated by a poorly functioning left hemisphere. Other awkward children who may evidence weakness on one side of the body may have been victims of cerebral incidents prior to, during, or after birth, similar to traumas experienced by adult stroke patients. These can include incidents occurring during early vascularization (the formation of blood vessels). Thus a slight stroke, that was not, and is not detectable, may have left a 'healed' lesions within either hemisphere of the motor cortex. The presence of a 'healed lesion' in one hemisphere or the other, may thus result in atypical asymmetrical movement pattern(s) appearing. If the lesion has occurred in the left hemisphere, right-sided coordination or strength problems may be observed; if the lesion has occurred in the right hemisphere, left-sided movement problems may be present.

IMPERSISTENCE AND PERSEVERATION

Impersistence and perseveration are contrasting movement qualities. Impersistence refers to the apparent inability to hold a positions, or to continue movements, for reasonable periods of time. Children deficit in this quality seem to lack the ability to sustain and maintain various body positions. Perseveration, in the other hand, refers to the inability to change a movement program when appropriate. Thus, a child who perseverates is one who repeats a movement excessively, and is apparently unable to change to other movements and tasks when it is appropriate.

Impersistence is thus the inability to maintain a movement, or position when it is desired. In contrast perseveration refers to the difficulty, some awkward children display when attempting to change a movement-program when it is appropriate and desirable to do so.

Perseveration

Perseveration has sometimes been studied among emotionally disturbed children. For example, some youngsters evidencing autistic-like qualities may appear to enjoy bouncing on a trampolin, as if in a trance, for excessive periods of time. Youngsters displaying these unwanted qualities may display other repetitive movements, including excessive ball bouncing. Some perserverating children apparently employ these rhythmic, prolonged actions as ways of removing themselves psychologically from what they may perceive as unwanted socially pressures. The child may thus be avoiding apparent pressures to communicate, and/or to interact with others, by exhibiting various forms of solitary perseverative behaviors.

Two types of perseverative behaviors may be seen in some youngsters and adults including:

(1) actions that are reasonably appropriate, such as ball rolling, and

(2) repetitive actions that are inappropriate or even self-abusive.

Perseveration in extremely disturbed populations of adults also may takes the form of holding statue-like positions. In obviously emotionally disturbed youngsters this kind of 'waxen flexibility' is seldom seen. Perserverative movements, if carried to extremes, are often labeled 'self-stimulation'. Their suppression and reduction are often important goals of those working with the retarded and/or emotionally disturbed.

Several methods may be used to evaluate perseveration. For example, a child may be asked to draw the capital letter S, several times in rapid succession (SSSSSS etc). Next the child is asked to change the S, in a reverse manner. Children who perseverate may have difficulty doing so, and after drawing one or two backward S', they may again draw an S in the way that was first required of them (S). Other methods may involves simply observing a child or adult during a day's activities to determine whether appropriate shifts are made from task to task.

Frequent perseverations by an awkward child may suggest that an emotional health evaluation is needed. Some poorly coordinated children may perseverate as ways of finding security in an otherwise threatening action situation when in a remedial setting. Their perseveration in a given task may suggest that they have found some momentary security in an action they can accomplish, and are anxious about terminating it, and starting a new task at which they may be less than successful. Thus perseveration is often a symptom that accompanies others undesirable behaviors, within the overall 'emotional overlay' that occurs among youngsters with poor physical coordination.

It may prove difficult for clinicians, including movement therapists, to interest a child in pursuing a new task, when the youngster frequently perseverates. Only by employing vivid stimulation, giving instructions in a loud voice, or rolling a ball toward them that requires an immediate response, may some perseverating children be 'broken out' of some favorite, repetitive movement task to which they have retreated. To reduce, or to eliminate, perseverative behaviors displayed by young clients during remedial programs, requires that high levels of teaching competency be displayed.

Impersistence

Impersistence is the inability of a child to monitor kinesthetic (and related) input, for reasonable time periods. Thus youngsters displaying this problem cannot maintain static positions for reasonable time intervals. Kinesthetic sensations emanating from held positions, seem quickly to fade away, as the sensory information from that position is apparently difficult to organize and act upon for reasonable periods of time. Thus impersistence may reflect the presence of sensory problems.

Clinical assessment of this problem may include: Asking the child to maintain a held position of the tongue. The youngster may be asked, for example, to 'stick your tongue out' . . . and then observations made as to how long this position may be maintained. Some children with a problem in motor impersistence may begin shortly to curl their tongue into their mouth again. The maintenance of an adequate 'tongue thrust' is of particular interest to speech pathologists. A child who cannot hold such a position may also evidence articulation problems that are partly caused by an inadequate awareness of the tongue's position.

Another clinical test of motor impersistence requires a child to hold both arms extended directly in front of the shoulders with the eyes closed. Next the child is asked to alternately open and close their hands. (alternately make fists). Impersistence is sometimes noted as these directions are given, when one arm may lower itself. If this occurs, the kinesthetic information from one arm-position seemingly becomes difficult to perceive and organize. This asymmetry of position may be amplified by the alternate fist-making actions that are requested. The arm that becomes lower, may afford a clue as to which side of the brain may be 'involved'. For example, if the left arm-hand lowers, there may problems in the right hemisphere. In contrast, if the right arm lowers, the sensory-motor area in left hemisphere may contain a slight lesion. This type of task is frequently employed in assessments given by pediatric neurologists.

Motor impersistence may be seen in a variety of contexts, as one works with physically uncoordinated children. Asking such children, for example, to assume various positions in class situations such as lining up, may cause them problems. Similar conundrums may be encountered as awkward youngsters are asked to assume some static positions, as when for example they are asked to begin an exercise. An awareness of this potential problem may help clinicians become more patient when working with awkward youngsters, and not assume that this kind of problem is volitional, and a sign of poor cooperation.

Difficulties when attempting to persist in continuous actions are also types of impersistent behavior frequently observed among awkward children. This problem may be evaluated by asking a child is to engage in a repetitive rotary movement of one limb, while the other limb remains at rest. This kind of is often placed in neurological evaluations, and is intended to measure what is termed 'diadochokinesia'. The task involves to asking a child to rotate one arm quickly, and repetitively, from a supinated (hand up) to a pronated position (hand down). Luria's clinical assessment task, involving asking a client to rapidly make a fist and then a 'ring' (touching the tip of the first finger to the thumb) in an alternate fashion, represents another test of this type. (Luria 1966).

Bonnevier (1968) formulated an apparatus test to evaluate this action quality. Often awkward children are unable to engage in this alternating action in a continuous fashion. Signs of overflow (synkinesia) may thus be measured in the resting limb. A child who does not execute this kind of action well is said to exhibit adiadochokinesia. Touwen and others have also included this kind of test in neurological instruments intended to evaluate children with minimal neurological deficits. (Touwen 1979).

HYPOTONIA & HYPERTONIA: TONUS ABNORMALITIES

Overview

Youngsters evidencing extremes of muscle tension are often found within groups of awkward children. Essentially they display what is termed 'residual', or resting, tension levels that are either in excess or less than those seen among groups of youngsters with average or above-average physical coordination. Either of these two conditions may be seen in all parts of the body, and potentially influence numerous tasks. The problems are assumed to be caused by deficits within the central nervous system. Often these youngsters display minor to moderate signs of either of two types of cerebral palsy. Those displaying an excess of muscle tension evidence mild forms of spastic cerebral palsy and children who are hypotonic are believed by some to evidencing a form of dystonic cerebral palsy. Both conditions present unique problems to those evaluating motor coordination then attempting to elicit change through remedial efforts.

Most youngsters evidence either of these conditions, and usually do not fluctuate between hypertonic and hypotonic muscular levels. However some evidence obtained in the 1980's among infants stressed with maternal drug use, suggest that some of these youngsters exhibit symptoms involving alterations of excessively high then of abnormally low muscle tone. (Lesser-Katz, 1982) (Cratty 1990). Infants stressed at birth with maternal drug use not only may alternate from hypotonic to hypertonia, during the first year of life, but recent conversations with caretakers suggest that these alternations persist among some into early childhood.

Hypotonias, Progressive and Benign

A hypotonic youngster displays levels of resting muscle tone throughout the body, that are less than that measured in normal youngsters. If one grasps their limbs, flaccid muscle tone may be felt. When observed they often appear both lazy and unfit. Sometimes this condition is termed dystonia, and may be accompanied by other problems, including postural abnormalities and obesity.

Progressive Hypotonia

Hypotonia may be either progressive, or benign. The condition may be progressive if a child's muscle tone seems lessens. Other behaviors may signal the presence of a progressive condition including falling, an increasingly slumped posture (due to the reduction of residual tone in the anti-gravity muscle groups), and by evidence of poor muscle tone in the face, eye lids, and limbs. If this symptoms of an increasing problem are seen, extensive and thorough evaluations are needed by several medical experts including neurologists and endocrinologists. These progressive problems may be covered up early in the life of a child by normal maturation, only to appear from the 3rd to 6th year. Progressive hypotonia is a symptom found within a variety of potentially debilitating and sometimes life-threatening syndromes, including muscular dystrophy as well as a variety of progressive ataxias. Several of these syndromes were discussed in Chapter 3.

Hypotonia in early childhood may also be a precursor of athetoid cerebral palsy, a dramatic condition marked by uncontrollable movements. A four-year old boy in our program several years ago passed through this progression of symptoms. These first consisted of general hypotonia, including a flaccid and ineffectual grip on a pencil, preventing him from making accurate and distinct marks on paper. His eye lids evidenced poor muscle tone, and remained half-closed. He tilted his head backward, perhaps attempting to see better, even when he was apparently awake and alert. A short time later obvious athetoid symptoms, appeared including wavering erratic movements of the lines made by his pencil when learning to print letters. Thus in this relatively rare case hypotonia in infancy was a precursor to an identifiable form of cerebral palsy.

Benign Hypotonia

Another type of hypotonia is labeled 'benign hypotonia'. These terms describe a condition that, while often apparent from birth, is not progressive. Not a great deal of literature is available on this condition, perhaps because its causes are not well known. (Eng et al 1979)

It appears to be caused by problems within the central nervous system within the mechanisms and centers that form and regulate resting muscle tension. The gamma efferent system within the brain stem has sometimes been cited as one of the main regulators of muscle tension, and thus this mechanism is suspect if resting (residual) muscle tension levels are below average levels.

During the past year I evaluated two young girls, both twenty-two months of age, who were unable to assume sitting positions without assistance. They had been diagnosed as evidencing benign hypotonia. Others we have tested recently could pull themselves to their feet, in preparation for walking, by mid-way through their second years of life. Hypotonic children have likely encountered a great deal of failure in physical activities, even in early childhood. Their below-average muscular strength is typically accompanied by in inactivity , sometimes resulting in excess body weight.

Several decades ago I encountered this condition in a teenage boy, participating in a high school class I was teaching. One day when he was confronted with a physical testing session, he could not even grasp the hi-bar and support his weight preparatory to performing chinups. At the time I assumed that he had been too lazy to exercise, that he was unfit, and thus he lacked character. I further assumed that he possessed undesirable personality traits reflecting poor ambition and low effort.

The assumptions I made about this hypotonic boy are commonly formulated by naive observers. These negative social judgements can thus cause them to experience marked problems, reflected in poor social acceptance and in other incidents that serve to lower their self-esteem. In truth their condition is caused by deficits in their central nervous system of which they have no control. It is not surprising that when hypotonia has been studied among neurologically 'suspect' children, associated symptoms (in factor analyses) have included social withdrawal and immaturity as well as fluctuations in mood states. (Nichols 1987)

Changing base levels of muscle tone in these children is not an easy undertaking. Exposure to vigorous exercise may not be immediately effective. Often it is only when they are given muscular tasks, whose intensities are gradually changed over a relatively prolonged period of time, that their abilities and muscle tone may improve. Even when this is done, it is possible that basic levels of muscle tone do not undergo dramatic improvement. They should be encouraged to exercise to their capacities, however, or their inherited hypotonia will combine with inactivity to produce even more pronounced decrements in strength and muscle tone.

Hypertonia

Hypertonia, an above average amount of residual-resting muscle tension, is often a sign of minor to moderate degrees of spastic cerebral palsy. Hypertonia is a main symptom in the 'tension syndrome' discussed in Chapter 5. Like hypotonia, hypertonic tensions usually occur evenly throughout the body and are of central nervous system origin. The usual cause of spastic cerebral palsy are descending pathways adjacent to the larger motor pathways. Often the reticular formation in the brain stem is seen as a mediator of muscle tone, and excess tonus might be attributable also to deficits in brain stem function.

Most hypertonic youngsters exhibit negative social-emotional accompaniments when attempting to learn and perform motor skills. Thus their problem becomes compounded, as the inappropriate functioning of centers in the central nervous system combine with socially induced tension, to detract from smooth coordinated actions attempted by these tense children and young adults.

General high levels of muscle tone plagues youngsters in several ways. Executing smooth, coordinated movements are difficult. As a hypertonic child reaches for an object, to give one example, the smooth and gradual lengthening of the muscles that flex the arm do not work in concert with the muscles that are extending the arm. Thus in this case, the arm may suddenly flex, when the intention has been to reach by extending the arm at the elbow.

When they begin to print letters, similar problems occur. When they try to draw a line of a given length, a 'motor program' when starting the line is initiated, but difficulty is encountered when the it is attempted to stop the line at the proper point. Thus frequent 'overshooting' (dysmetria) in such tasks often occurs. When printing the hypertonic child becomes particularly tense, and often seems to be trying to initiate and inhibit a movement at the same time.

I often notice that hypertonic youngsters in my program are unable to throw balls short distances with accuracy. The catcher (sometimes me!) may be struck in the face with a too-rapidly projected missile. When they attempt to lessen force when throwing, they shorten the arcs through which they move their arms, rather than continuing to move their arms through long arc, in a relaxed manner, while slowing the speed of their upper limb. Their tense motor programs, when throwing a ball, seemed capable of expressing only one level of speed and force. Thus to reduce the velocities of their arm-hand, as they release an object, they apparently have to move their arms through short arcs. In contrast normal youngsters are able reduce the force and speed of their throwing arms, while keeping the length of the arc through which their arms move, almost the same.

Associated, synkinetic movements, discussed earlier, tend to be marked in hypertonic children. In hypertense children associated movements may occur in a wider variety of body parts and with greater intensity, than is true among children whose muscular systems do not display these too-high levels of residual tension. In addition spinal reflexes, when elicited in a neurological evaluation may be exaggerated. The excess tensions seen throughout the body are also likely to detract from efforts to formulate smooth sequences of action. This excess tension may also make it difficult for these children to perform in biomechanically efficient ways, and to present themselves socially to others in a relaxed and competent manner. Various forms of hyperactivity may also accompany hypertonus.

This condition may be assessed through the use of expensive laboratory equipment that can include measures of electrical activity recordable in various muscle groups, using an electromyograph. Observational scales are also available through which resting muscular tension may be evaluated. Schilling and Poppen (1983) for example, have formulated a rating scale containing ten behaviors which, when observed and rated reflect the presence of excessively high levels of muscular tension. These signs of muscle tension include movements of the body when reclining; whether or not the lips are slightly parted in the middle as the face relaxes, and if the feet and legs rotate outward when the child is on his/her back. This type of observational data has been found to correlate well to electromyographic evidence of levels of muscle tension. This observational assessment permits evaluations of levels residual muscular tension present in youngsters before, and after, exposure to various kinds of relaxation training (Cratty 1989a).

Efforts by clinicians to reduce this problem may include the imposition of relaxation training, as well as using cognitive behavioral therapy, both of which are described elsewhere. (Cratty 1985b) Often the hypertonic child begins to exhibit increased muscle tone when various events, during programs of games and sports, that prove exciting and emotionally arousing. Thus, when working with hypertonic youngsters, relaxation training should often be interpolated between activities that prove too excitable. Of particular importance is to adjust the child's level of activity and hypertonicity at the completion of a program of motor activity. If this is accomplished than subsequent parts of the school's program may be entered in a relatively relaxed manner. I have had teachers plead with me to encourage physical educators in their school to apply this kind of relaxation training, before returning them to their classes.

Optimum effort directed toward remediation and relaxation of hypertonic youngsters may be result in moderate to minimal overall changes in the resting muscle tension displayed. Some of these children may require medication, as well as instructions in the modification of skills to help them to accommodate to the problems they encounter when attempting to move accurately. Attempts should also be made to adjust the demands of their environments so that their hypertonicity does not interfere with their academic and intellectual functioning. Their teachers, for example, may be asked to reduce the quantity of their writing assignments given to them, or/and to substitute verbal responses for written ones when giving tests.

TREMORS, AND UNSTEADINESS

Cyclic, low amplitude tremors, and irregular unsteadiness, are displayed by some physically awkward youngsters. These symptoms may constitute signs of mild to moderate forms of cerebral palsy, and can stem from mildly pathological developmental histories that may include low birth weight (Lesny 1980). A slight and regular tremor may be a sign of cerebellar dysfunction, and may be a mild form of cerebellar ataxia. Various kinds of unsteadiness when trying to balance and when walking and engaging other locomotor tasks may also be symptoms of cerebellar dysfunction.

Difficulties can also occur when trying to replicate alternating-cyclic movements as when asked to alternately and rapidly supinate and pronate the arm and hand. This problem is termed *dysdiadochokinesis*. Further 'cerebellar signs' can include difficulties when attempting to execute movements for prescribed and precise distances, as when attempting to print block letters. When block-printing is attempted, for example, a child with this problem may produce a movement that is too short. On the other hand he/she may 'shoot past' an intended ending point, evidencing what is termed *'dysmetria'*. Other more marked cerebellar symptoms can include the decomposition of regular, rhythmic and smooth actions into disjointed ones.

All normal people evidence normal tremors in various parts of their bodies. These normal low-amplitude fluctuations are not usually not apparent to an observer. These tremors occur, for example, at the rate of about ten-a-second in the fingers and hands, and in slower fluctuations of body sway. In contrast, however, some awkward children evidence tremor rates, as well as unsteadiness in gait and balance, whose amplitudes far exceed those of normals. A awkward child may exhibit tremor symptoms reflecting a mild cerebellar syndrome that are apparent even to casual observers. These symptoms can consist of fluctuations of the hand the limbs and of trunk.

The overall 'motor programs' of these youngsters may be relatively intact. For example, they may draw an accurate triangle when asked to do so, or when given a model to copy. However the quality of the line in the triangle may contain evidence of tremors occurring in the hand and arm. Letters may be reasonably well-formed and legible, but in the lines making them up slow amplitude and rapid tremors may be seen.

Unsteadiness may also occur within actions engaged in by the lower limbs. After the support phase of the gait occurs the leg may be seen to bounce and extend, rather than to display a relaxed flexion or clawing action typical of the gait cycle normal youngsters display.

These tremors, and signs of unsteadiness, may be general, and evidenced in activities involving the upper limbs including drawing, as well as walking. On the other hand they be confined to either the upper or to the lower parts of the body. Specific portions of the cerebellum mediate precision and steadiness of movement in localized body parts. Thus a lesion in a single portion of the cerebellum may influence imprecision of movement in a specific body location. Therefore, a child may display either an overall ataxia, or one in which only tremors in the upper or the lower limbs occur.

Often these children evidence normal to above-average intelligence quotients. The part of the brain that is apparently involved, the cerebellum, mediates fine precise movements, and controls rapid pre-programmed movements. The higher centers used for associational and memory processes are independent of cerebellar functioning.

Important movements of the eyes may also be influenced negatively by cerebellar dysfunction. These include the rapid saccades (throws) the eyes make while reading. Precision of these same saccades is necessary when tracking and extracting data from moving balls and from other objects in games. Thus a moderate cerebellar ataxia may be associated with imprecision of the eye movements needed in reading, as well as with precise saccades needed when intercepting incoming balls.

Practical Implications

Completely eliminating these subtle signs of neurological dysfunctions in awkward children may prove difficult. More helpful are the interposition of task modifications that can help the child to function better, and to reduce the amount of tremor and the inaccuracies that result from this problem. For example, we worked with a five year old who evidenced this problem after one year of learning to print her letters. We found that she was not keeping her writing hand, wrist and arm in contact with the page when printing. When she was aided to better anchor her upper limb, by resting her wrist on the table, it was found that the tremors were less disruptive to her efforts.

THE INTEGRATION OF MOVEMENTS

Frequently poorly coordinated children are unable to smoothly integrate the sub-movements of a desired action. They evidence a inefficiencies of both effort and accuracy, that may be occur in one or more forms. They may have trouble transmitting force from one side of the body to the other. They may also have difficulties integrating the top of their body with its lower parts, as when throwing for example.

Force transmission problems

Awkward youngsters often cannot smoothly transmit force from one body part to another when it is desired to do so. This may be seen when they attempt to throw, and it becomes necessary to transmit (to summate) forces and velocities from the ankles, through the legs and trunk to the shoulders and finally to the arms and hands. Their throwing action appears fragmented. A step and even a weight shift may be taken, but the appropriate movements of the upper body occur later, so that force is lost, rather than passing from the lower body and trunk to the upper body parts.

Similar problems are seen when a child evidencing this type of problem tries to create force by putting body actions together. When executing a standing broad jump, the leg extension is not likely to occur when the arms extend upward and forward. Both when jumping forward or upward, the legs may be seen to extend after the arms thrust, or the leg extension may never be accompanied by a useful thrust of the arms.

Integration of rhythmic movements

Often a movement series involves reasonably complex series of movements. Clumsy children often have difficulty in smoothly putting together the rhythmic movements needed in jumping rope, as well as in alternately hopping from foot to foot. Even simpler problems may plague an uncoordinated child. Most children, for example, by the age of about six to eight years of age are able, when encountering a flight of stairs, to quickly observe their height and width, and then quickly formulate an appropriate and precise motor program that permits them to rapid ascend or descend. In contrast many awkward children often have difficulty in this situation, and must either constantly watch their feet when walking up stairs, or suffer the consequences, and fall or stumble. At times this kind of motor problem, is diagnosed as a symptom of a visual perceptual difficulty reflecting poor depth perception. However in many cases stair climbing problems have motor, not perceptual, origins.

Cyclic, continuous motor programs cannot be formulated well in children evidencing this kind of problem. Thus an action that requires the integration of the lower limbs, alternately hopping from foot to foot for example, are seen to occur in "jerky", stop-and-go patterns. Instead of a continuous foot to foot action taking place, the child must stop and take time to re-program the movement as each cycle is reached.

Riding a bicycle, to cite another example, may prove difficult for several reasons. One of these is the inability to sustain a rhythm in an automatic way, without constant thought being given to the alternating movements of the legs and feet. Secondly bike-riding may prove difficult because the child cannot transfer a program from one side of the body to the other in a rhythmic way as the pedals are alternately pressed down. Bike riding may also be dangerous because the child cannot quickly catch his/her balance when the bicycle tips off center, by placing one leg-foot or the other to the side, stopping the bike's fall.

These types of integration problems may be associated with the poor motor planning, the apraxic behaviors discussed previously. Their remediation takes the major portion of a program intended to remediate or reduce motor awkwardness in children. Often visual feedback, or the addition additional cues including verbal and auditory stimuli are helpful. The opportunity to view video-taped practice sessions during which difficult movement have been attempted may be useful. Standing on a small tilt platform when throwing may be helpful. As the platform tilts, additional auditory and vestibular cues, accompanying the desired weight shift, may contribute to a better throwing pattern. The use of mirrors may also be helpful. Watching himself in this manner, the youngster may better observe the proper sequences of a complex movement as it is executed.

OTHER MOVEMENT QUALITIES

Several other movement qualities may be found in associated with motor incoordination, and are found on lists of neurological soft-signs. However most of these other types are not as pervasive as are those discussed earlier. Additionally, both the neurological and behavioral significances of these other symptoms, are not always clear.

For example, choreas (from the Latin 'to dance') consisting of spasmatic, jerking movements occur among neurological suspect children. Rasmussen and his colleagues found these prevalent in a group of one-hundred and forty-one awkward children they studied in Sweden (Rasmussen et al 1982). Choreas may be present in various groups of muscle including those in the eyes. The usual way to elicit choreas clinically is to ask the child to stand as still as possible, with the arms elevated and stretched to the front; the eyes are closed and the fingers spread. (Prechtl 1987). The spasms, if they occur, are often observed among neurologically suspect children including those exhibiting signs of awkwardness. These actions were first described, as a type of neurological soft sign, in 1959 by Prechtl & Stemmer (1962). Their possible significance has been recently surveyed by Prechtl (1987).

Like associated movements, choreas (Choreiform or Choreatiform movements) occur in body parts not directly involved in a task, and/or in body parts upon which the child is not concentrating. A chorea may be felt in a child's grip when some of the fingers twitch, and all the digits do not exert the same constant pressure at the same. Choreas are also may be seen when a youngster is asked to maintain a position, as when evaluating motor impersistence. However there are many variations in clinical tests for choreas (Rutter et al 1966).

Choreas (sometimes labeled choreiathetoid movements) are seldom seen in children before the age of about two years. However, after that age these spasmatic-jerking actions have been observed to inhibit early writing efforts, as they often occur in the hands and fingers (Prechtl 1987). The relationships of these spasms, however, to other behavioral indices are often not clear-cut. (Prechtl 1987) Choreiathetoid movements are seen among infants whose mothers used abusive substances, including cocaine during pregnancy, and also in groups of awkward children (Rasmussen et al 1983). Their possible neurological significance among drug-stressed infants has been discussed in a recent publication (Cratty 1990)

OVERVIEW

In this chapter several movement qualities were surveyed. These included poor motor planning behavior (apraxia and dyspraxia), distortions of muscular tonus including hypotonicity and hypertonicity, movement tremors and similar irregularities, distortions in motor programs including the inability to move from action to action (perseveration), and the inability to maintain a program or posture when appropriate (impersistence).

Two types of functional asymmetries were also described. These included normal hand and foot preferences, and also atypical functional asymmetries that appear in the form of muscular weakness, or poor coordination, on one side of the body. The meanings of overflow, or associated movements, were also discussed. These unwanted actions often impeding the execution of sports skills, included those that overflow in space, appearing in body parts not directly involved in the task. Also discussed were actions that persist in time, flappings and other apparently involuntary movements that continue to be seen in some awkward children, past the time an intended action is usually terminated. Other qualities reviewed in this chapter included the inability to integrate body parts well and to summate forces. In each section the possible clinical significance, etiologies, and remedial efforts related to each of these varied movement qualities, were discussed.

The implications that these generalized qualities have for planning program content were also presented. It was suggested that some of these qualities may be modified through direct practice and intervention. Others, it was pointed out, need to be dealt with by modifications in task demands. For example, a dyspraxic child may be helped when dressing, by laying out in order they are to be put on, the articles of clothing he or she is about to wear. Still others of these unwanted movement qualities, it was pointed out, need to be circumvented by presenting the child with choices of alternative motor activities in which these unwanted qualities may not interfere.

The clinical and neurological significance of several of these qualities are still unclear, and the subjects of further investigation. However the presence of these qualities is a fact, and they often present obstacles with which the awkward child should be helped to deal.

QUESTIONS FOR DISCUSSION

1. What in daily tasks might be disrupted by a child evidencing ideational dyspraxia and ideomotor apraxia?
2. What does benign hypotonia mean? What symptoms may be present in a child with this diagnosis?
3. What kinds of abnormal and normal functional asymmetries might be assessed in groups of youngsters suspected of possessing motor problems? What kinds of tasks would you use in this assessment?
4. What is diadochokinesia? How might its presence be evaluated?
5. What variables might influence the outcomes of tests of dyspraxia given to a group of children from 5-12 years of age?
6. How might tests for the various motor qualities discussed in this chapter be integrated into a traditional battery of motor ability tests?
7. How might you assess overflow in (body) space, and overflow in time among a group of neurologically impaired children.
8. What is trunkle apraxia? Are the symptoms and behaviors similar to, or different from evidenced by a youngster said to be suffering from a spatial agnosia?
9. How might a score be derived from a test of the facility with which a child evidences the ability to integrate various parts of the body?
10. What possible neurological implications are suggested by the presence of various types of excess neuromotor overflow in a youngster?

Chapter 7
Dysgraphia

INTRODUCTION AND DEFINITIONS

Dysgraphia is a broad label that includes various types of disturbances seen when printing, writing and drawing. Dysgraphia may include difficulties with the execution of single letters and words, problems with spelling and/or confusion when writing sentences. O'Hare and Brown have broadly defined dysgraphia as the "retarded development or an abnormality in the skill of writing" (1989a). Both awkward children and adult stroke patients often display symptoms of dysgraphia.

Two types of dysgraphia are described in the literature. One form appearing in childhood is called *'developmental dysgraphia'* Dysgraphia resulting from cerebral strokes, has been labeled *'stroke-related dysgraphia'* (Cratty and DeOliveira 1989).

It has been suggested by some, that children evidencing developmental dysgraphia have suffered neural insults prior to, during or after birth, similar to those occurring in adult stroke patients (Margolin 1984) (Temple 1988). The available literature usually discusses *Stroke-related dysgraphia* using neurological models (Margolin 1984). *Developmental dysgraphia,* in contrast, is frequently considered within educational and psychological contexts. (Freischlag 1973) (O'Hare and Brown 1989 ab).

Writing letters and words is the last type of communicative behavior to emerge in developing youngsters. Letter printing is usually accomplished several years after spoken language appears (Myklebust 1973). Thus symptoms reflecting various types of dysgraphia may appear well after the acquisition of earlier linguistic-communicative behaviors that may have been mastered in a normal fashion by a growing youngster.

Dysgraphia is prevalent among poorly coordinated children. It may be accompanied by the inability to engage in coordinated acts involving the larger muscle groups. However, dysgraphia in children may also present itself as a separate condition, appearing in youngsters possessing either average or superior gross motor skills.

Dysgraphia is frequently seen among the learning disabled. In a learning disabled populations we recently surveyed, this problem was found to occur in from 30–40% of those assessed. (Miyahara,

Cratty, and Goldman 1990) Dysgraphia, however, may also be unaccompanied by other academic problems. For example, in a recent investigation of children with writing and printing difficulties, it was found that about one-half of the youngsters surveyed evidenced dysgraphia without the presence of other learning disabilities. (O'Hare and Brown 1989). Dysgraphia, unaccompanied by other academic difficulties, has itself been labeled a 'specific learning disability' by Brown (1981) and others (Myklebust 1973).

Neural Modeling

Historically dysgraphia was believed by clinical neurologists to be due to lesions among stroke patients occurring within the parietal area of the brain. The left middle gyrus, and the angular gyrus were among the centers cited initially as responsible for mediating written language. (Henschen 1922) (Exner 1881). Later Goldstein suggested that there are two types of neural mechanisms responsible for written language functions including those that mediate language and those controlling motor output (Goldstein 1948).

Contemporary models depicting dysgraphia, are often based upon the location of pathway disturbances and/or lesions, accompanying written language disruptions, within groups of stroke patients. These models have attributed various forms of dysgraphia to numerous neurological sites, including areas controlling speech (Wernicke's and Broca's areas) centers mediating motor output (Exner's Area), structures associated with visual spatial functions (non-dominant portions of the parietal area) and to sites mediating auditory functions (Heschl's gyrus) (Roeltgen and Heilman 1985).

In addition. disruptions in inter-hemispheric communication involving pathways in the corpus callosum have been hypothesized as disturbing adequate written language. Roetlgen and Heilman (1985) in their comprehensive model point out that there are probably three levels of inter-hemispheric communication that support written language:

(a) verbal-motor pathways,

(b) visual-kinesthetic connections, and

(c) linguistic information passing from hemisphere to hemisphere. Hypothetically lesions in several regions of the brain, and among more than one inter-connecting pathway, may thus result in dysfunctional printing and writing in developing children. However clear-cut relationships between damage to various neural sites and pathways, and disruptions in youngster's attempts at written language, have not been well established.

Written and Expressive Language

The close alignment of neural centers mediating expressive language, to those controlling graphic areas, typically results in parallel disturbances in both written and expressive language, among both children and adults. For example, aphasic children whose speech is disturbed, or may be nearly absent, often evidence similar problems in written communication (Raychev et al 1984).

Similarly, when adult stroke patients are asked to write a sentence, they have struggled to vocalize, difficulties are typically seen in their written attempts of the same sentence. In one study, for example, it was found that 486 out of 500 stroke patients evaluated, evidenced their disturbances in written language closely paralleling problems in spoken language (Chendru and Gerschwind 1972).

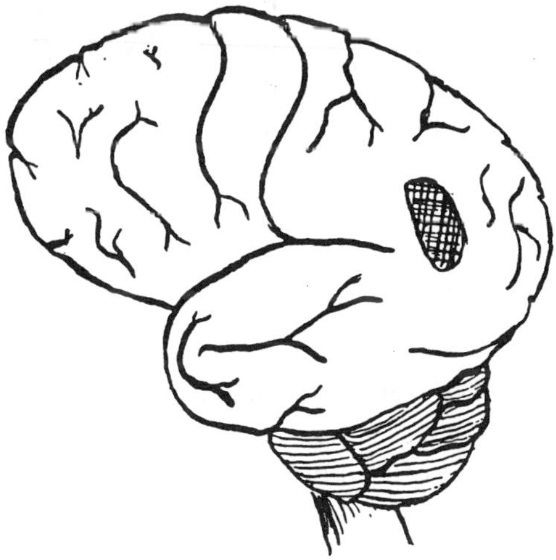

Plate 7-1. The neural basis of some types of stroke-related dysgraphias usually damage to the left angular gyrus, as shown, is said to cause both dysgraphia, as well as the inability to recognize words in stroke patients. In children however, different types of dysgraphia may be due to problems in this area, as well as in other structures, including the basal ganglia, and cerebellum.

Central Programming

Most disruptions in the execution of letters, and of numbers, in both printed and written form have been hypothesized as caused by subtle deficits within programs in the central nervous system (Edelman and Flash 1987). Most dysgraphic symptoms thus are not due to peripheral difficulties such as hand-muscle weaknesses, or the mechanics with which a pen or pencil is held.

Several examples illustrate the probability that printing and writing are mediated by programs in the central nervous system. For example if a child is asked to produce an A using cursive writing at the blackboard, employing large arm and shoulder muscles, the resultant letter will be similar in shape to the same a written on the desk with smaller muscle groups. The two A's will also be likely written at the same speed! This comparison is shown below.

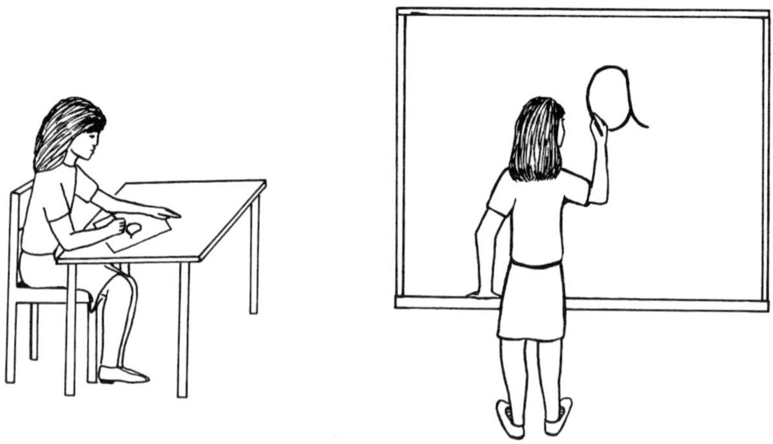

Plate 7-2. A letter written with different body parts

The hypotheses that central nervous system programs play major roles in mediating printing and writing is also illustrated by the writing samples seen below, from a 1977 study by Raibert. In this investigation highly similar shapes were produced both in individual letters and in words, when the investigator wrote with various body parts. He used both his dominant and non-dominant hands. He also wrote with a pen taped to the foot, when his wrist was immobilized, and even while holding the pen with his teeth! Thus in this case also the kind of peripheral mechanics and/or musculature involved did not significantly alter the various letter and word shapes apparently produced by highly similar programs within his central nervous system.

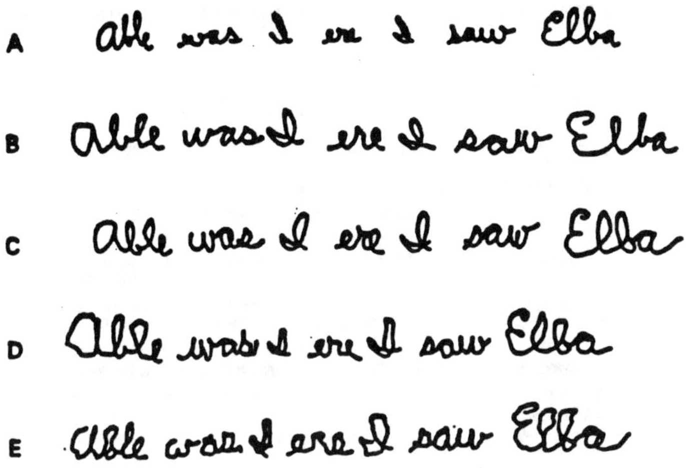

From Raibert M.H., (1977) Motor Control and Learning by the State-Space Model, Ph.d. Thesis Artificial Intelligence Laboratory, Massachusettes Institute of Technology. AI-RI 439, Cambridge Mass. with permission of the author.

Plate 7-3. Illustrating a central programming theory of graphic behavior. In these samples by Raibert, the same sentence was written by (a) the dominant hand, with (b) the non-dominant hand, with (c) the pen taped to the foot, and (d) with the wrist immobilized, and finally (e) with the pen held in this teeth.

CAUSES OF DYSGRAPHIA

The following chart further illustrates the complicated nature of graphic behaviors, and the difficulty in identifying the potential causes of dysgraphia. As shown, various sub-vocal, and cognitive-perceptual processes are involved in the production of clear and coherent written languages. These processes include both visual and auditory perception, as well as thoughts that aid in the formulation of internal speech, forming concepts that undergird the production of written language. Recent literature further emphasizes importance of various cognitive qualities important to adequate writing behaviors (Sovik et al 1987). Thus writing is not only a motor skill, but is sub-served and contributed to by numerous perceptual and intellectual abilities.

The chart further indicates that if multiple causes of sgraphia are identified, specific and individualized remedial strategies should necessarily follow. Even the numerous types of problems illustrated on the following chart (7–4), do not exhaust all the possible difficulties that may underlie various types of dysgraphic behaviors.

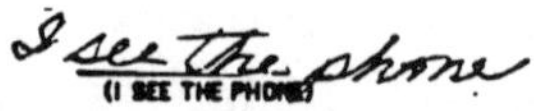

(I SEE THE PHONE)

CAUSES, CONDITIONS	NEURAL BASES	EXAMPLES	REMEDIATION
MOTOR CAUSES			
APRAXIA	BASAL GANGALIA	I ESE HET OHPNE	SEQUENCE WORK
ATAXIA	CEREBELLUM	TREMOR IN LINES	ANCHOR HAND, USE GUIDES
SPASTICITY	EXTRA-PYRAMIDAL PATHWAYS, BRAIN STBM	EXCESS TENSION, AND EFFORT	RELAXATION TRAINING,
ATHETOSIS	BASAL GANGALIA	IRREGULAR LINES	GUIDED PRACTICE
AUDITORY PERCEPTION			
ANOMIA, DYSNOMIA	AUDITORY CODING AREAS	I SEE THE BOOK..??	RE-EDUCATION
FORMULATION APHASIAS	PARIETAL AREA	WE HIT THE PHONE	RE-EDUCATION
AUDITORY SEQUENCING	PARIETAL AREA	SEE PHONE I THE	RE-EDUCATION
RE-AUDIBILIZATION	CODING AREAS	I CE THA FON	RE-EDUCATION
VISUAL PERCEPTION			
VISUAL MEMORY	OCCIPITAL LOBE	I....PHONE ??	EDUCATIONAL THERAPY
VISUAL SEQUENCING	FRONTAL AREAS	SEE PHONE I	RE-EDUCATION
VISUAL ORGANIZATION	OCCIPITAL AND FRONTAL LOBES RIGHT HEMISPHERE	LETTER REVERSAL , UPSIDE DOWN ETC	EDUCATIONAL THERAPY
COGNITIVE PROBLEMS			
BROCAS APHASIA	BROCAS AREA	JUMBLED WORDS	COGNTIVE THERAPY
WERNECKE'S APHASIA	PARIETAL AREA	JUMBLED WORDS OUT OF SEQUENCE	COGNITIVE THERAPY
SHORT-TERM OR LONG TERM RECALL, AND RETRIEVAL	ASSOCIATIONAL AREAS	GAPS IN SENTENCE	COGNITIVE THERAPY

From Cratty B. J. and DeOliveria, (1989) Modifying Printing Behavior in Children, Seven Case Studies, Unpublished Monograph, Children's Enrichment Center, 2959 South Sepulveda Blvd. Los Angeles, CA 90064

Plate 7-4. Causes, neural bases, and remediation

THE DEVELOPMENT OF GRAPHIC BEHAVIORS

The first primitive graphic behaviors typically emerge during the second year of life. Infants become fascinated upon finding that some of the objects they hold and swing through the air make marks when accidentally striking surfaces, including walls, floors and table tops. If these first efforts are rewarded by the approving statements of others, and prove satisfying in and of themselves, further attempts will be made to scribble using pencils and other markers. As the months pass youngsters properly stimulated, will likely increase both the intensity, and the variety of scribbles they produce.

Rhoda Kellogg after collecting and analyzing thousands of children's graphic efforts, identified twenty basic scribbles (Kellogg 1969). She contended that these early scribbles represent parallels to rudimentary infant speech. Kellogg thus suggested that these first primitive markings, composed of twenty basic scribbles, constitute early "motor babbling", and are thus important sensory-motor precursors to more coherent graphic efforts that later will appear. A fisted grip is used initially to hold the marking implement. Thus these first efforts are made by moving the whole arm and shoulder, and the pencil may be grasped inefficiently at its upper end (Saida and Miyashita 1979).

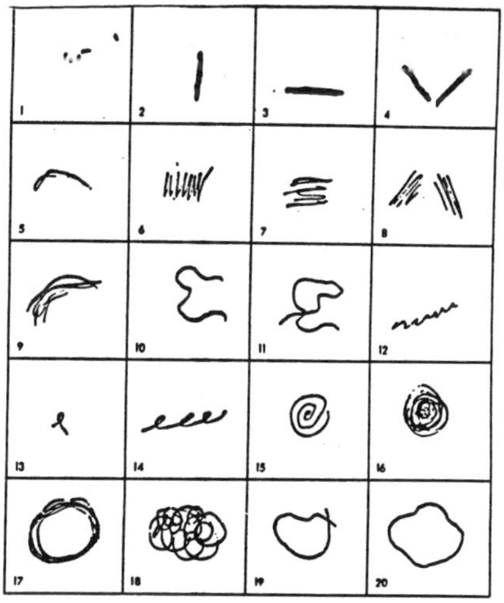

From Kellogg, R Analyzing Children's Art, 1969 National Press Books, Palo Alto California with the kind permission of the publisher.

Plate 7-5. Twenty-basic scribbles, from Kellogg

Further opportunities to use implements that make marks, plus the encouragement of others, results in the formation of several types of rapid, ballistic scribbles. Later these marks begin to slow down, at about the third year of life, and more controlled circles emerge, together with simple patterns that include early attempts at designs.

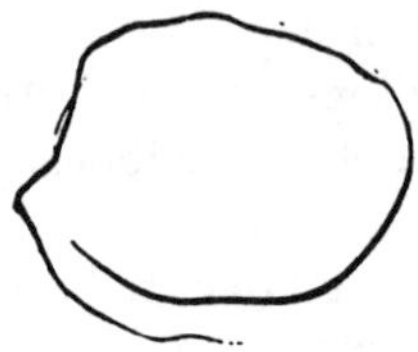

Plate 7-6. (A) Early graphic behaviors

Later simple line crosses may be drawn together with sun-like objects called 'mandellas'. These early figures have been found to appear among children within numerous cultures throughout the world. At about this same time other figures appear, that Kellogg has labeled, combines and aggregates. The grip used to hold the marker also matures. The writing implement begins to be guided more with finger action by the fourth year, rather than with the cruder movements of a fisted hand, seen earlier.

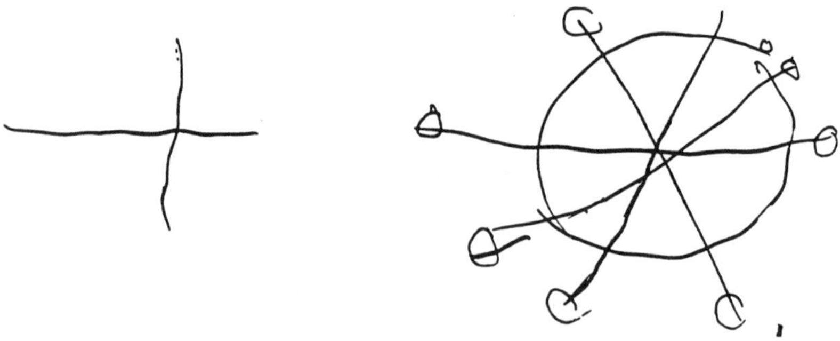

Plate 7-6. (B) Early graphic behaviors

In many cultures, by the fifth year, if all goes well, the child begins to print block letters about 2″ high. During the year that follows letters are gradually refined, and made smaller preparatory to printing lower case manuscript letters. Squares are able to be copied accurately (Broderick 1987). In some countries at this age children are first guided toward acquire cursive writing, rather than encouraged to engage in block printing.

The child will be seen to continue to draw shapes and pictures, whose quality may be largely independent of efforts to draw letters. Thus it is possible that a child will be labeled 'creative' by parents, based upon their observations of artistic efforts, despite the fact that there is emerging evidence of dysgraphia by the same child. This independence of traits, may be because graphic-artistic behaviors are likely mediated by spatial-motor programs within the right hemisphere; while in contrast, letter and word reproduction may be a left-hemisphere function.

Usually by six years of age, children in most countries evidence a relatively precise and mature grasp of the pencil guiding the implement more and more with the fingers rather than with movements of the arm and wrist. (Saida and Miyashita 1979). At this same age triangles are able to be reproduced, and by eight years diamonds are often copied accurately. (Broderick 1987).

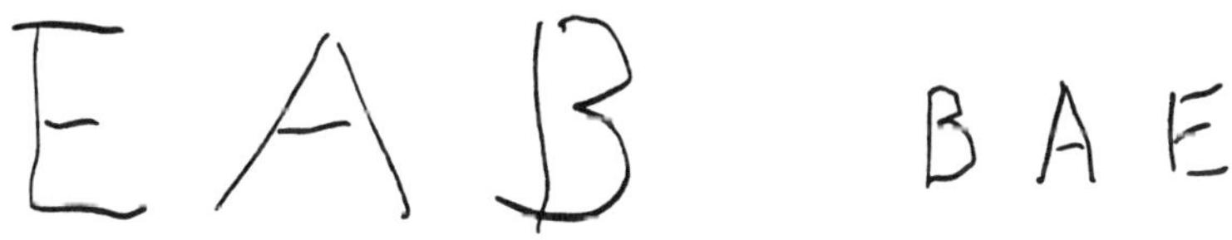

Plate 7-7. First printed letters

Youngsters in the United States are usually introduced to cursive writing at about eight years of age. However in other countries, including those surrounding the Mediterranean and in Central and South American, children are introduced only to cursive writing as they enter school at about five to six years of age. Thus youngsters in many parts of the world, and are never confronted with the task of acquiring the ability to print manuscript letters.

For many children in these latter countries cursive writing proceeds easily, as "handwriting" is difficult to reverse, and involves rhythmic actions that are easy to reproduce and to retain. Some schools for the learning disabled within the United States also encourage cursive handwriting rather than manuscript printing.

However if youngsters are required only to write cursively, they are thus reproducing letters which are unlike the printed letters they must first read.

At times, however, "things" do not go well, during these formative years. Some children may struggle when first attempting to print or to write letters. The unhappy results may include poorly executed letters (dysgraphia), or a complete absence of letter production (agraphia). These difficulties are inevitably accompanied by emotional overtones, as frustrations are encountered in school, producing excess muscular tension that further impedes attempts to write and print.

For many children this is the first time that they have felt inferior to others when doing anything. Thus many dysgraphic children first begin to experience a lowering their self-esteem, as they perceive that they are failing to match the printing and academic performances of peers in their pre-school, kindergarten, or first grade classrooms. Some otherwise intelligent children at this age, with high verbal I.Q.s, may become so frustrated that they de-value printing, and give up altogether attempting to graphically reproduce letters and words.

A few months before this chapter was written three dysgraphic children, ranging in age from 9–10, were tested in our clinic. They had begun to refuse to do any work at school, and had begun to exhibit marked symptoms of poor emotional health. All three evidenced severe school phobias, and depression due to the inability to match the academic production of their peers because of their poor writing efforts. The happy outcome of these cases, however, was that all three evidenced measurable improvement in about three months, resulting in satisfactory adjustment in their classrooms. Additionally the teachers of all three agreed to test each one orally, rather than requiring them to write their tests. These perceptive mentors also agreed to reduce the length of their written homework assignments.

CLASSIFICATIONS OF DYSGRAPHIA

Ogel was one of the first to attempt to classify various forms of dysgraphia and agraphia in stroke patients 1967). Observers evaluating the efforts of dysgraphic children to write, over the past several decades, have also identified various sub-syndromes and categories that that lie within the general label of 'developmental dysgraphia'.

These include sub-groups include several closely paralleling the sub-syndromes, reflecting gross motor coordination problems, covered in chapters 5.

Some of these sub-divisions were based upon observations that the poor printing may reflect symptoms of the presence of mild to moderate forms of cerebral palsy. Other categories they formulated reflected either cognitive problems, or neurological-structural anomalies. Among the contemporary classification systems been proposed is by O'Hare and Brown (1989). They divide dysgraphia into two main categories. One is labeled *specific dysgraphia;* and includes three motor coordination sub-groups, and a fourth reflecting spelling problems. A second main classification they called *non-specific dysgraphia*. This classification, they suggest, includes writing problems caused by cognitive and experiental variables, difficulties typically seen within mentally handicapped and culturally deprived populations.

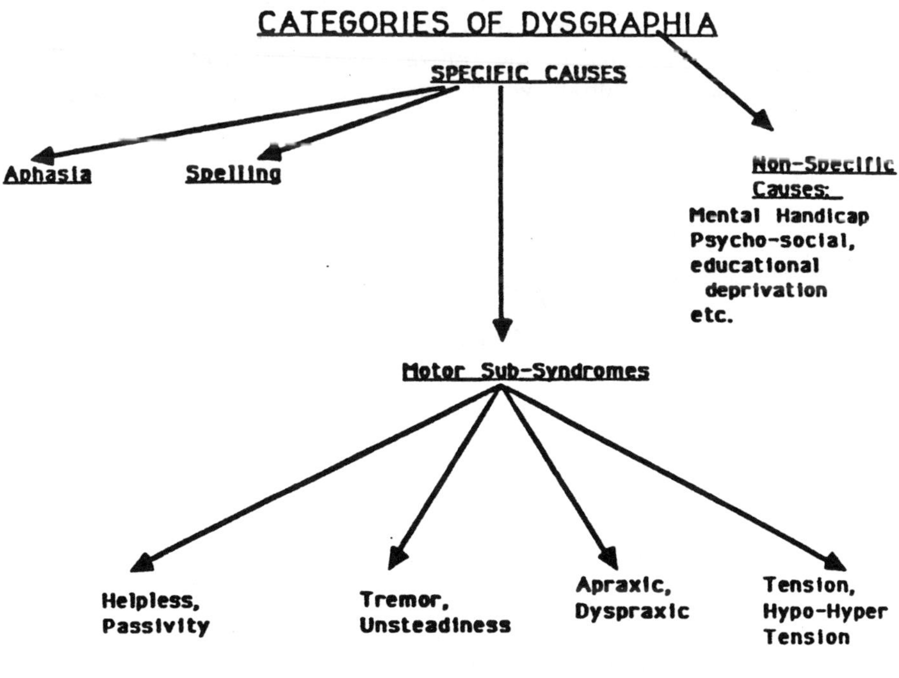

Plate 7-8. Categories of dysgraphia

In the model shown above, several motor components, in ,addition to those identified by O'Hare and Brown (1989), have been included. These were formulated by observing youngsters dealt with over the years in our clinical program. Overall the components of the motor sub-division include:

Tension-Syndrome

This child's printing evidences a spastic-like condition, characterized by excess tension. Difficulties in stopping lines when they should be terminated, and over-shooting ending points are also experienced. The heightening of muscular tension in dysgraphic children has been documented by O'Hare and Brown (1989b)

The presence of this condition causes difficulties when a child begins to try to print block letters. Often as this child matures writing, efforts continue to be accompanied by excess tension. The child may often appear to be attempting to simultaneously both initiate, and also time to stop, strokes necessary in both printed and cursive letters. Relaxation training is often an important accompaniment to the writing lesson when working with this type of problem. Additional discussion of the general characteristics of youngsters evidencing this syndrome when executing gross motor skills is found in Chapter 5.

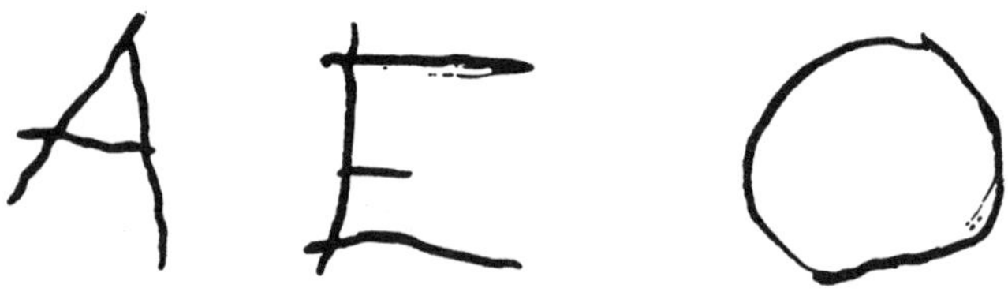

Plate 7-9. Tension syndrome

Tremor-Ataxic Syndrome

Youngsters displaying mal-adaptive behaviors within this problem area draw lines that are characterized by regular and low-amplitude tremors. This unsteady print out may be due to minor and healed cerebellar lesions, and may be accompanied by ataxic symptoms in gait, and posture. The result often is that the general form of the letter (or geometric figure) drawn may be reasonably well executed, while lines making up letters and figures evidence tremors. When the line quality produced evidences an irregular quality, rather than tremors of a regular amplitude and frequency, some kind of mild athetoid condition may be also present.

These problems are exaggerated when the child fails to properly anchor the arm and wrist when writing. Thus part of the remedial strategies employed may involve aiding the child to stabilize the write and arm, while the pencil contacts the writing surface.

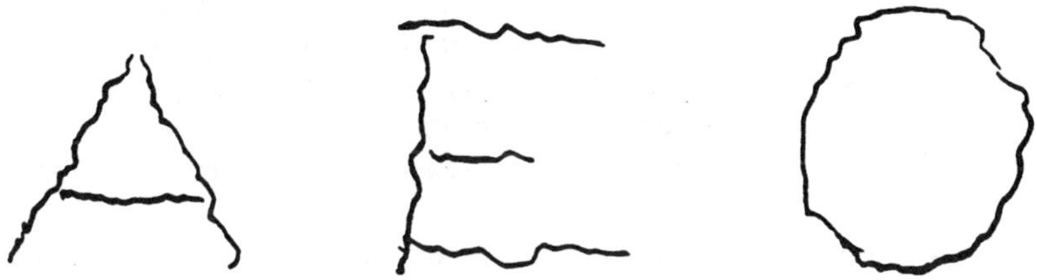

Plate 7-10. Tremor syndrome

Helpless Syndrome

Learned helplessness' is pervasive among clumsy and/or learning disabled children. youngster evidencing this type of problem when writing and printing, evidences apparent difficulties when attempting to exert adequate pressure inward on the pencil, as well as downward on the paper. The output is thus often a sketchy, unrecognizable effort, as the child seems to be saying . . . "see I am helpless, and cannot do this kind of thing".

This type of mal-adaptive graphic effort may be caused more by the presence of negative psycho-social conditions factors, than by faulty neuromotor mechanisms. These negative social conditions may include overly permissive parents, or caretakers who ignore the child's efforts. This child may also be surrounded by parents, or teachers, who are too punitive, and who frequently express anger over the child's ineptitude. This ineffective child may also have spent a great deal of time with a nanny or maid who has not stimulated early graphic efforts. This condition may also be caused by caretakers who produce helplessness by catering to the young child's every need, and who have failed to encourage the display of adequate independence and effort when the youngster has been confronted with a variety of important developmental tasks.

Negative social-emotional feelings of helplessness often interact with neurologically based symptoms, described elsewhere in the text. For example, 'learned helplessness' is typically accompanied by benign hypotonia, a condition involving lower-than-average resting levels of muscle tension in various parts of the body. Other neurological conditions, including those producing excess tension or dyspraxia, may have also served to render the child 'helpless', after early efforts at printing have failed.

Sometimes these "helpless" children hold the pencil in a passive grip, hook (flex) the wrist and make ineffectual swiping movements toward the body, as they attempt to print letters or simple geometric figures. These children usually need to be offered simple success experiences in various kind of pre-writing tasks. Then instruction should be given in how to hold, and exert pressure with a writing instruments.

Continuous positive social reinforcements, and also concrete rewards, need to be offered when signs of even minimal improvement is evidenced. Moreover retaining (and dating) practice efforts obtained during each lesson, will enable these children to observe improvement as their program progresses. Parental reactions which have produced, and that is continuing to promote and support helpless grapho-motor behaviors, requires modification by a family counselor.

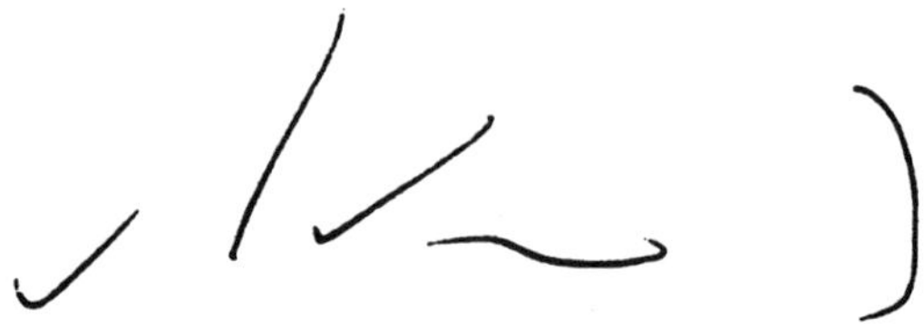

Plate 7-11. Helpless syndrome

Dyspraxic Syndrome

Dyspraxia, poor motor planning, is seen in printing efforts of some youngsters. This symptom is observed as child attempts to integrate several lines together, while trying to draw letter strokes in the correct order. This problem may also surface when youngsters attempt to learn the complicated sequences within upper-case cursive letters. Efforts to print numbers also often appear disjointed, and unconnected.

Often frustration in graphic tasks is seen as the child visually inspects a letter just drawn, whose components may not be well integrated. This frustration evidenced by many dysgraphic children, upon looking at their poor attempts to draw letters strongly suggests that many possess intact visual perceptual abilities. The poor printing and writing efforts by many young dysgraphics, are mainly attributable primarily to coordination problems encountered when attempting to integrate and sequence components of the required motor programs.

Luria (1966) and others have in the past, focused a great deal of attention to this type of graphic problem in adult stroke patients. In some literature this difficulty is classified as a type of 'construction apraxia.' This syndrome has been examined more recently by O'Hare and Brown (1984). They found the condition pervasive in stroke patients with lesions in the dominant parietal lobe. Head (1926) was one of the first neurologists to explore this condition among children. He labeled this type of dysgraphia, apraxic agraphia. As is often the case among youngsters within other dysgraphic sub-groups, an overlay of tension accompanies dyspraxia in printing and writing. (O'Hare and Brown 1989a)

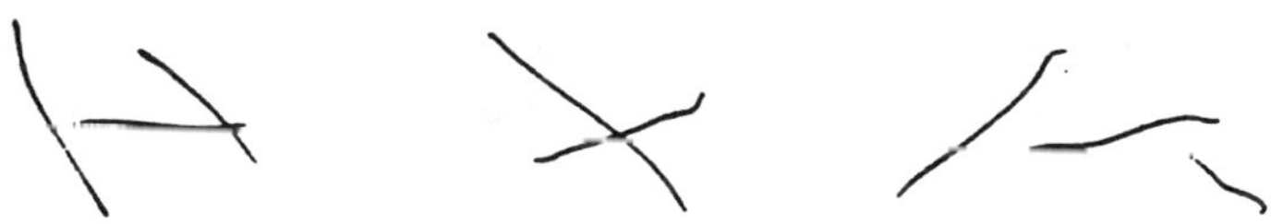

Plate 7-12. Dyspraxic syndrome

Spatial Agnosia

Difficulties in the organization of space also results in defective printing and writing. These children exhibit an undue number of letter and number reversals, and may confuse the proper order of letters in words. Letters may be slanted laterally across pages, rather than following horizontal lines, which are provided. This problem has been labeled "spatial agraphia" by Marcie and Hacean (1979) and others. Among stroke patients it has been associated with lesions in the non-dominant parietal lobe.

In children this problem may be part of a more global spatial agnosia syndrome (due to the presence of a right, or non-dominant, for speech) hemispheric lesion. This kind of dysgraphia may also be reflected in the inability to manage their bodies while moving though space. Thus participating in games or simply moving around the room may present problems. Thus is type of dysgraphia may be one, of several symptoms, reflecting the presence of a general spatial agnosia (*See Chapters 5 and 8*). However some children evidencing spatial disorientation when printing and writing do not evidence confusions in other spatial-motor tasks, including those requiring accurate, sequential movements of their limbs, and bodies.

HAND PREFERENCE AND DYSGRAPHIA

At times various models of dysgraphia have alluded to anomalies in hand, and eye preference as causes. However relationships between hand preference and both written and verbal communication are often difficult to determine. Moreover many contradictions exist in the writings of those attempting to clarify the meaning of relationships hand-preference and hemispheric dominance for speech and language.

It is probable that mixed dominance (lack of concordance between eye and hand preference) is not more prevalent among dysgraphic children than among groups of youngsters with normal printing-writing abilities (Armitage and Larkin 1991). However, It is a consistent finding that left handers are over-represented among dysgraphics (O'Hare and Brown 1989b). Left handedness is not only inherited (*inherited left-handedness*), but also may occur because some kind of neurological trauma (*obligate left handedness*) has detoured hand preference from right to left handedness due to subtle modifications in the hemispheric control of both written and expressive language. Thus it could be hypothesized that some dysgraphic children may both evidence left handedness and also have problems with graphic behaviors because of a subtle neurological "incident" taking place prior to birth, or because of a mild trauma occurring during, or shortly after birth.

Dysgraphic left-handers encounter special problems when attempting to print and write. Moreover those attempting to remediate the graphic behaviors of left handers should follow several basic principles (Cratty 1987). For example, left handers tend to cover their written work with their writing hand, and thus may need additional feedback about success or failure when attempting to print sentences, words and letters.

Left-handers may either hook their grip (writing with a their left hand-wrist in a cramped and flexed position, or they may keep their wrist and arm in alignment angle the paper, so that they are writing up-hill and away from their body. This second type of compensation is usually preferable, and is usually encouraged by effective therapists. These types of compensations may be represent efforts by the youngster to better view his/her work when printing and writing is taking place.

There is little evidence however that left-handed dysgraphics have more difficulties learning to print than do their right-handed peers. However cultural sanctions placed upon using the left hand in printing efforts differ markedly from culture to culture. For example, in The People's Republic of China and in other Asian countries, children are prevented from using their left hands when printing. In these cultures the left hand is assigned to less uplifting self-care tasks. Therefore in some cultures and countries numerous youngsters who may have inherited left handedness, or who are obligate left handers, may be forced to employed their non-preferred right hands, and as a result evidence various degrees of dysgraphia.

MANIPULATIVE MOTOR PROBLEMS ACCOMPANYING DYSGRAPHIA

Dysgraphia may be aligned with immaturities of manipulative behaviors, as well as with sensory-losses in the hands and fingers. For example, a fisted grip persisting into the 5th and 6th year is usually a sign of poor sensory feedback from the fingers. The child is likely having difficulty obtaining tactile information about the pencil's size and location. This is usually a sign of digital agnosia (Chapter 8)

Inability to reduce the size of block letters, and/or to reproduce lower-case manuscript letters may be caused by difficulties executing precise finger movements. When writing well finger movements need to be made, independent of hand-wrist actions. Thus poor manipulative abilities, such as those detected in a finger-opposition task, present problems for some dysgraphic children.

These types of sensory-motor problem require the child to move the wrist and fingers as single unit when printing larger block letters. Thus the reproduction of small letters is difficult or impossible for some dysgraphic youngsters. Often extra help with manipulative behaviors, including work with clay and finger painting, may heighten sensory awareness of the fingers and hands and can also improve the manipulative abilities that are needed in the adequate production of letters. These strategies may help some dysgraphic children change from a fisted grip at the end of the writing implement, to a grasp of the pencil permitting them to guide their efforts more accurately. Thus accuracy is gained as they become able to employ finger actions when writing, movements relatively independent of the less precise movements of which the hand and wrist are capable. (Saida and Miyashita 1979). The following is a sampling of several kinds of grip-grasp problems, together with the picture of a mature grip.

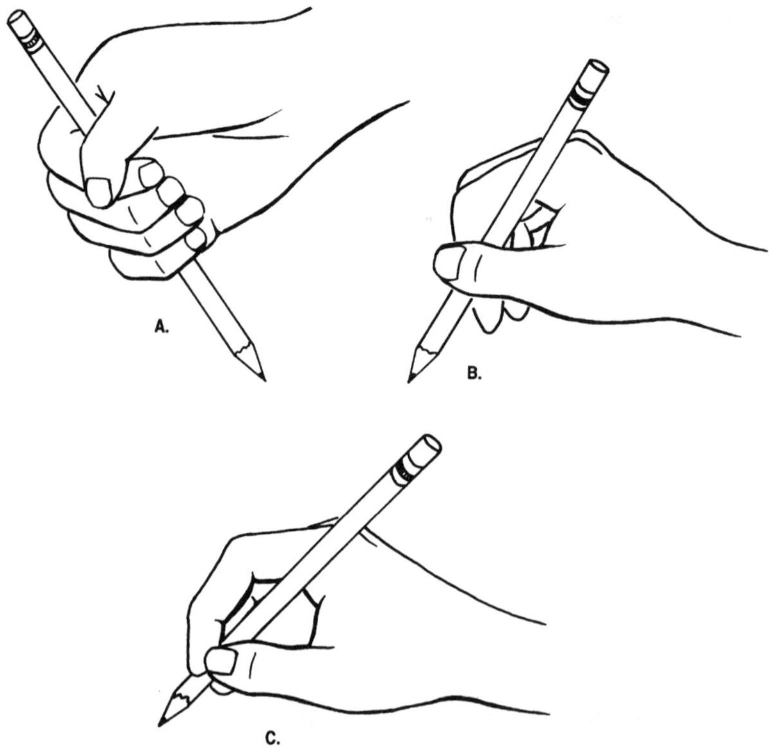

Plate 7-13. Various grips seen in developing children including (A) a fisted grip, often seen early. At about 2–3 years. A semi-fisted grip (B), and a mature grip (C) in which the fingers move independently of the hand and wrist

Other Symptoms

Numerous other problems, acting alone or in combination, may cause poor writing efforts, in addition to the motor difficulties emphasized within this chapter. These include difficulties in thinking, the formulation of sub-vocal speech, as well as confusions caused by faulty auditory and visual perception. Acquired or congenital structural abnormalities of the hands, wrist, and fingers may also cause graphic problems.

Problems with visual-perceptual organization often impede youngster's first efforts to print letters. This kind of difficulty is often evidenced when the youngster tries to connect dots while making lines, in vertical horizontal as well as vertical directions. Later difficulties are encountered when trying to print capital letters havingh slanted lines (the X,V, Z, K, and the like), by youngsters displaying this kind of problem. These visual problems can include accommodative error. Recently I observed a child attempting to print while holding the printing arm-hand in an extended position to the far left of the body, while seated as far as possible to the right of the printing surface used!

Auditory-perceptual difficulties can also plague a child in ways that may produce dysgraphic behaviors. These problems can include auditory sequencing, re-audibilizing words, and the matching of sounds to letters and words. If defective these difficulties can result in the incorrect ordering of letters in words, and the production of improper letters when a word sound, or sounds, are heard and then must be replicated in writing. The effective formulation of paragraphs, and the blending of paragraphs into stories, may also be impeded by auditory perceptual difficulties. This type of difficulty among dysgraphics has been referred to as *syntatical problems* (O'Hare and Brown 1989a).

MIXED SYNDROMES AND MULTI-SYMPTOM DYSPRAXIA

Other problems are found among dysgraphic children, some of which interact with the more common syndromes discussed above. Margolin (1984), and others, has postulated the existence of "*multiple component agraphia*", caused by the interaction of more than one factors. It is common to find a child with more than one type of problem interfering with efforts to write and print. These youngsters with mixed syndromes pose special challenges both when evaluating their efforts, and when designing remedial strategies.

REMEDIAL STRATEGIES

Research dealing with the efforts of children write and to print was popular during the first decades of this century. Included in this literature were efforts to obtain norms, to explore improvement strategies (Anderson 1966) (Askov et al 1970), and to formulate evaluation instruments (Otto et al 1969). However by the late 1970s more emphasis began to be placed upon understanding the neurological and psycho-educational causes of dysgraphia, and upon the formulation of classification systems (O'Hare and Brown 1989ab). Recently the use of computers has been advocated as a tool for improving writing behaviors (Glazer and Curry 1988).

A thorough review of methods to improve handwriting and printing would encompass a book larger than this one. Many popular remedial strategies focus not only upon improving the motor coordination of printing and writing, but also include efforts to modify poor spelling, faulty sentence and paragraph construction, as well as other syntax, and composition problems.

Essentially the strategies employed need to be matched carefully to the symptoms seen and the type of factors(s) that are believed to underlie poor efforts at written language. Remedial efforts should also be accompanied by

(a) efforts at circumventing the problem, providing the dysgraphic child with an opportunity to type, instead of insisting on cursive writing and

(b) lessening the pressure to produce a lot of written work by shortening written assignments, as well as by providing opportunities to substitute verbal responses for written ones, when giving examinations. Some of the examples of matching symptoms to educational strategies include the following.

Apraxia

Apraxia or dyspraxia in printing reflected in difficulty in motor planning, results in problems integrating, and placing letter parts in proper spatial perspectives. Dysgraphic children who evidence dyspraxia also may have problems arranging the strokes of a printed capital letters, and/or correctly integrating the lines making up large-capital letters in cursive writing.

Remedial Strategies

Efforts to improve this problem could include encouraging the child to verbalize the nature and directions of the strokes while drawing a letter. Multi-sensory approaches often prove useful. For example, the apraxic child should be encouraged to gain a wholestic visual-impression of the letter shape, before printing it, by first drawing it with a finger in sand, cutting it out of paper, or forming it with ropes of clay.

Fading techniques are also useful, in which the child is first provided with strong visual supports, and then the visual cues are gradually reduced until they are eliminated. Using this method the child first traces over a whole letter, and then later is guided only by lines of dots. This approach is seen has been formulated in materials by the author (Cratty 1987). When teaching difficult-to-execute cursive letters (or block letters), an additive method may also be used. In this method a total letter is formed after working on its parts. Using this approach each component is acquired and then added to the whole, until the whole letter-form becomes replicable.

Tension Symptom: Excess tension when printing

This symptom can be seen when undue pressure on the pencil is exhibited, resulting in early fatigue when a child attempts to complete long writing assignments. Other signs of this symptom can include over-shooting the ending of block printed letters, as well as tension exhibited downward on the paper when trying difficult-to-form letters.

Remedial Strategies

Relaxation training may usefully accompany lessons when dealing with a child whose is overly tense when printing. A judgmental-free environment should be employed in which more encouragement than criticism is used. Efforts should be made initially to give the child relatively easy printing and drawing assignments, in which success is assured, before presenting more difficult printing jobs for completion. Reducing the length of writing assignments is usually indicated.

Helplessness-Infantile Printing and Drawing

This group of symptoms is accompanied often by learned helplessness, hypotonia, or dystonia. The young pre-school children exhibiting these produce produce figures, or scribblings that are often from 1-3 years less mature than peers of the same chronological age are seen executing.

Remedial Strategies

Initially a great number of accomplishable drawing tasks should be introduced. Finger painting, as well as clay work can prepare children exhibiting this symptom to begin to use their hands. In some cases the child should be encouraged to copy the therapists efforts to produce numerous scribbles.

The therapist also should encourage the child to expand both the number of scribbles produced, and also to assist the "helpless" youngster to begin to exert increasing control by drawing some scribbles slower. Drawing shapes with the use of templates and grooved surfaces are useful pre-printing activities in which to engage. Later the fading technique, described earlier, may provide a useful way to introduce the printing of block letters to such youngsters. This technique is seen used in the case studies which follow.

Letter reversal

Reversal of asymmetrical block and lower case manuscript letters, (Ee, Gg, PpFf, Jj, Kk, Rr, etc.) and the misplacement of letters-order in words. (Substituting WAS for SAW etc. marks this problem. Facing asymmetrical numbers in the 'wrong' directions is also seen among children exhibiting confusions of this type.

Remediation

This problem if persisting after the 6th or 7th birthday, may be assisted with remedial efforts that may include (1) helping the child determine what is the left and right side (hand) of their own body, using verbal cues, and visual ones (placing a red cuff on the right hand), and then (2) helping the child find out which is the left and right sides of the page, and which letters open, or somehow relate to these two sides. The sides of the page may be clearly labeled "left" and "right" to facilitate the acquisition of important spatial ideas about individual letter reproduction, the proper letter order, and where to begin to print and to read sentences.

CASE STUDIES

The following seven case studies are taken from a monograph completed in 1989 depicting the problems and progress of seven children brought to our clinic for remedial of dysgraphic tendencies as well as other gross motor problems. In general they represent several of the sub-syndromes discussed in the previous sections. (Cratty and DeOliveria 1989)

Case Study 1

The first are Tommy's attempts to copy a line cross, circle, and square.

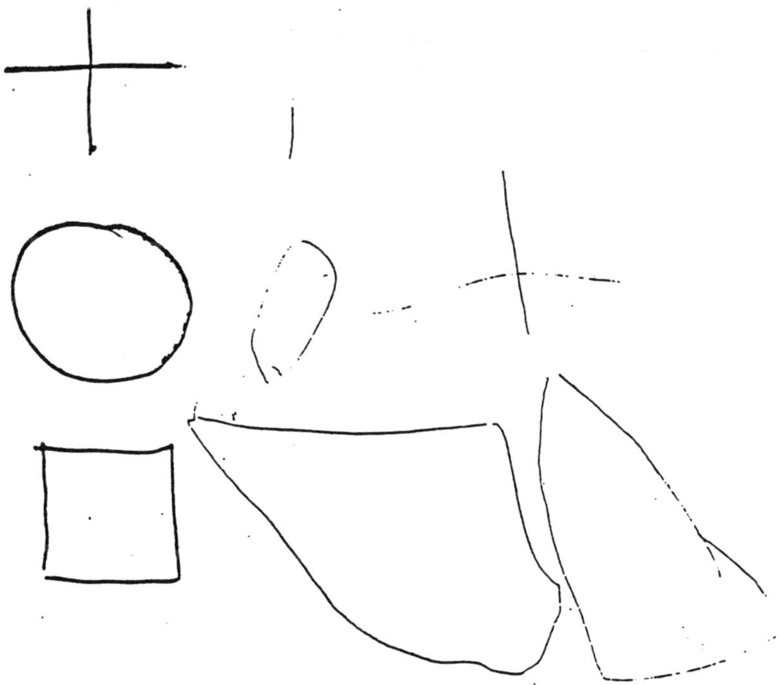

His efforts to copy capital R, P, K and C, resulted in the following efforts, during this initial evaluation.

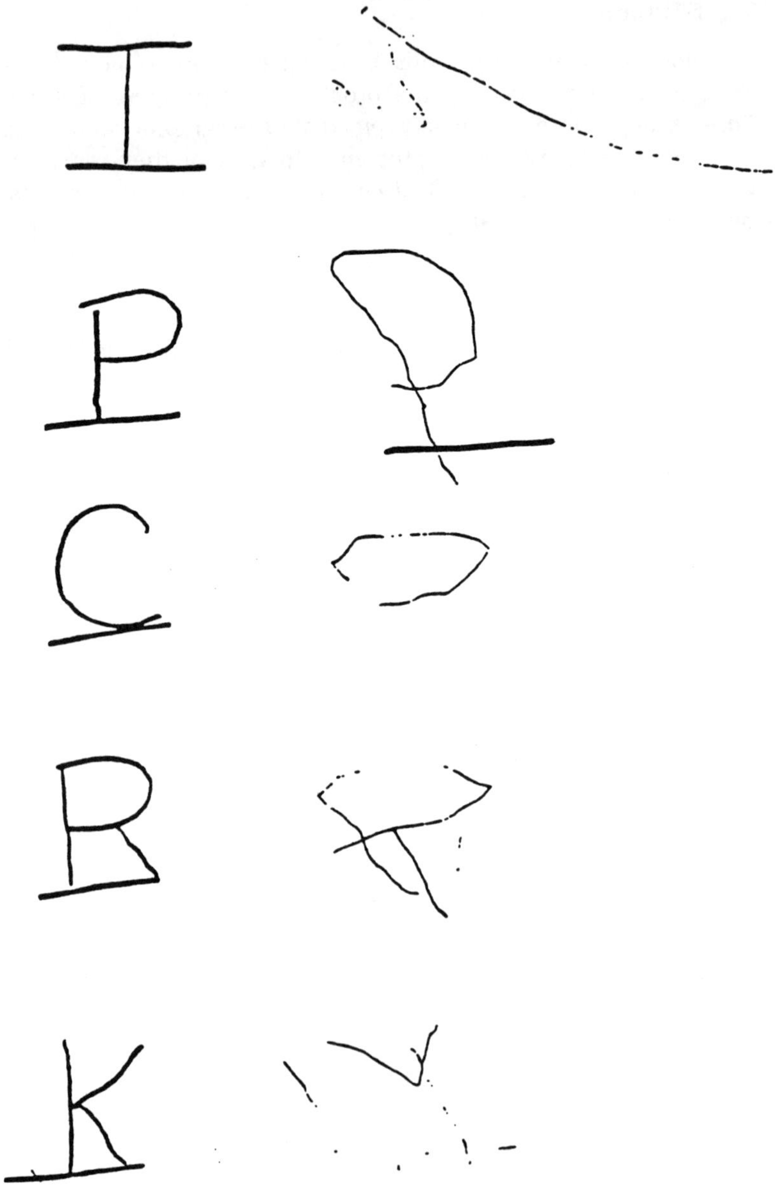

During the first weeks, efforts were made to aid him to begin to draw coherent, and related lines, in order to form letters Moreover the verbal identification of letters were encouraged, and at the end of the third week he could identify the capital FTPACILH. Using 'fading' techniques, block letters containing right angles were worked on, however letters formed from circles were still difficult for him to execute, as shown.

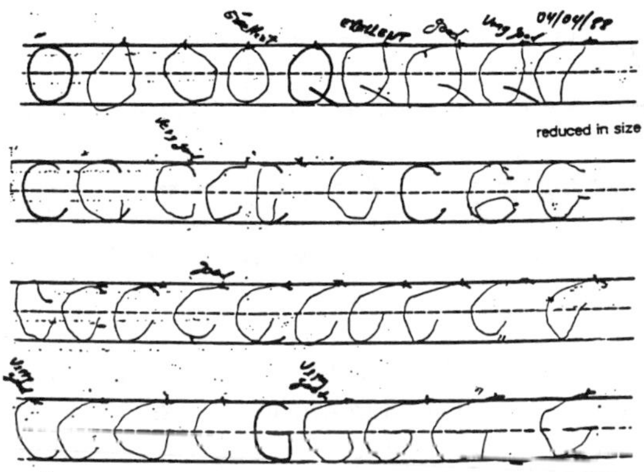

Midway through the second month he was evaluated at a private religious school, to ascertain his readiness for entrance into kindergarden. He seemed to continue to show a disinterest and/or ability to execute figures, as he copied a radiating mandella in the following manner. This kind of drawing behavior, together with the school's observation that he apparently had a short-attention span when in a group, resulted in their declining to admit him.

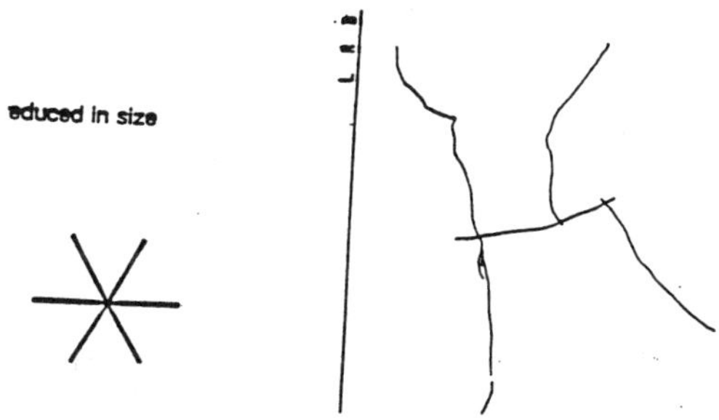

Toward the end of the second month of therapy the formation of block letters had considerably improved, and his verbal identification of all his block letters had neared completion.

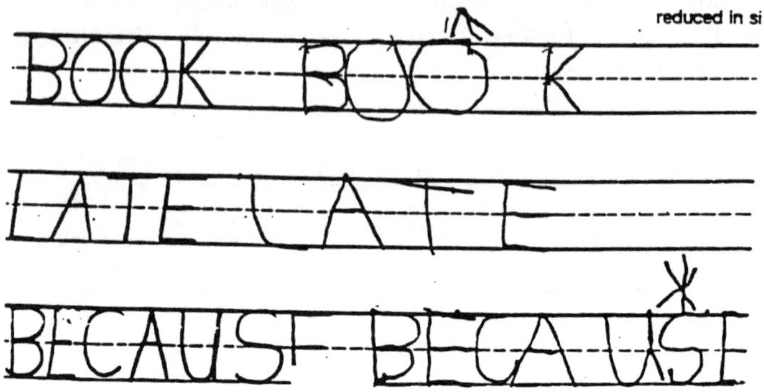

Tommy learned to identify and to print the large block letters after three month work. He was then introduced to lower case letters, and also work on printing numbers was begun. Within about three weeks he had made considerable inroads on these latter two task areas, and was able to print all his numbers accurately and without reversals together with eight lower case letters which were also formed well. These lower case letters are shown below. During this same time he was aided to attach sounds to various letters, in preparation for reading.

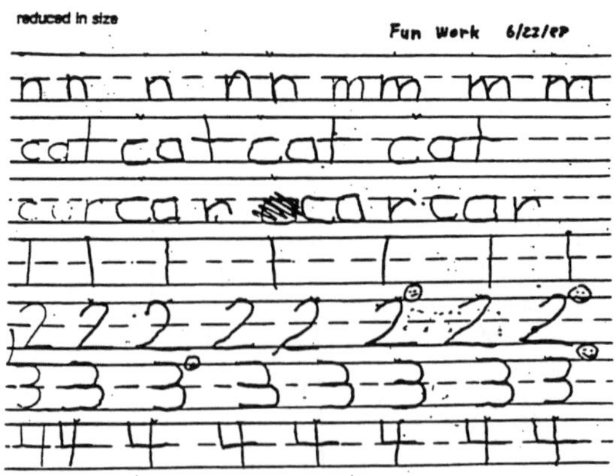

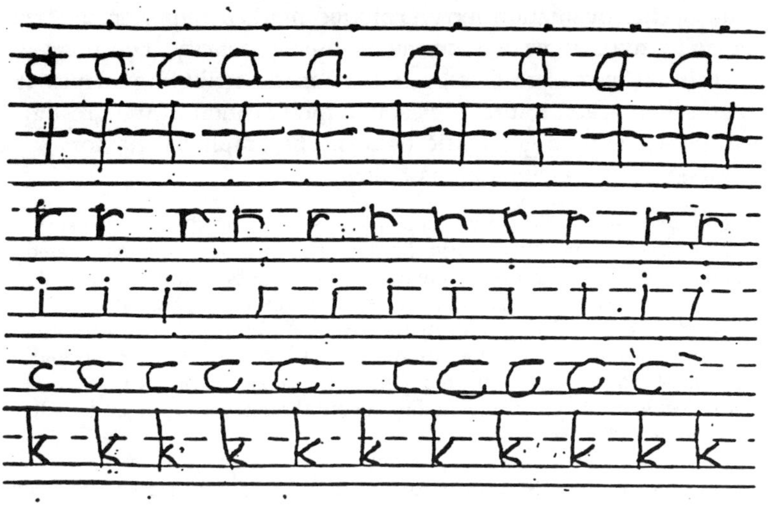

Thus in summary, within a period that lasted slightly over three months Tommy had progressed from a child who could not recognize, x print any letters well, to mastery of both upper case letters, numbers, and some lower case letters at a level usually seen in boys of about six years. The developmental change within this 3.5 month period was approximately 2 years.

It should be noted that Tommy's initial problem may have been more attitudinal, than motor. As was noted, he did not exhibit any signs of neurological dysfunction reflected in any kind of central nervous system disorder. Initially he seemed to have other priorities that we more important to him than were printing or writing. Bugs, flowers, and nature, for example, seemed to attract him more than did things he could draw. When these priorities were re-arranged, and combined with remedial help, the depicted improvement was the result.

Case Study #2 Tension and Aggression

"Jerry" was referred to our program by the administrator of a pre-school which he had been attending. He was described by her as evidencing poor coordination, and also as exhibiting aggression to other children at play. At the time of his evaluation he was 4 years 5 months old.

During the evaluation Jerry exhibited marked hypertension, coupled with hypertonia amounting to mild spasticity. He grasped a pencil in an immature fisted grip, and made scribbling swipes at a paper, when asked to draw lines, in a modification of the Frostig, or to duplicate simple geometric figures. His graphic behaviors were described on the evaluation as follows.

> "His manual skills were poor and he evidenced poor sensory-awareness in his hands and fingers. His printing and associated behaviors were extremely immature and resembled those of a child about two years younger (2.5 years) than his chronological age. He had problems with figure-drawing, and even had problems coping a simple line cross (+). Most of the time he could not exert enough pressure downward with his pencil to make marks. Circles and squares were beyond his ability, even though he appeared well-motivated."

Samples of his attempts to draw and write obtained in this first evaluation, are shown below. Most of the lines he produced were so faint that they had to be re-drawn in order to make them replicable. Essentially his effort in this type of task involved barely perceptable and inaccurate scribbles.

Jerry also exhibited obvious and marked problems when attempting to execute gross motor skills including those requiring the handling of ball, balance, and locomotion. His responses on a questionaire-type self-concept test (A modification of the Piers-Harris) indicated that he felt badly about his social acceptance and his relationships with peers.

Jerry's graphic behaviors in his first evaluation resulted in the following.

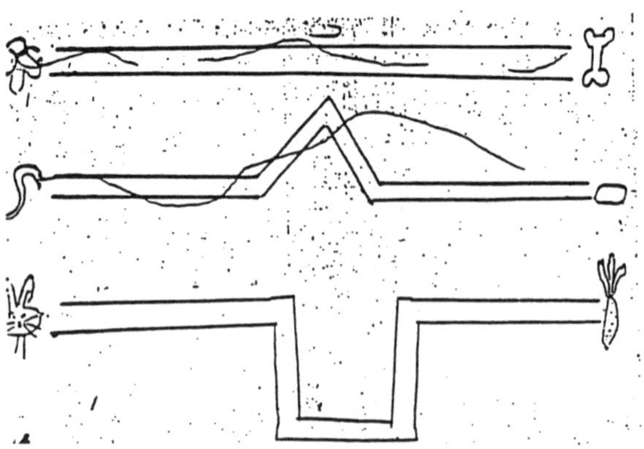

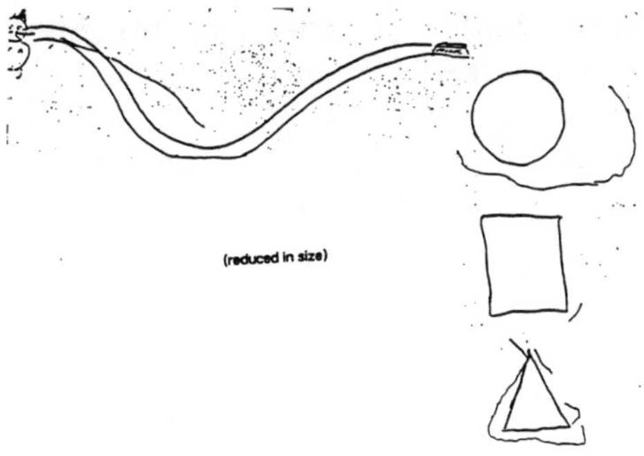

Progress was slow during the first several months. Not only was Jerry hampered by obvious motor problems but also by a-low self-concept that was reflected in frequent verbal outbursts reflecting frustration. For example, he frequently shouted "I can't' when a difficult letter was attempted. The therapist encouraged him to substitute positive statements when this occurred ("I can, if I try hard"). He was rewarded when he succeeded, as well as when he spoke in positive ways about effort and success.

Often 'fun work' (homework) that was assigned was not completed. He arrived at the therapy site upset with the fact that he had not completed his work. The therapist was frustrated because he only came once a week.

First goals included helping Jerry to hold a pencil reasonably well, and to make marks. Templates and grooves were used to draw in, in order to guide a pencil that simply seemed to refuse to obey commands issued from Jerry's central nervous system.

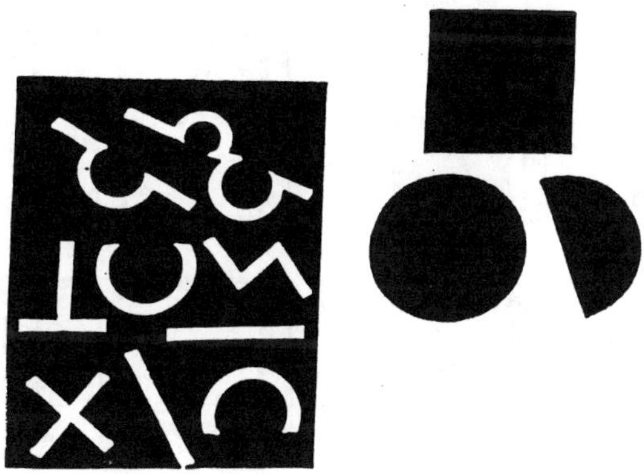

After a difficult six months, however, Jerry began to improve and to take pride in his work. Help was given in other manual skills including the cutting of paper with scissors. Additionally he began to guide his pencil with more accuracy and became able, with help, to trace over letters and numbers as shown below, using 'fading' techniques as shown.

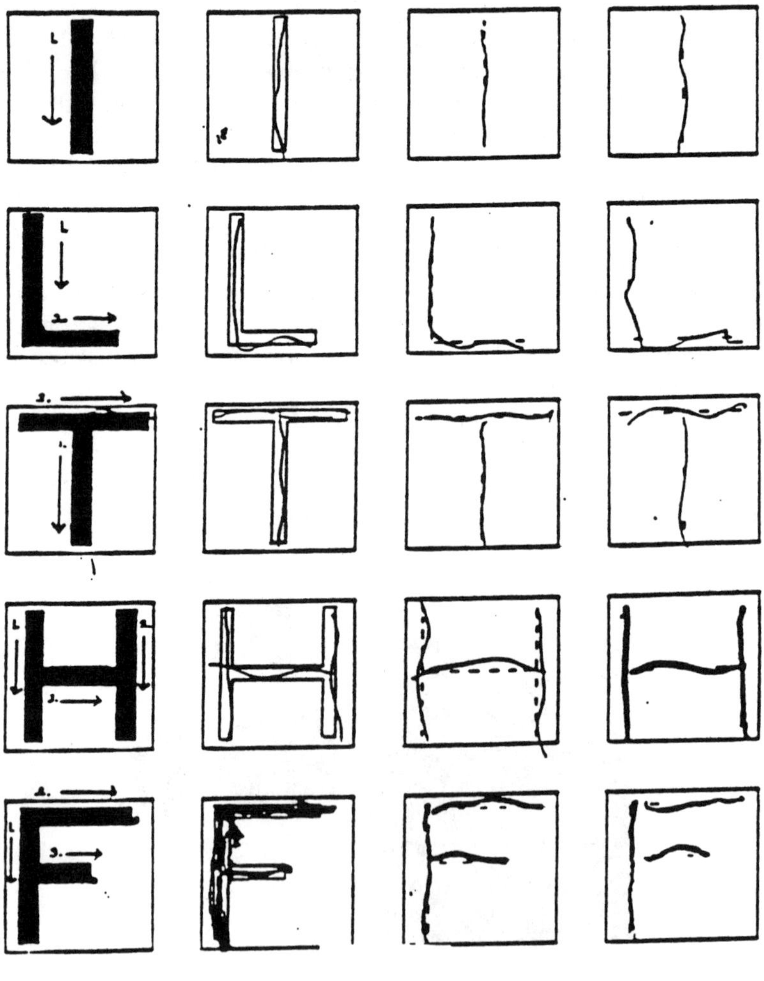

A month later Jerry was given lined paper and began to replicate block letters with increasing accuracy, and with fewer visual guides (dots etc), and with less prompting by the therapist.

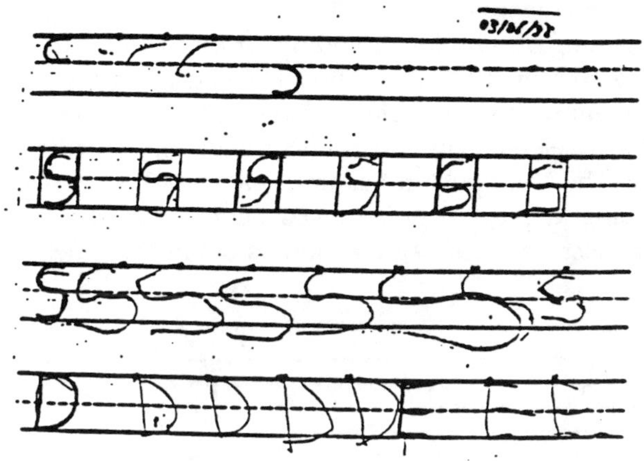

Fading techniques continued to be used, however, with the following results.

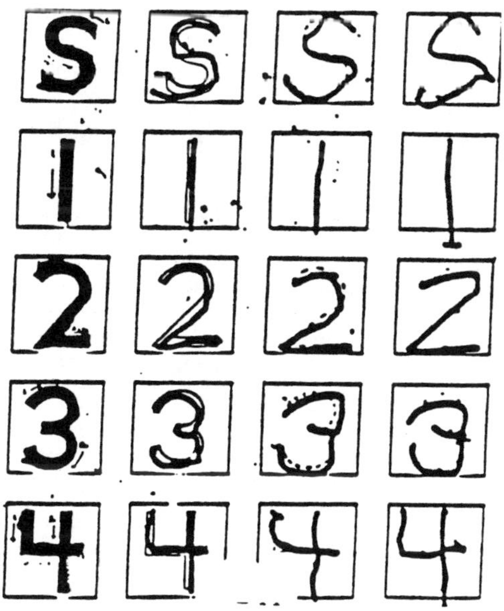

When Jerry mastered the block printing of large upper-case block letters, it was becoming apparent that he was not only quickly learning to name all his letters, but also could attach sounds to most of them. Soon, with little prompting and encouragement, he began to read simple words.

The printing of both lower and upper case letters, about a month later, pleased him and his therapist. He quickly learned to name and to print them with reasonable accuracy, at the same time his reading seemed to accelerate. His efforts on a standardized reading test given at school (The Metropolitan Reading Readiness Test) revealed that he was reading at the 3rd grade level; quite a remarkable finding as Jerry was just five years and 4 months old at the time!

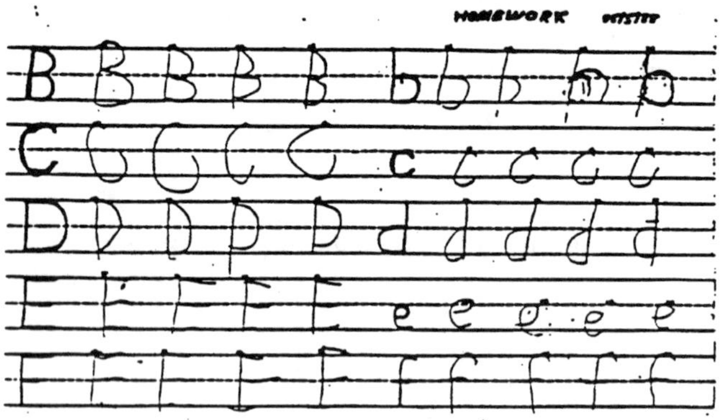

(reduced in size)

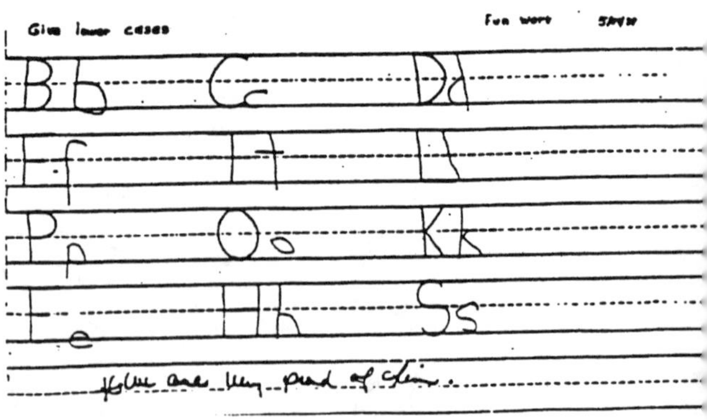

Thus in about a year Jerry's improvement was remarkable. From a start that did not include making legible marks on paper he became able to print both upper and lower case letters, his numbers, and upon attaching sounds to letters and letter combinations he became able to read.

Jerry's progress was attributable to several variables and conditions. He is extremely intelligent, and his progress was quickly perceived by him, resulting in a shift upward of his self-concept. His intelligence enabled him to participate in weekly goal setting, and to monitor his own progress carefully. Success in this area seemed to generate greater emotional stability and placement in a new pre-school resulted in more social satisfactory adjustments with his peers.

Jerry's hypertonus remains, and motor development therapy is continuing. His gross motor skills remain below those of his peers; while his printing is executed with above-average tension. Help with self-administered relaxation training is proving useful at this time, together with continued work on ball skills, balance and locomotor activities.

His graphic behaviors in a 14 month period improved from about the 2.5 year old level to those resembling the efforts of a child of six years.

Case Study #3 Infantile-Helplessness

"Bobby" was referred to us for evaluation by specialists from a private school. He was currently finishing a pre-kindergarden grade and it was felt that he evidenced immaturities in his motor behaviors. He was almost five years and two months old at the time of his evaluation. During the evaluation it was found that he evidenced minor to moderate problems in both fine and gross motor skills. The results of his attempts to draw accurate lines between channels are shown below. Similarly his attempts to reproduce geometric figures and the letters of his name were difficult for him, as also depicted below and next page.

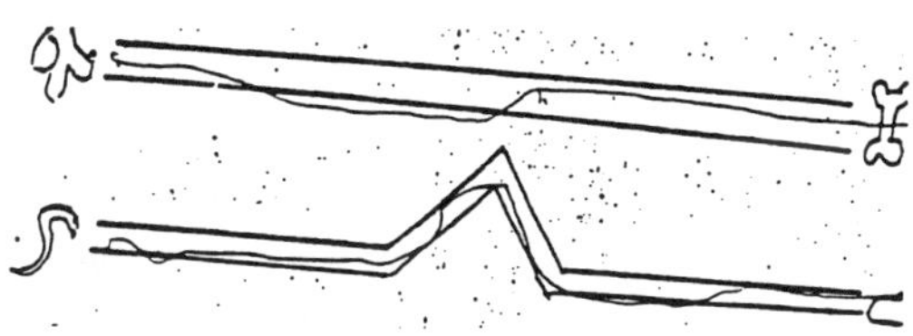

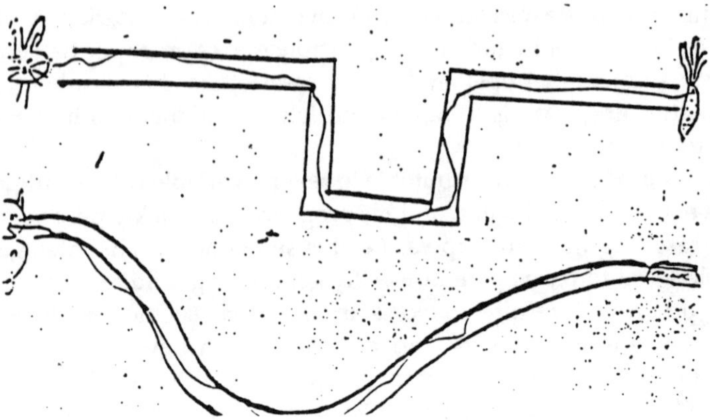

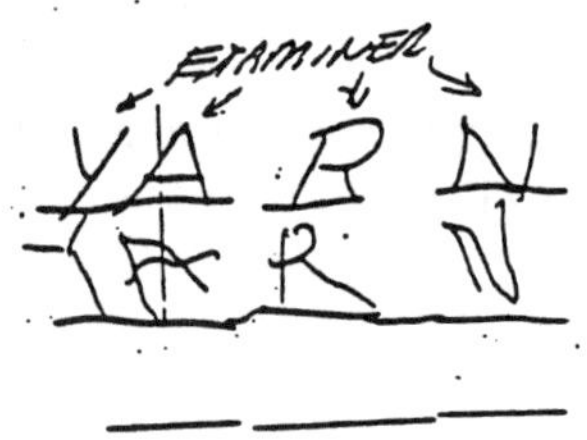

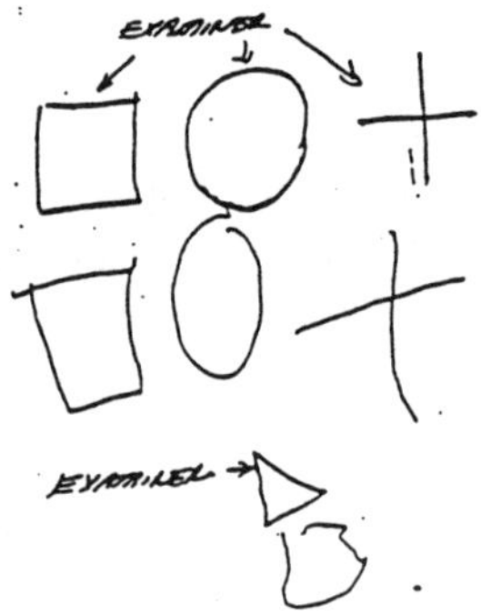

Bobby's skills were summarized in several paragraphs within the written summary of his evaluation.

> "("Bobby's") written printing-drawing skills were immature. Squares and circles were drawn inaccurately, while a triangle was impossible for him to execute. This kind of difficulty was seen in letter reproduction which was labored and inaccurate. Special remedial help is suggested in these and related skills in order to prepare for effective functioning in kindergarten and the first grade." ("Bobby") appeared to be right-hand."

In general Bobby evidenced similar immaturities in ball skills, and in locomotion. Lateral movement was difficult for him, while he threw and caught balls poorly for a boy his age. Moreover he evidenced motor planing problems that involved observing a demonstration and then reproducing three or four movements in a series. It should be emphasized, however, that Bobby's problems were not marked, and may have been partly due to inexperience, he is an only child. Moreover his appeared to display no subtle signs of neurological dysfunction. His balance, for example, was within normal ranges.

As a result of his evaluation Bobby was placed in a twice-a-week program of remediation. Each session consisted of an hour that was divided between work on fine and gross motor skills. He approached some of the sport skills tentatively at first, but within a week began to perform vigorously. Additionally he appeared to find great pleasure in doing the 'fun' work that was sent home after each lesson. One evening, for example, Bobby was discovered at the dining room table completing his 'fun work' even though the rest of the family had gone to bed!

During the first month Bobby engaged in various activities including drawing basic figures, over lines and dots (using the 'fading' technique in which the stimuli guiding him were gradually faded out). Later during this period he began to draw over letters in the same manner. As is true of many children this age, Bobby held a pencil in various ways when printing letters. When a constant and appropriate 'grip' was acquired by him, his printing skills improved in a parallel fashion.

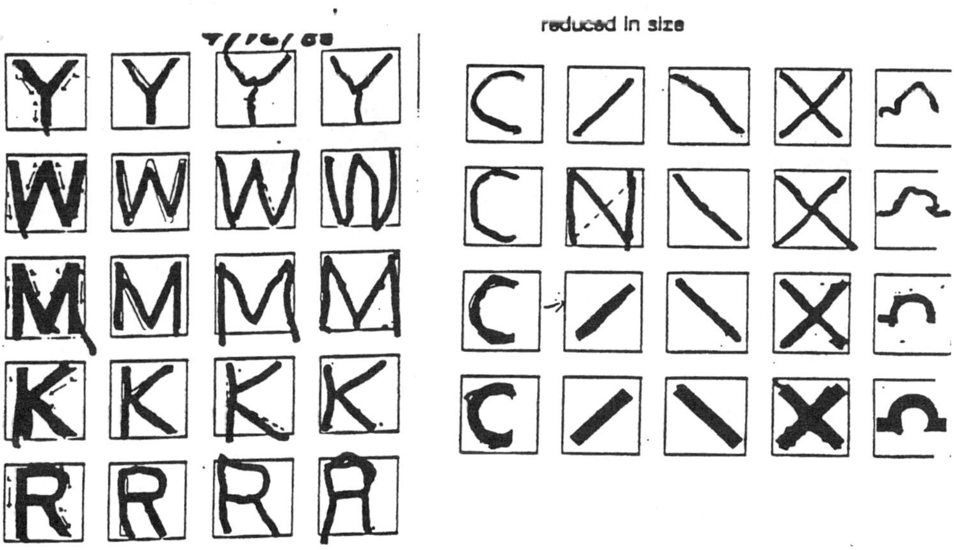

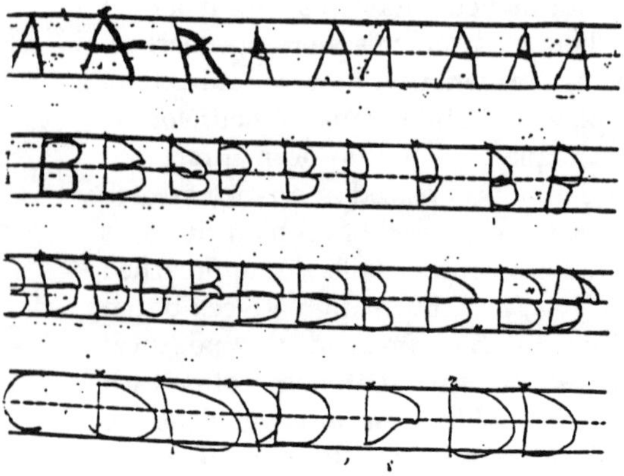

reduced in size

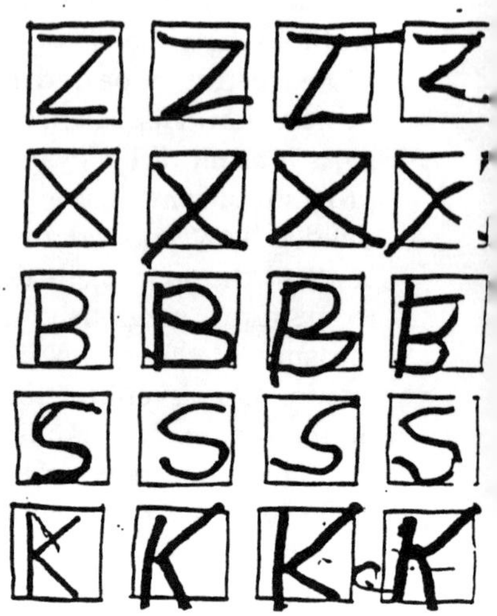

As is sometimes the case Bobby began to draw free-hand better when the letters to be reproduced were placed into small squares, about 1''/ × 1'' in size.

At the end of the second month Bobby began to drawn letters free-hand, within lined paper as shown. Toward the end of his 2.5 month program he also began to draw numbers as shown below. When he was first exposed to asymmetrical letter and number he had to be given clues as to which way a given figure 'faced', as is necessary with most children. However, Bobby evidenced little problems when learning assymetrical letters and numbers.

At the termination of his program, Bobby was beginning to attach sounds to letters, and appeared ready to learn lower-case manuscript letters. It appeared that he was easily read to begin work in an academically-oriented kindergarden toward which he was headed. Moreover his improvement in sport skills was obvious and he approached them in a vigorous manner, seeking activity instead of avoiding it.

In general, Bobby represents an optimum set of factors that result in positive changes in graphic behavior. He was young, he did not display obvious neurological "soft-signs", and he was highly motivated to do well, always completing his brief 'fun work' assignments between twice-a-week sessions.

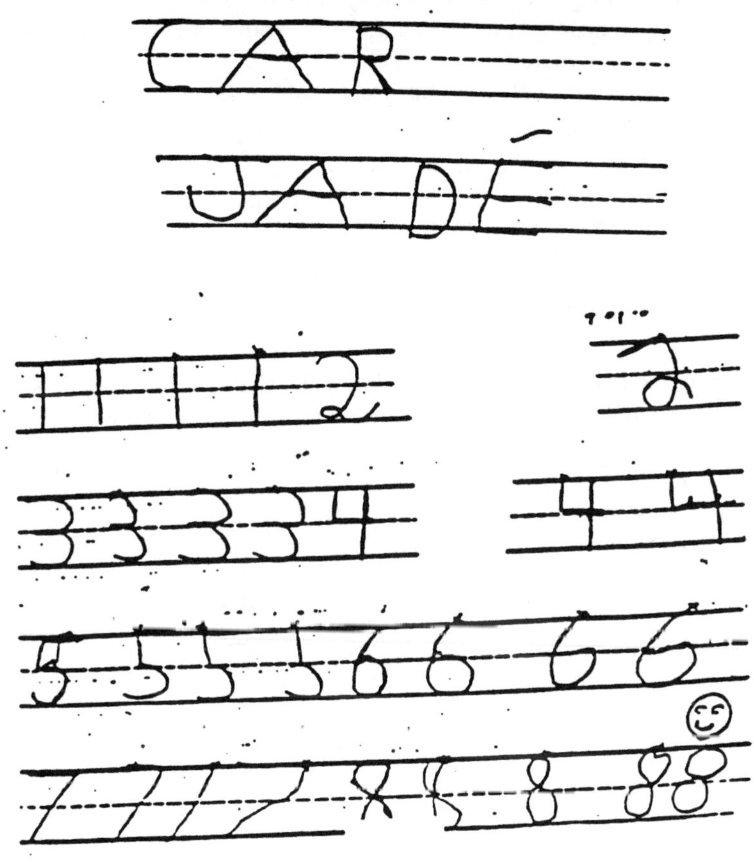

Case Study $4 Hypotonia

Larry was evaluated when he was five years, two months of age. He was referred to us by his mother, who stated that he was in need of help in the printing of his letters prior to entering kindergarten. Larry proved to be big-boned and heavy, evidencing moderate problems in gross motor skills including ball skills and locomotor activities including lateral movement. His balance was adequate, however, he was slightly hypotonic (displaying less and average residual muscle tone). In the self-concept test he was administered (a modification of the Piers Harris), he admitted to being 'sometimes' clumsy, however most of his responses indicated that he believed himself functioning more than adequately both socially and physically. Larry was the oldest of two sisters, and a third sister was born during the period he was being remediated.

The paragraph describing his graphic skills in the initial evaluation was as follows.

> 'Larry's drawing and attempts at printing letters are immature. Help is needed to enable him to begin to draw letters in correct perspective (without reversals) and to help him with the more difficult-to-print letters like S C, and other containing lateral lines. He confuses upper and lower case manuscript letters. He held a pencil with various grips, usually with his right hand. Remediation of this kind of task would be helpful.''

Samples of his efforts on this initial evaluation are shown below. As can be seen the circle, square, and even the line cross were drawn poorly.

tester's samples

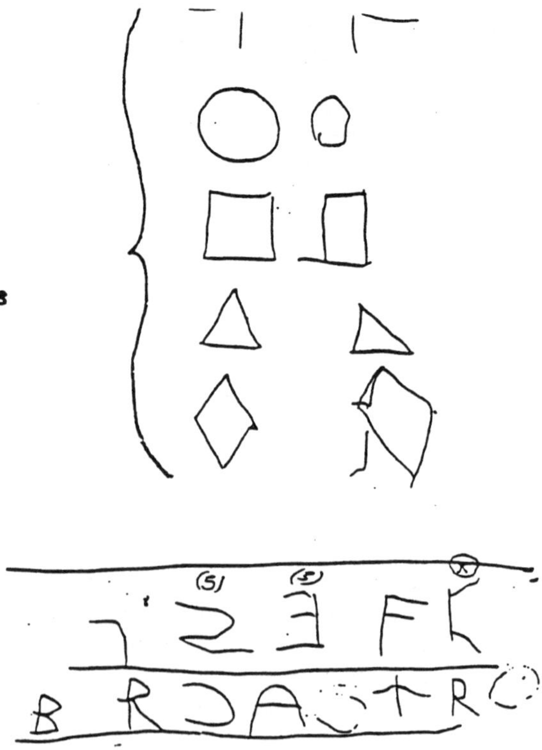

The first month, Larry engaged in sessions lasting one-hour each twice a week. Half of which was devoted to improvement of printing behaviors. Progress was made easy by the fact that Larry easily recognized all his letters. However he evidenced a mild athetosis in his printed efforts. As a result Larry needed to exert a great deal of tension to overcome the irregular movements that seemed to dominate his hands, when he attempted to print accurate horizontal, vertical, curved and lateral lines that make up block-printed letters. Thus, as can be seen below, he was given simple mazes to execute, and dots to trace over using fading techniques.

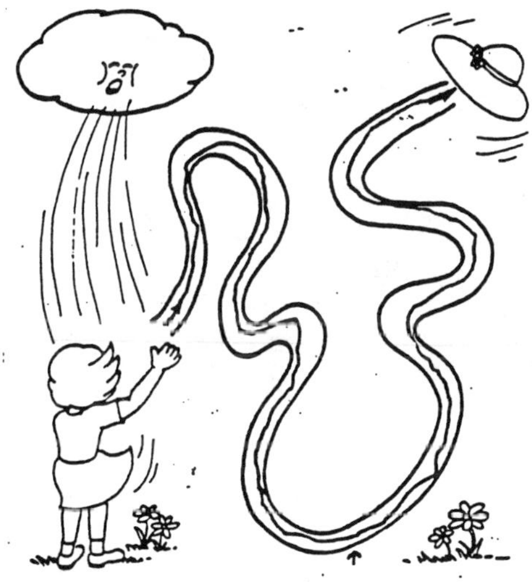

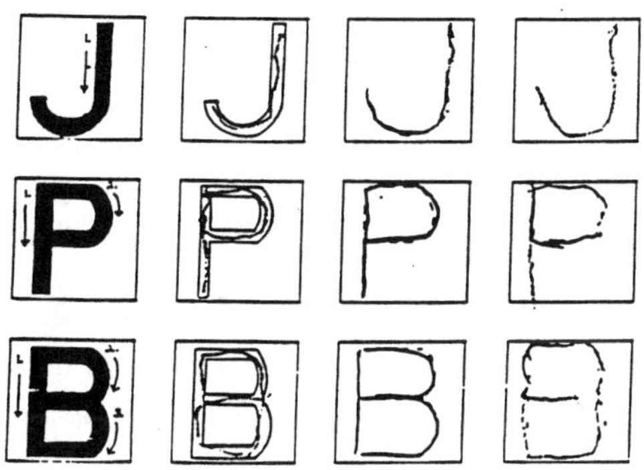

During the second month Larry was able to copy most letters without using dots to guide his efforts. However, he was reluctant to do and return short-home work assignment, and only did so after being denied presents that normally accompanied the termination of remedial sessions. The grip he used became more consistent, and his hand and fingers began to relax more when printing.

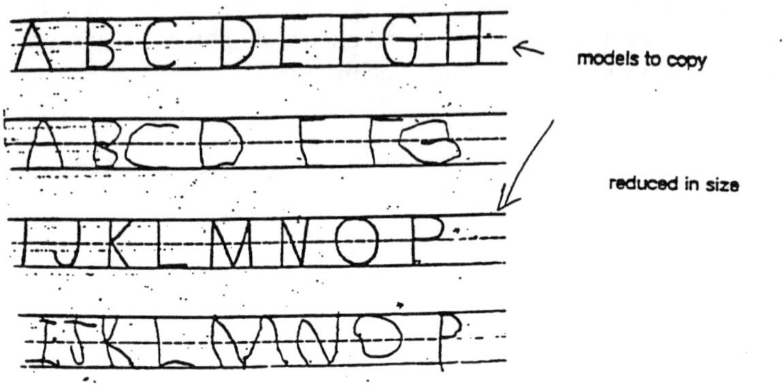

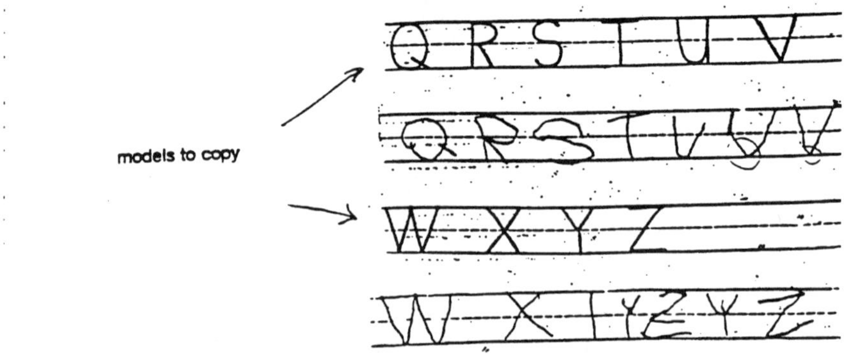

During the final sessions (he participated in about 20) Larry improved measurably and began to work on numbers, most of which were difficult for him to draw. He terminated the program as he was becoming ready to learn to print lower-case manuscript letters, after having acquired a few. His mother believed him to be ready to enter a kindergarden in which moderate demands would be made of his printing skills, and we generally agreed.

His final efforts are shown next page.

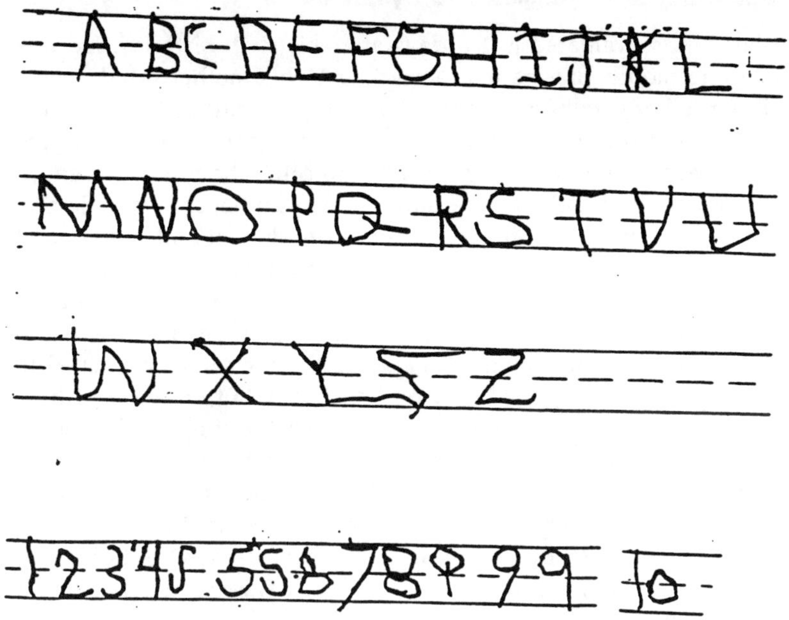

In general Larry evidenced moderate improvements in graphic behaviors due to remediation (and perhaps maturation), from his 62nd month to his 65th month of age. Improvement was enhanced because of his above-average intelligence that enabled him to easily identify all the letters quickly; he also worked hard during each therapy sessions, while under supervision. The therapist's efforts were somewhat blunted because of the presence of moderate neurological soft-signs, and because of his apparent lack of ability to self-monitor his own efforts when not present in the therapy sessions (when faced with his 'fun work' to do at home).

As can be seen in Larry's final efforts, more improvement is needed. He still printed with excess tension present, and with obvious inaccuracies. It will be helpful if his kindergarden teacher does not pressure him for a large quantity of written work, enabling him to relax and to improve his efforts. His tendencies to reverse letters and numbers initially seen, and common in five year old boys, seemed to be well under control during the final weeks of his therapy sessions.

Case Study #5 Tension and Dyspraxia

"Mark" was evaluated just 8 days after his sixth birthday. He was born one month pre-mature, according to his mother. Mark was a thin tense body, tall for his age, and with poor muscle tone. He was simply terrified of incoming balls, and chringed when the approached him and thus was unable to catch them. He evidenced other gross motor delays, including problems in locomotion. He also evidenced motor planning deficiencies, finding it difficult to first observe a simple three part movement, and then copying it.

Graphic skills were delayed. A Loose grip on a pencil almost prevented him from making legible impressions. He also seemed to have difficulties perceptually organizing the forms he was asked to copy. His mother reported that he had had about one-year of help in these tasks, prior to the evaluation. Even the simplest figures on the evaluation were drawn poorly, as shown below. His ability to print letters was almost absent. He held a pencil in his right hand. According to the results of a previous psycho-metric evaluation, based upon his performance in the Berry Development Test of Visual Motor Integration, his abilities kind of task was approximately 1.5 years delayed.

"(Mark's) graphic behaviors appear to be markedly delayed. He had difficulty drawing lines accurately (in a modification of the Frostig). Circles and squares were difficult to execute. He attempted a triangle, and it came out a thin rectangle. He declined to attempt a diamond. He produced a recognizable capital B, and E, while the A and C were fair. He could not execute a capital S, while the R and Y were unrecognizable. Although his mother reported that he had been taught lower case letters, he only produced large block letters during the evaluation. He drew a crude number 1, and reversed the number 4. He declined to try other numbers, except the 6, 7, and 9 which were executed poorly and were barely recognizable.

(Mark) appears to be right-handed, and his work methods vary greatly when printing. For example, at some points the correctly anchored his writs and arm (on the table), while at other times his arm and hand floated above the page, making the tasks difficult for him. Attention both to work methods as well as to letter-number execution appears important at this point."

Samples of his efforts in this initial evaluation are shown next page.

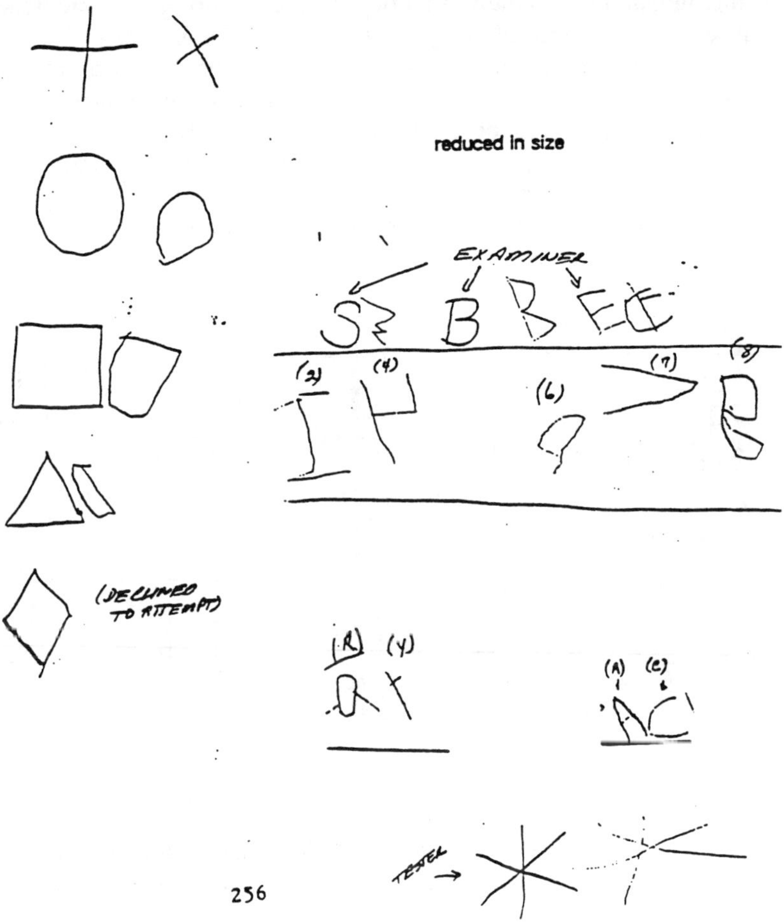

Mark began on a twice a week program, in sessions lasting approximately one hour, divided between activities intended to enhance his gross motor abilities, and graphic behaviors. During the part of the session devoted to gross motor behaviors his insecurities manifested themselves in compensatory verbal behaviors, usually not connected to the task. This kind of anxious task-avoidance compensation is common among youngsters with motor delays, when they are confronted with the need to exhibit their ineptitude. During the first sessions his recognition and recall of letters were evaluated, and it was found that he could recall (bring from memory, without the presence of cues), nine letters of the alphabet.

The activities in the first sessions began very simply, concentrating upon block letters, and using 'fading' techniques during which visual guides (usually a series of dots) was gradually withdrawn. His work methods were also given attention. For example he was taught to anchor and re-anchor his hand-armwrist properly when attempting to draw a letter. By the third session Mark began to execute several letters without the presence of visual cues, as shown below.

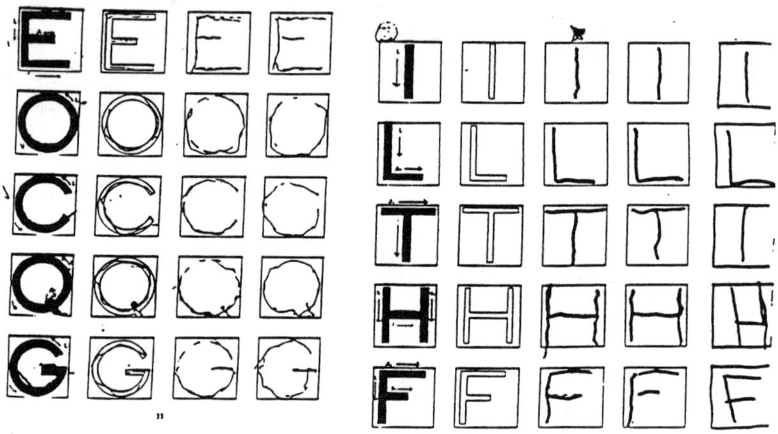

A month later Mark was able to copy all the letters of the alphabet, as shown. The compound curves in the S were still difficult for him, as were some letters containing slanted-lateral lines (K, V, N, etc). It was also found that he often could do better, when the size of the area in which a letter was to be reproduced, was made smaller.

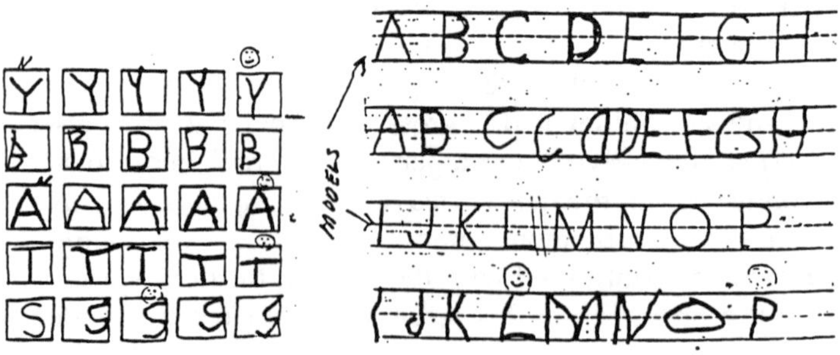

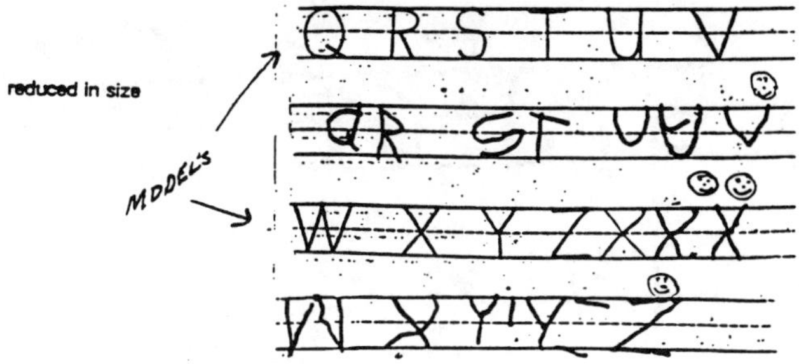

After about two months of remedial sessions, Mark is proceeding well. He can execute all the letters of the alphabet in recognizable forms. He continues to have some problems in the memory-retrival process, prior to printing several letters, and this is currently being addressed. His verbal behaviors extraneous to the task has been markedly reduced both when working in both halves of the therapy session, while he is taking obvious pride in his progress. His mother reports that he is willing and able to engage in unsupervised effort when doing the 'fun (home) work' that he takes with him after each session.

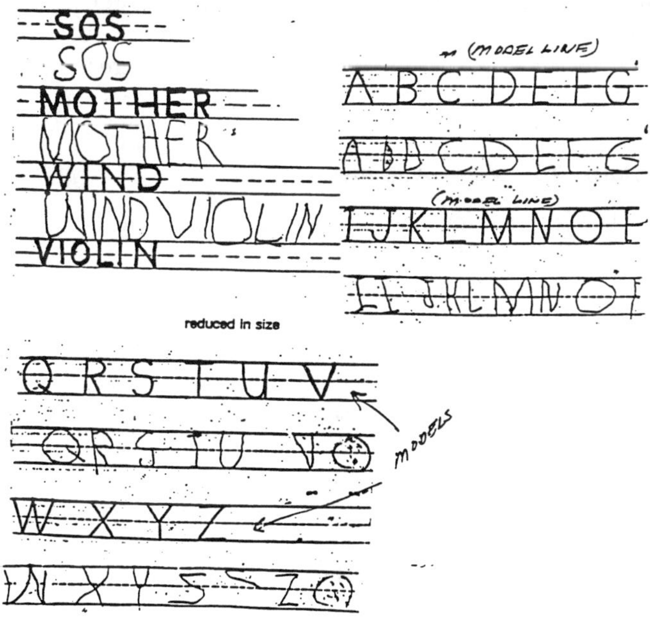

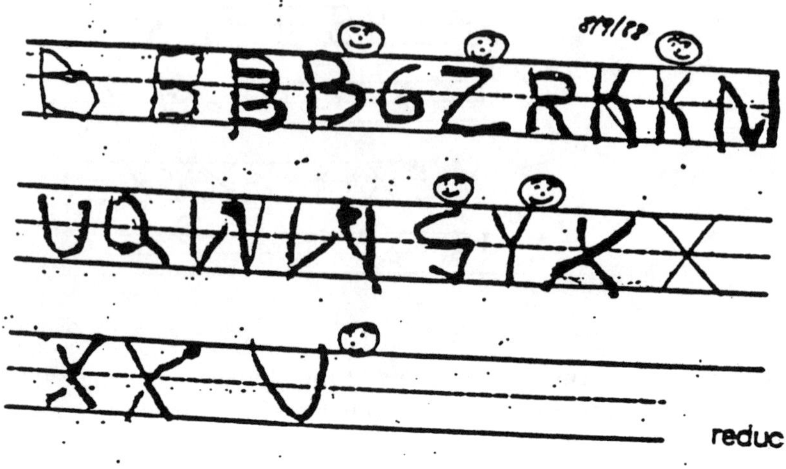

Mark continues to attend motor improvement sessions. He is working on the better execution of block letters, and their perfect recall. His work methods, reflected in the holding of a pencil are more consistent, and mature. His physical strength is improving, while he has made some inroads in the throwing of balls. Intercepting balls, continues to need help, and he remains tense, and thus ineffective in catching incoming missiles. As he gains confidence there is a marked diminuation of the shrill verbage that was initially used by him to block instruction in both fine and gross motor skills.

Case Study #6 Minor Athetosis

"Sally was evaluated four months before her sixth birthday. She was a tall attractive child, whose cognitive abilities seemed intact. However, she evidenced 'typical' signs of minimal neurological dysfunction including problems in the execution of gross motor skills, as well as difficulties when printing and drawing. Motor planning was difficult for her, and replicating a three or four part movement, (given one part a second) proved stressful. She evidenced particularly difficulties when attempting to intercept balls.

Emotionally Sally appeared quite happy, and her responses on a self-concept test reflected this state of mind. She stated that she was happy most of the time, that liked herself, and that she had no trouble making friends. She also stated, however, that she was clumsy and "fell a lot", additionally she said that she had trouble making things with her hands, and that she was the last to be chosen in games.

Sally's graphic behaviors were delayed. She had difficulty drawing letters as shown below, while her attempts at replicating simple geometric figures were poor. She held a pencil in her right hand, but with a grip that varied from moment to moment. Even a simple line cross (+) was difficult, while a square was impossible for her to draw well.

When describing her manipulative and graphic behaviors on the summary of her evaluation the following statements were made.

> Finger opposition (touching each finger, in order, to the thumb of the same hand) was labored and immature, reflecting problems in manipulative behaviors. She drew with her right hand, producing immature circles and a line cross. A square was impossible for her to replicate, while line drawing (in a modified form of the Frostig) was poor. (Sally) consistently used her right hand in these kinds of tasks, and her grip varied from a fist, to one using several fingers to hold the pencil. Enrichment is needed in this area, starting with work on template drawing, and proceeding to letter reproduction using lines and bars to guide her movements. She currently draws recognizable P's, H's and E's, but other letters were not replicable, or not attempted.' (She refused to attempt an R, and an S).

Examples of Sally's efforts on this initial evaluation are shown below.

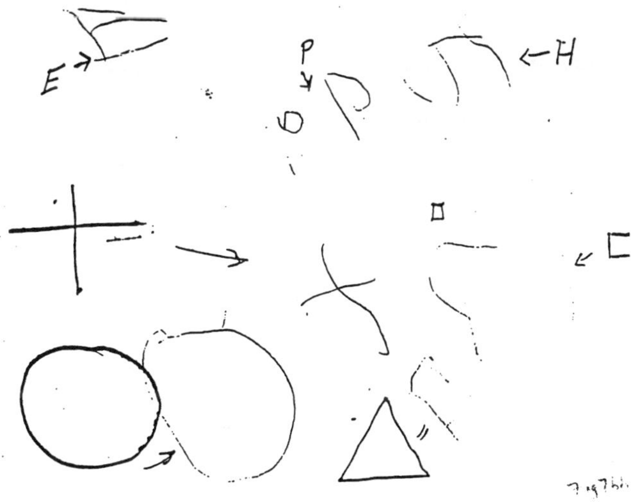

Sally began by simply drawing through grooves and tracing around both inside and outside templates. As improvement in these simple activities progressed, she was exposed to visual guides, and asked to execute simple block letters, containing right angles (H I T, L, E and F). Examples of these initial efforts are shown below.

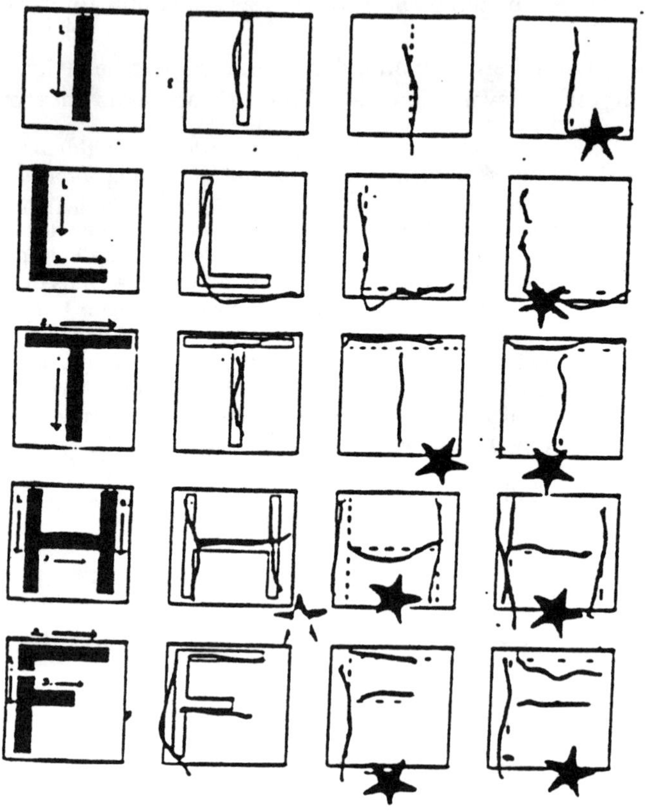

After a month Sally 'graduated' to the replication of letters containing curves and slanted lines. These proved particularly difficult for her, and she often evidenced letter reversals on such letters as a C. The compound curve of the letter S, gave her great difficulties, while the slanted lies in the letter Z was also difficult. However, she and her mother worked hard to improve these letters.

Fading techniques were also employed during the second month, with the results as shown below. She became able top replicate letters using these visual cues, (bars, and dots to draw over), however when she was asked to draw letters unaided by such guidelines the task proved far more difficult.

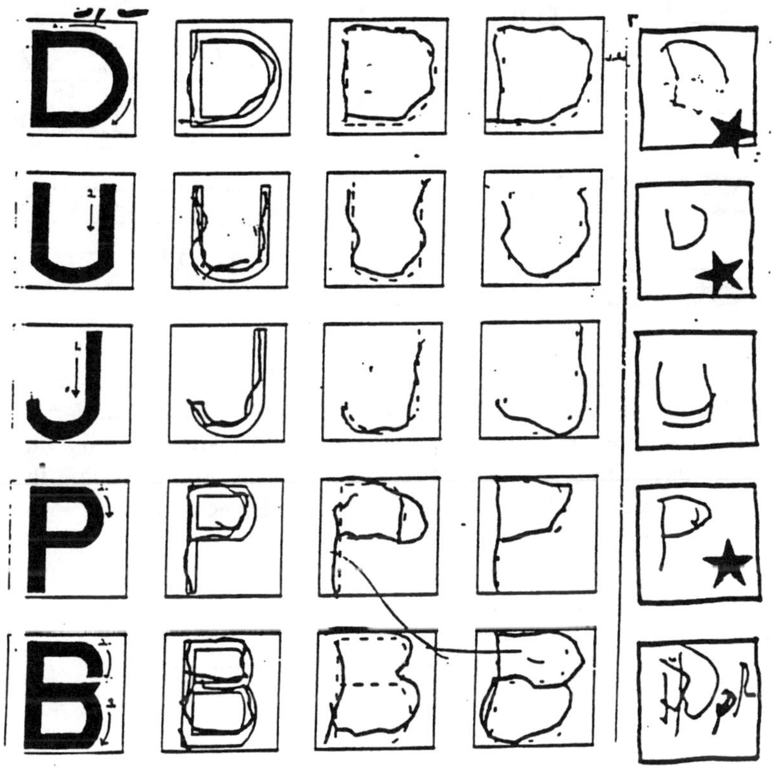

However with additional work a month later, Sally evidenced improvement in the freehand drawing of letters as shown below. Numbers were also introduced, and she experienced some difficulty with asymmetrical numbers, often reversing 4's, 5's, 6's, 9's, and 7's. The curves in the number 5 was difficult for her, as it resembled the vexing S. Sally, however, worked hard both at our sessions and with her mother. Aiding her progress was apparently a good intellect, and thus memory strategies for the replication of letters was accompanied by useful verbal formulas. At times impeding her was the presence of moderate hyperactivity, she often required some pressure, and high levels of reward (happy faces, and colourful stickers) to continue tasks that proved frustrating to her.

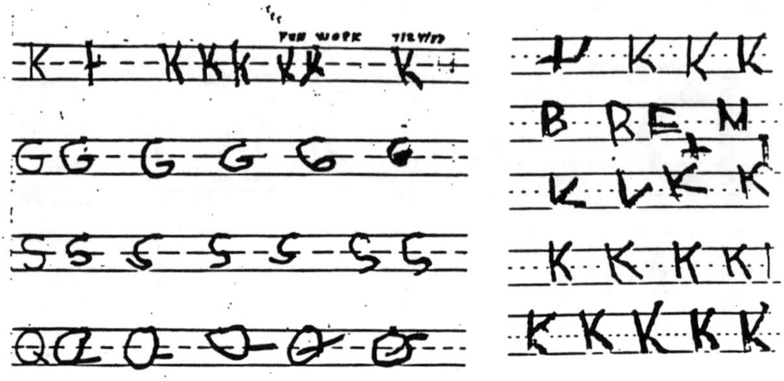

During the 3rd and 4th month additional progress was made, and Sally became able to replicate reasonably accurate numbers and letters, without the use of visual guides. Moreover various games were played that enhanced her letter reproduction, including those that involved finishing the letters and similar activities.

Her more recent results are shown below.

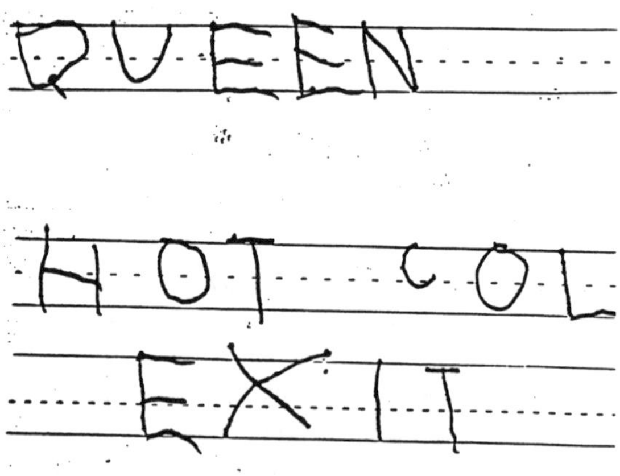

Sally's work and progress continues into the 5th month. She is becoming more relaxed and motivated when printing.

Case Study $7 Helplessness

"Judy's mother was referred to our program by a clinical psychologist who had examined her. She proved to be a shy girl, extremely short and with a delicate bone structure. At the time of the evaluation her chronological age was five years five months. She was the second born of fraternal twins. Her twin brother, her mother reported, was quite a bit larger, and functions physically at normal levels. We haven't seen her brother at the time of this report. Judy proved to be left-handed, and evidenced marked delays in both gross and fine motor abilities. Her graphic behaviors consisted mainly of circular scribbles, typical of a child of from 24–36 months of age. A history of partial deafness, now corrected, has apparently resulted in delays of expressive language; while receptive language was apparently more intact.

The statement concerning her fine motor abilities, appeared as following on the summary of her initial evaluation.

> (Judy's) graphic and drawing skills appeared markedly delayed. She was unable to copy a simple line cross (+), while the request to copy a circled resulted scribbles. A square was also responded to with a scribbled circle. Marked inaccuracies were seen when she was asked to draw accurate lines, either down channels of various widths, or from point to point. If the points were located too far apart (over 10°) she was apparently unable to organize the entire problem, and instead drew circular scribbles around each of the points she was to connect. Letters appeared impossible for her to attempt. She held the pencil with her left hand, but her grip varied widely from task to task. She appears to have neither consistent work methods, nor consistent grips, when trying to make marks and to draw.

Judy, although shy, appeared to have no obvious mental delays, and could identify most of the letters of the alphabet, when they were presented. Other motor delays, however, involved problems in motor planning, in gait (running was unaccompanied by a cross-extension pattern), and in ball skills which were typical of a child of about three to three-and-a-half years of age. She appeared to have no severe postural problems, although her muscle tone was below average.

Judy immediately was placed in a twice-a-week program of therapy, in which each session was split between tasks focusing upon graphic behaviors, and those intended to improve her gross motor functioning.

Examples of her graphic efforts in the initial evaluation are show below.

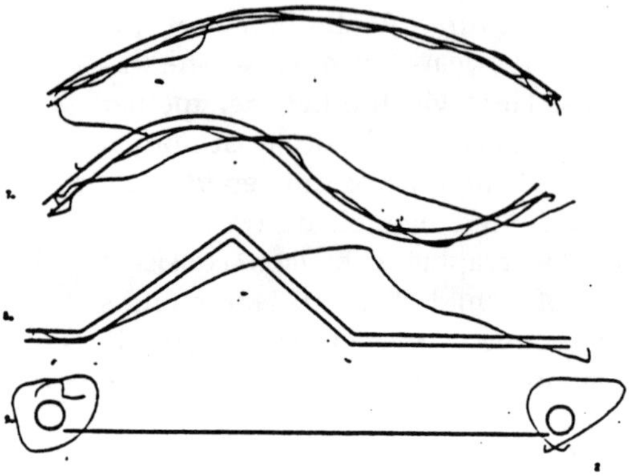

reduced in size

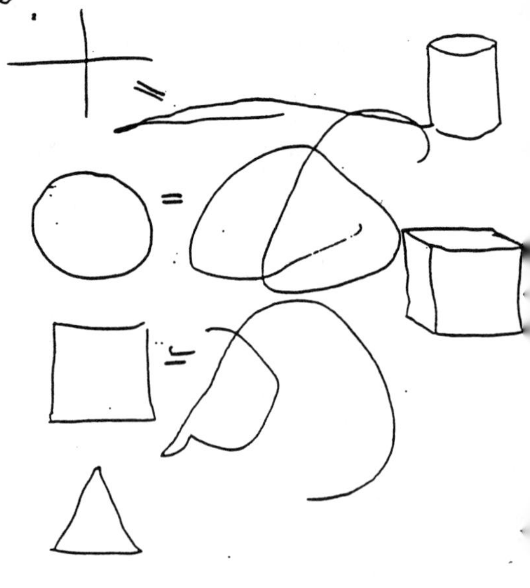

Judy's work at first consisted of tasks to help her exert sufficient pressure on the pencil so that they would make an imprint. Her shy, retiring nature seemed to be reflected in the tentative manner in which she would use a pencil, or felt pen. Simple coloring exercises were also used as shown below. She also spent time drawing in grooves, so that she could carefully monitor her own actions.

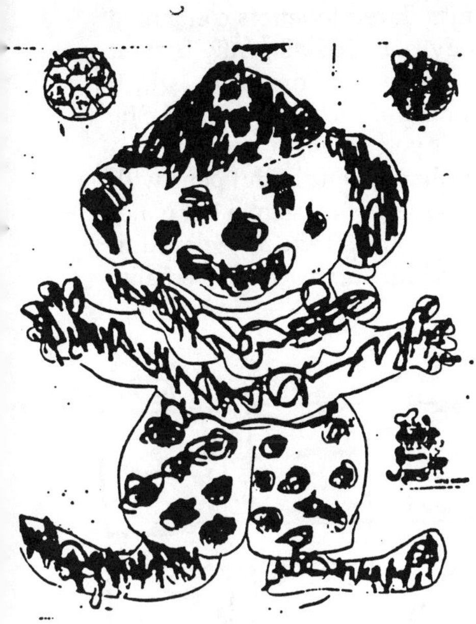

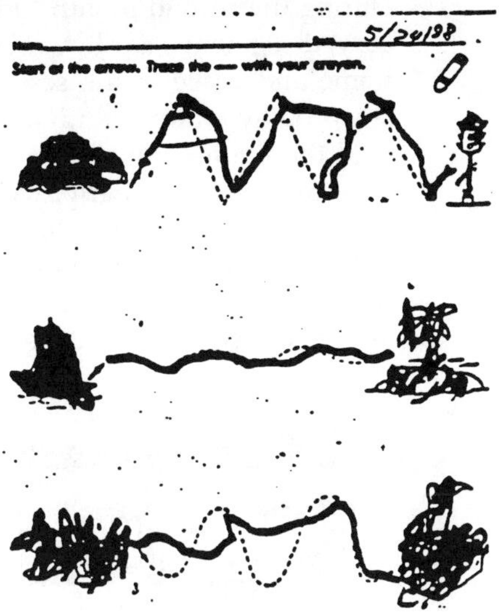
5/24/98
Start at the arrow. Trace the — with your crayon.

reduced in size

After several weeks, she graduated to attempting to draw over visual guides that guided her toward the formation of various letters, as shown below.

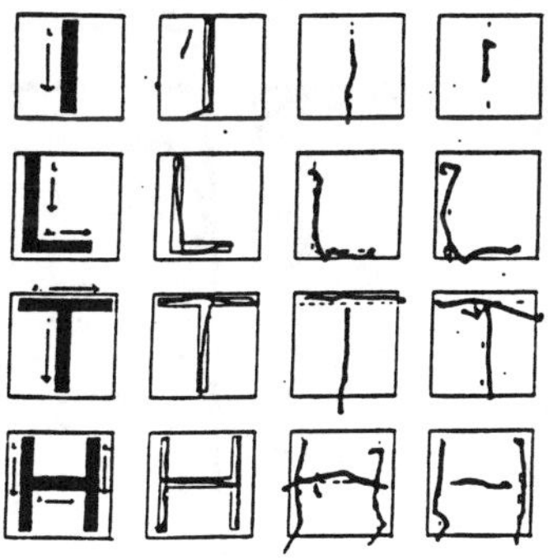

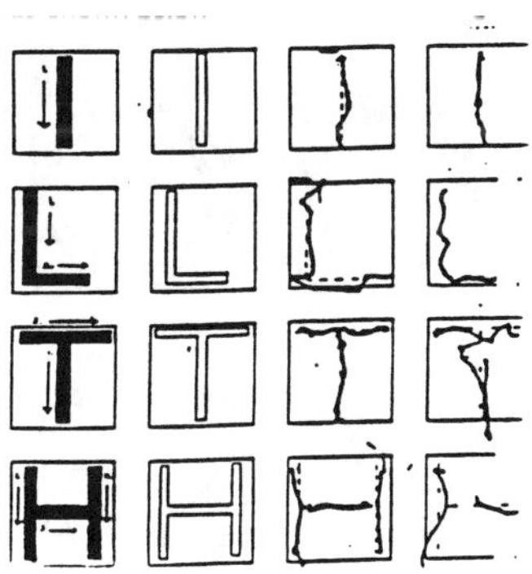

During the second month Judy was introduced to letters containing curved segments, as shown below. Judy practiced diligently both at home and while in the sessions, completing her 'fun work' which she proudly returned with at the beginning of each new session. She held the writing implement (usually felt pen having a large circumference) in a hooked grip, with her left hand. Pencils and pens with smaller diameter seemed to create a great deal of tension in her hand, at times resulting in tremor. Gross motor games were also played in which she jumped in the various letters, identifying them verbally, as she landed on each one.

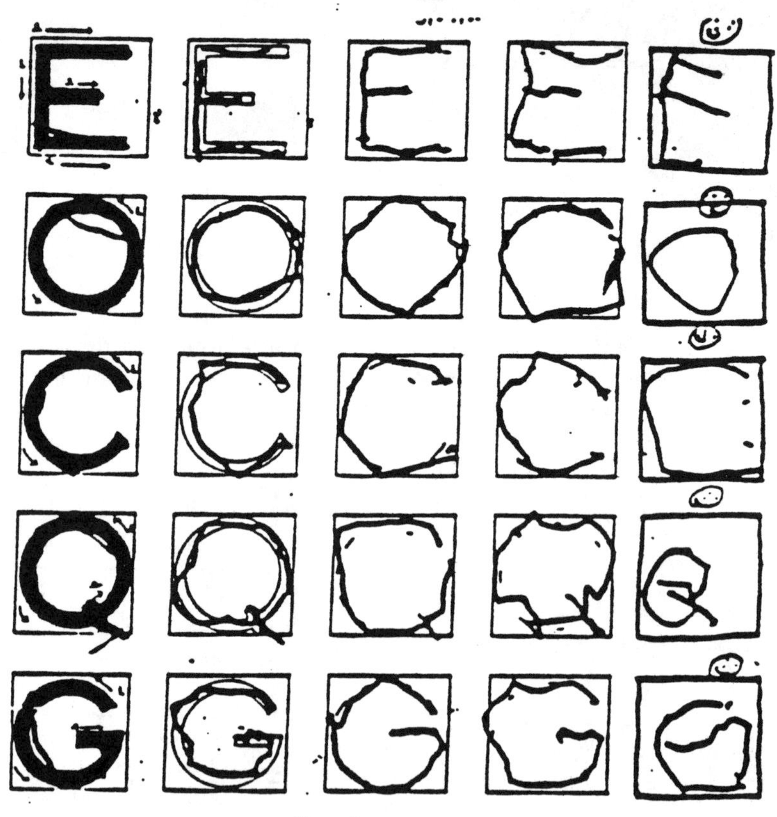

By the beginning of the third month she began to attempt letters, in a dot-to-dot fashion, and then later freehand, as shown. More and more she appeared to organize the directions of lines, and their interrelationships in letters with increased accuracy.

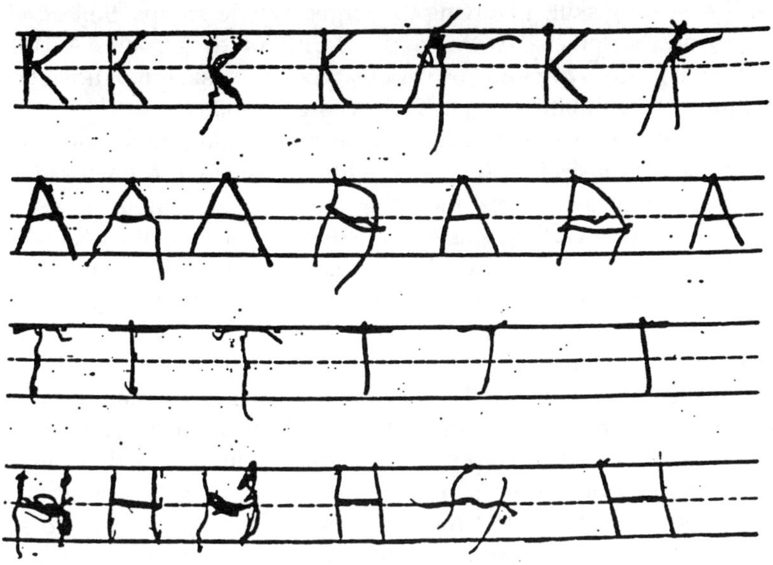

Judy is continuing to work with us, and emphasis is being placed upon independent self-monitoring for increased periods of time. Judy is responding well both to the work on her graphic skills, as well as work on her gross motor skills. She now, for example, shifts her weight when throwing, and employs her arms correctly when running. Exercises using slight resistance, is apparently increasing her muscular strength, having her perform 'risky' Tumbling activities has seemed to improve her self-confidence in physical tasks. Judy is proving to be highly creative, and this creativity together with her good mental abilities are being put to good use when introducing her to new letters, and when otherwise engaging her in both fine and gross motor activities. As the result of her progress she is being enrolled in a regular kindergarden class in the fall, one month after this report is being written.

SUMMARY AND OVERVIEW

Developmental dysgraphia is commonly found among groups of children identified as awkward or poorly coordinated. Some dysgraphic children may evidence concomitant learning problems including dyslexia. Some dysgraphic youngsters also evidence problems executing skills involving the larger muscle groups. Still others may only be afflicted with various forms of dysgraphia. A child displaying only symptoms of various types of dysgraphia, however, it said to be exhibiting a specific learning disability.

There are numerous types of dysgraphia, ranging from those with psychogenic causes including learned helplessness, those with identifiable motor symptoms including apraxia, and mild forms of cerebral palsy including spastic-hypertension, ataxia, and athetosis. In addition other types of dysgraphia may reveal faculty cognitive, as well as deficit auditory and/or visual perceptual capacities. Several causes are often present, resulting in what has been termed a 'mixed type' of dysgraphic.

Printing letters is the last of several linguistic-communicative behaviors to emerge in human children. Developmentally printing emerges from earlier graphic efforts that include scribbling. Seen later are production of simple figures, and then appearing are attempts to produce block letters, at about the age of four to six years. Often a child has evidenced no other problems until confronted with the task of reproducing the language in printed or written form. Thus a severe loss of self-esteem may occur when a child cannot keep up with the written efforts of his/her peers in a kindergarten or first-grade classroom.

Remedial efforts should include the use of imagery, visual-guides, as well as preparatory pre-printing activities including clay modeling, finger painting and simple drawing. Moreover efforts at change should be individualized taking into account motor difficulties, inhibiting social-emotional characteristics, as well as perceptual and cognitive problems found within various dysgraphic subpopulations. Educational interventions should also provide carefully sequenced activities, presented in a relaxed environment, in which success is likely to be acquired and rewarded.

QUESTIONS FOR DISCUSSION

1. Differentiate between stroke-related and developmental dysgraphia. In what type is one likely to obtain neurological confirmation of insults to the structures causing the type of dysgraphia observed?
2. Does developmental dysgraphia mean that the child will likely outgrow the problem? Explain.
3. How do the various sub-syndromes outlined in this chapter on dyslexia parallel the sub-syndromes discussed in Chapter 5? In what ways do the two classification systems seem to differ?

4. What kinds of remedial efforts seem useful to assist the child with dyspraxic dysgraphia? Can you formulate others, based upon you experience, readings, and/or your observations of remedial specialists?
5. What kind of symptoms might be exhibited by a child with a mixed type of dysgraphia?
6. How might digital agnosia influence the precision with which child writes small manuscript letters, or cursive writing?
7. Discuss how visual and auditory perceptual difficulties might interfere with coherent written communication?
8. What are symptoms of syntatical dysgraphia? What types of disabilities might cause this problem? How might the difficulty be assisted?
9. What symptoms might a child with a spatial-type of dysgraphia evidence when playing group-team games on an athletic field? Deficits in which neurological sites may cause this type of problem?
10. What strategies might be employed to assist a child with a tremor-type of dysgraphia, another with the tension-type of dysgraphia, and one who evidences "learned helplessness?"

Chapter 8
Sensory-perceptual Deficits

INTRODUCTION

Following the Second World War the terms perceptual-motor and sensory-motor, (and even motor-sensory) began appearing in books and articles dealing with learning disabilities, motor learning and related topics (Cratty 1964). Sometimes these words were employed to indicate that precise, voluntary movements are invariably accompanied by various sensory and perceptual processes. Others employed these hyphenated terms to indicate that they believed there were *causal relationships* between accurate movement and various kinds of perceptual and sensory qualities including those that required accurate visual organization. Those holding this latter view believed that a variety of perceptual processes, including reading, might be improved simply by exposing children to various movement tasks. Fortunately at this time only the most naive believe in the existence of simple causal relationships between movement capacities, exercise, and motor skill and various sensory and perceptual abilities.

There are, however, numerous ways in which various sensory systems, and perceptual judgements are woven into the ways youngsters move their bodies and its parts. The historical background of interest in the sensory and perceptual underpinnings of motor activity among clinical and experimental neurologists, may be surveyed in the book by Luria. (Luria 1966).

The linkages between perception and motion, include pairings between muscular coordination and vision and hearing. Sensory cues from components of the balance mechanism also influence accurate movement. Neural pathways and organs monitoring touch and pressure form other important bridges to muscular coordination. Finally kinesthetic receptors in the tendons and joints, affording information about the location and movement of the limbs, provide important contributions to accurate motor control.

As indicated on the following diagram (Plate 8-1), the sensory and motor cortexes are closely associated, across the central sulcus. Neuronal connections between a movement and the sensations that contribute to that movement lie in adjacent areas. These close neural

FIGURE

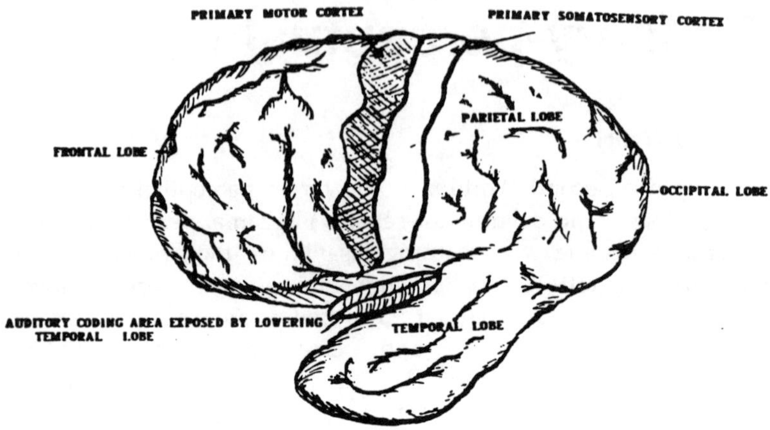

Plate 8-1. Body perception and movement. As shown the primary somatosensory cortex that responds to stimuli applied to various parts of the body sends axons to neurons in the primary motor cortex that move muscles in the same part of the body. Thus this close association accounts for the close relationships between sensation and motion when handling objects, and using the limbs in gross motor skills. These neurologically closely aligned areas also account for deficits in skills that are accompanied by corresponding sensory deficits

associations reflect the correlations often found when measures of sensory and motor abilities are contrasted.

In Plate 8–2, schematic look is taken at hypothetically how a motor program may formed and expressed. This schematic also reflects the manner in which sensory information flows continuously into to the structures contributing to the production and execution of motor programs. In addition sensory information and perceptions produced by the movement itself enables subsequent and successive attempts to become more refined and improved.

The associations between sensory-perceptual qualities and movement capacities may be viewed in several ways.

(1) Deficits in several sensory systems, and sensory end organs may cause motor inaccuracies. For example, partially blind children often do not move well.

(2) Some perceptual problems, contributed to by sensory and/or motor deficits, may cause a child to exhibit coordination prob-

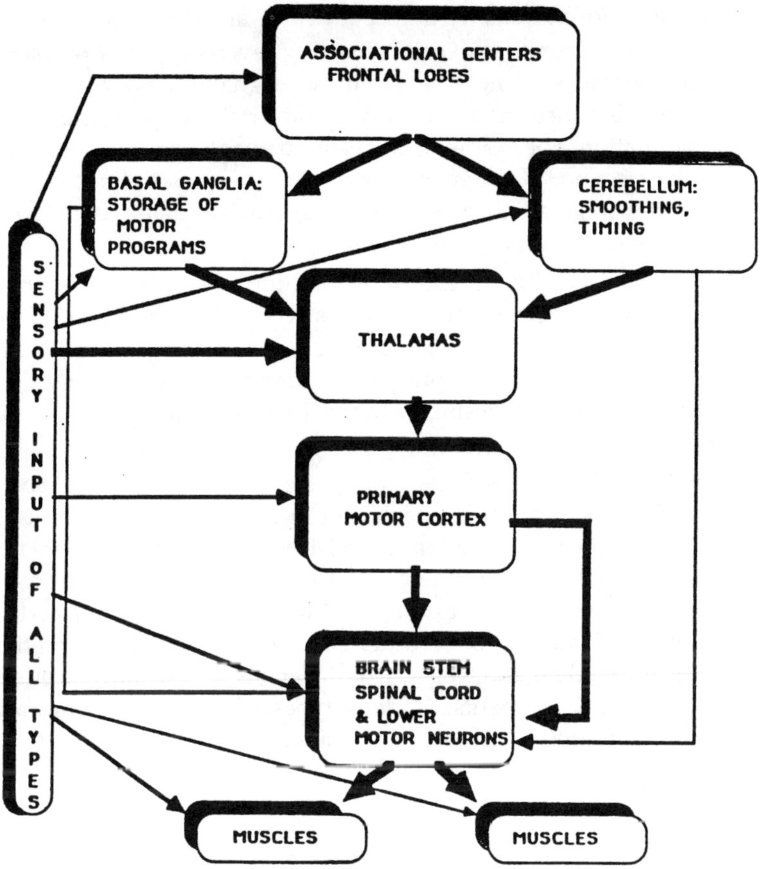

Plate 8-2. Interactions of the central nervous system

lems. For example, youngsters whose motor components of their visual systems do not provide accurate information about clarity, depth, and/or distance of moving and stable objects are likely to have problems in ball games. Inaccurate motor adjustments that change the size and shape of the eye's lens (accommodation) may result in difficulties dealing with objects in distant space, as well as when printing and writing in the proximal space field. Poor control of the muscles that move the eyes upward downward and laterally may contribute to problems tracking balls.

(3) Damage to various neural pathways and/or specific nerve centers may result in deficits reflecting several types of problems simultaneously. These may those signaling poor sensory-perceptual functions and also symptoms reflecting atypical motor coordination. For example, cerebellar damage may cause balance problems and, if extensive, may result in disruptions of the saccades (regular 'throws of the eye) that are made as the eyes move across the page when reading.

(4) The visual system functions at optimum only when numerous intricate and coordinated motor acts occur within and around the eye. Disruptions in brain structures mediating visual-motor functions, as well as the presence of tumors adjacent to, or in, the optic chiasm, may result in motor incoordination of the larger and smaller muscle groups.

(5) Sensory deficits involving the perception of the total body, including its location in space, and the kinesthetic awareness of its parts and their location are all frequent accompaniments to motor incoordination. These can arise from tumors or lesions in the somatosensory cortex, adjacent to the primary motor cortex, as seen in Plate 8-1, or on other structures receiving information from the body's surface, or from changes in tension placed on tendons and ligaments. Various types of motor awkwardness seen in children who evidence bodily agnosias are discussed in a following section.

Sensory-Perceptual Problems Among Awkward Children

In general clumsy children have been found to evidence problems in the overall processing of more than one kind of stimuli including both visual-perceptual as well as kinesthetic information. (Smythe & Gencross 1986). It has also been found that awkward children often have problems forming correct matches between kinesthetic information and visual-perceptual stimuli. (Hulme et al 1982). Also it is frequent to find parallel deficits in both the sensory and coordination qualities within the same parts of the body.

There are pervasive types of sensory and perceptual-motor difficulties that are commonly found among various sub-categories of awkward children. For example, it appears more likely that a child who is learning disabled and awkward will display a larger number of perceptual deficits than will be present when an academically average or superior child is evaluated.

The learning disabled child who is awkward may display visual-perceptual problems that limit his or her functioning in fast-moving playground games, as well as reading. Various functional relationships, found in awkward children, between perceptual functions and motor incoordination has encouraged several scholars to study kinesthetic awareness among this population. (Hulme et al 1984, 1987).

The apparent importance of visual information, when attempting to execute intricate motor tasks, has prompted some to describe clumsiness as "visual-motor incoordination" (Wilson 1974), and as a "visual-motor disability" (Brenner et al 1967) (Dare & Gorton 1970). The importance of Kinesthetic-perceptual information when moving accurately has encouraged many to incorporate sensory measures into tests. Clinicians have also used strategies to heighten sensory abilities within remedial settings.

Data from investigations involving, two general classifications of sensory-perceptual mechanisms are reviewed in this chapter. First the visual perceptual system, is surveyed, with regard to how some of its components interact with coordinated movement. In the final part of the chapter selected types of 'body agnosias' are discussed. Among the types of sensations contained within this broad category are those reflecting both tactile and kinesthetic awareness of the body, and of its parts. In this second section the ways in which deficits in body awareness may produce incoordination are also considered.

VISUAL-PERCEPTUAL ABILITIES & DISABILITIES

Overview

From birth vision is closely aligned with movement capacities. Early in life neonates become fascinated with watching both their hands and feet passing within their visual fields (Cratty 1989b). About the same time close visual attention is given to the interesting faces of adults hovering over their cribs. By early childhood hand-eye adequate coordination becomes essential in the mastery of self-care skills, and when the printed letters are first attempted. By middle childhood visual demands placed upon youngsters as they are required to organize the trajectories of balls, and of other children, both moving rapidly in games.

Simply stated the visual system consists partly of groups of muscles that place the eyes, and their components, in positions enabling them to look at, register, and organize components of the world. Muscle groups within the eye aid to coordinate the actions of both eyes, and adjust the lens and the shape of the eye ball to permit a clear picture of the world to pass to the retina.

Microscopic neurological and biochemical mechanisms are also important in producing adequate vision. For example Chemical processes within the retina result in the reception and impregnation of incoming pictures, that are then transmitted through neuro-electrical impulses to several portions of the brain (including the posterior occipital area).

Brain structures and connecting pathways then enable the individual to organize, interpret, store, and later retrieve what has been seen. These latter processes are usually labeled visual-perceptual activities. Physical awkwardness may be caused by a breakdown or defect in any, or several, of the steps within these complex processes. Some of the symptoms of these 'breakdowns' are surveyed in the following section.

Visual Stability and Balance

Balance and vision are closely aligned both behaviorally and neurologically. A child's whose visual system performs poorly is unlikely to balance well, either in static-stable positions, or while moving. Several atypical visual behaviors may contribute to balance problems in children. For example, an unstable gaze reflected in the inability to quickly locate and then to easily fixate both eyes on immobile and moving objects, will usually disrupt the youngster's attempt to maintain a stable, balanced position in space.

In both children and adults there are marked individual differences in how quickly and efficiently the eyes 'settle down' upon an object that it is desired to look at. Sometimes the eyes of a person quickly come to rest on an object, while at other times the eyes move irregularly, both prior to, and when apparently coming to rest on the target. Individual differences in the structures that mediator gaze and fixation influence similar differences in balance and in various coordinated tasks attempted. These centers include, nuclei within the associational-frontal areas of the brain (Area #45). These differences may reflect problems when attempting to look at things for reasonable periods of time, and thus also result in differences in maintaining prolonged attention to tasks.

The close pairing of gaze qualities and balance should be taken into account when evaluating balance. However few standardized tests of balance do so. For example it will be found that better balance scores will be obtained from youngsters who are asked to 'look at a point just in front of you', in contrast to balance scores from children who are not given this kind of instruction to stabilize their gaze (Zernecke, Gregor and Cratty 1982).

It may be found, however, that when evaluating the balance of a few awkward children, whose visual control is poor, *better scores* may be obtained when asking them to close their eyes, than when they leave their eyes open The sudden improvement of balance when these youngsters are given instructions to close their eyes, illustrates the possibility that unstable visual fields are detracting from their attempts at maintaining stable balance. In contrast when they rely solely from feedback from their motor systems, and exclude disruptive visual information by closing their eyes, they become better able to balance. Thus when assessing static balance, it is important to determine whether the balance problem arises primarily from the visual or motor systems by varying the directions given relative to the use of vision. The evaluation of balance is covered further in Chapter 11.

Defects in the visual system may result in other abnormalities including strabismus, and the presence of various kinds of nystagmatic movements (twitching-vibrations of the eyes). Visual-motor problems can also include poor ocular control of the two eyes as they attempt to fixate on stable objects or to follow a moving object accurately. Thus when evaluating balance using traditional methods, what often is observed is only the indirect evidence of difficulties that may be caused several possible ocular mis-functions. Assessing these anomalies is best left to eye-care professional, individuals well-prepared to both test and interpret what may be signs of serious and progressive visual conditions.

Visually Tracking Movement

Intact visual and interpretational-perceptual qualities are needed when attempting to track moving objects. The eyes move in slow arcs (ramps) when slower moving objects are looked at. However when ocular system is exposed to faster moving objects (transcending visual arcs of 50–70 degrees a second), the eyes begin to jump in a series of 'throws' the eyes make. These rapid jumps are called saccades. The well functioning visual system may makes the objects seem to 'stop', as saccades occur, helping the individual to extract information from the missile(s). The person then must quickly interpret the information obtained. The mechanism that is believed responsible for visually 'stopping' the object is labeled the opto-kinetic reflex.

The eyes thus periodically stop on the moving object in a series of saccades, similar to the short stops and jumps used when reading as the eyes pass rapidly over immobile words. However the efficiency of these rapidly occurring and complex processes vary markedly from child to child, and are likely deficient in many awkward youngsters exhibiting difficulties in ball games. In contrast, superior batters in major league baseball are probably fortunate in the nature of the good visual systems they have inherited.

Data from our research (Cratty, Apitzsch, and Bergel 1972), and that of others point to several important findings relative to the efficiency with which the developing ocular system engages in this visual-perceptual 'stopping' of moving objects. It has been found, for example, that this quality improves with age. Younger children are not as adept at predicting the pathways of objects and of extracting information as are older youngsters.

Marked individual differences have also been identified, in how well children engage in this reflex-like process. A few five-year olds we tested, evidence adult-like capacities. These we labeled velocity resistant youngsters, meaning that they were relatively resistant to increases in object speed, when required to make visual-perceptual judgements about information the objects contained.

The ocular systems of other young children's evidenced marked immaturities. These youngsters we labeled velocity susceptible . . . This meant that these latter children became unable to make visual-perceptual judgements about moving objects, when target speed was increased. It is likely that many youngsters evidencing problems in ball games possess visual systems that fall within this second category.

Some research surveying jumps, or saccades, the eyes make while reading indicate that many dyslexic children do not quickly obtain information as their eyes briefly come to rest on the printed page (Breitmeyer & Ganz 1976). A similar problem may beset some children who fail to quickly obtain information from rapidly moving objects. These the visual systems of these velocity resistent youngsters have difficulty both intercepting and extracting information during the time each fast saccade briefly stops their eyes on moving targets.

Our research, and that of others, also reveals that measures of dynamic acuity, are unrelated to measures of static acuity. The child who reads the letters and word clearly from a wall chart, cannot necessarily be depended upon to function well visually and perceptually when trying to perceptually interpret the pathways taken by fast balls and by rapidly moving people during various games. Thus there are apparently inborn individual differences in the important reflexes function within the visual systems of children mediating how well movement is seen and interpreted. Awkward children may evidence poor visual qualities, and subtle deficits within the neural mechanisms controlling these qualities, necessary to carry out this kind of task well. The apparatus we used to evaluate dynamic visual acuity is shown below.

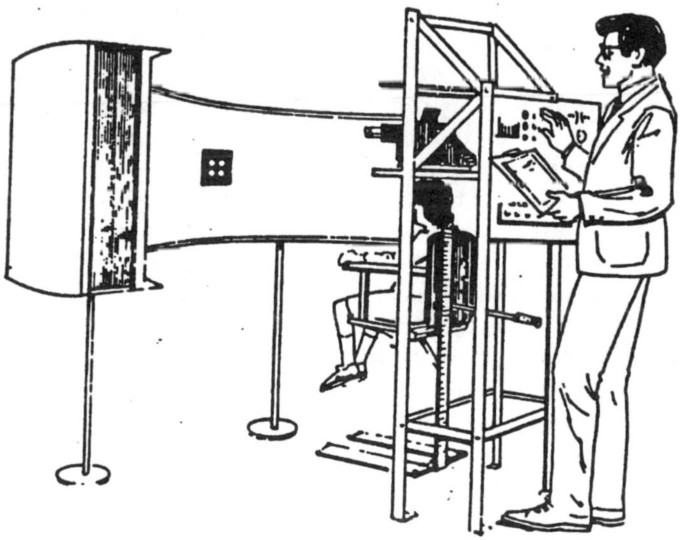

Plate 8-3. Evaluating dynamic visual acuity in children in the apparatus depicted, a standard visual target was made to pass 180 angular degrees around the frontal visual field of youngsters of various ages. Target speed, as well as target size, could be varied. The child-subject, was required to indicate by their hand in which corner a checker-board pattern was placed during each pass of a target.

A lack of ability to track balls well may be a symptom of serious visual and medical problems. For example, tumors located at various points on the branches of the optic chiasm may restrict the size of a youngster's space field. Thus a child afflicted with a tumor in various locations will have great difficulty tracking balls, because the time and space within the visual field, in which the tracking may take place, is limited. To such children, balls suddenly seem to appear abruptly within a constricted amount of space, rather than passing through the larger spatial 'window' available to normal youngsters viewing incoming missiles. When it is found that a child does not catch balls well, referring the youngster to an appropriate medical specialist is sometimes desirable. Problems encountered in ball games thus may not be attributable only to mechanisms necessary to visually track missiles, but may be caused by serious tumors or lesions that impede the transmission of impulses along essential visual pathways to the centers necessary to adequate peripheral and central vision. It is important that those educated primarily to detect overt motor problems, including physical educators and motor therapists of various kinds, should refer children with tracking problems to proper visual-medical professionals, in order that the possible causes for such problems may be validly assessed. Such a child is likely to benefit from a 'field-of-vision test' in addition to other components of through visual evaluation administered and interpreted by qualified medical personnel.

The lack of ability to track balls well may be a symptom of serious visual and medical problems. For example, tumors located at various points on the branches of the optic chiasm may restrict the size of a youngster's space field. Thus a child afflicted with a tumor in various locations will have great difficulty tracking balls, because the time and space within the visual field, in which the tracking may take place, is limited. To such children, balls suddenly seem to appear abruptly within a constricted amount of space, rather than passing through the larger spatial 'window' available to normal youngsters viewing incoming missiles. When it is found that a child does not catch balls well, referring the youngster to an appropriate medical specialist is sometimes desirable.

Problems encountered in ball games thus may not be attributable only to mechanisms necessary to visually track missiles, but may be caused by serious tumors or lesions that impede the transmission of impulses along essential visual pathways to the centers necessary to adequate peripheral and central vision. It is important that those educated primarily to detect overt motor problems, including physical educators and motor therapists of various kinds, should refer children with tracking problems to proper visual-medical professionals, in order that the possible causes for such problems may be validly assessed. Such a ild is likely to benefit from a 'field-of-vision test' in addition to other components of a thorough visual evaluation administered and interpreted by qualified medical personnel.

The ability to track moving objects proceeds developmentally in predictable ways. This emerging ability has sometimes been labeled 'perceptual anticipation'. At five it is poorly developed, by six and seven improvement usually measured. This quality, however, is not fully developed, even under optimum conditions, until late childhood or early adolescence (Williams 1972). This ability has also been incorporated into tests for children with perceptual-motor problems. (Bruinink's 1978)

Numerous reasons, acting along or in combinations, may thus account for why a child intercepts balls poorly. These range from the defects in neural mechanisms referred to above, maturational lags, lack of experience, motor ineptitude reflected in poor lateral movement of the body, and a slow reaction time reflected in not placing the hands rapidly into proper position for the catche. Thus both motor as well as visual-perceptual problems may detract from adequate ball skills, and from participating well in games that require such judgements and actions. It thus appears that faulty perceptual judgements, reflecting limited abilities to organize moving space field, are more closely associated with motor awkwardness, than are scores from tests designed to simply measure static acuity. (Lord & Hulme 1987).

Social Modeling and Coordination

Clear vision, and adequate perceptual abilities, are important contributors to adequate coordination in children. Conversely lack of clear vision, or total blindness, may prevent the developing youngster, from looking at and copying appropriate actions of other children. Illustrating this point are data obtained twenty years ago in a study contrasting the coordination, and other qualities, in a pair of 10 year old twins, one of whom was totally blind. (Cratty and Williams 1968). The blind twin was found to be functioning in a superior manner in many aspects of life, including the exhibition of good academic and social skills. It was only when physical skills were compared, that the blind twin was found to be deficient.

The blind twin lacked the opportunities to see, and thus to model and to copy, appropriate arm-leg coordinations needed in effective jumping, ball throwing and in similar skills. The findings of this study as well as others (Cratty 1970) of the visually impaired illustrate the point that some children lacking adequate perceptual and/or visual abilities may perform awkwardly at play because they cannot visually organize, and thus replicate, the movements of their peers .

Visually organizing, and remembering demonstrated movements can also cause problems in the quick acquisition of tasks. This kind of problem was also discussed in Chapter 6 in the section dealing with apraxia and dyspraxia. It has been clearly demonstrated that awkward children, when compared to normal youngsters, are likely to have difficulties when attempting to chain together and remember activities that require sequentially presented pieces of visual information. (Murphy & Gliner (1988). Thus awkward children appear to have problems, not only in the sequencing of complex visual-motor activities, but also when attempting to organize visual information contained in demonstrations of skills.

Figure-Ground Perception

Among the various kinds of perceptual problems encountered in life, include the necessity to select a single object out of a complex background. This can occur in the auditory mode, as a guest tries to listen to a single conversation at a noisy cocktail party. Visually the task of 'central selection' is needed in sports and games as well as when reading. When looking at a printed page the child must select a word or phrase from background information, and extract meaning.

When engaging in various games a this selection process is important. Balls must be tracked, selected out, and then struck in tennis, or caught and baseball, when complex backgrounds are present. Opponents, a hostile crowd as well as other confusing and irrelevant visual information may prevent a basketball player from accurately "zeroing in" on the basket's rim, when attempting to make a free throw. These confusions often plague perceptually handicapped children, within populations of awkward youngsters, as they attempt to participate in sports and games.

Accommodation

There are numerous other types of visual perceptual problems that interact with coordinated movement. Among the most important is near-point fusion, an accommodative ability needed when the child first starts to attempt to print letters and numbers. This action of the eyes is termed a type of dysjunctive movement, meaning that the eyes are required to move in opposite directions, in this case turn inward to focus. If a youngster, at age four or five, is struggling to focus both eyes together on the page about 10″–16″ away, problems will likely be encountered when trying to pair the motor coordinations and sequencings needed to reproduce the shapes of both the letters and numbers. Accommodating at near-point is a relatively recent evolutionary task imposed upon the human animal. Accommodation requires far greater effort by the muscles that turn the eyes inward, than is necessary when focusing upon objects several feet away.

At our clinic we recently worked with a child whose accommodative problems at near-point were so great that he was forced to place the page, upon which he was attempting to print, at arms length and to the side, while struggling to focus upon his efforts. Fortunately accommodation is one of the few qualities usually amenable to well designed training, as well as to the application of corrective lens.

Overview & Implications

Physical awkwardness may thus occur because of the presence of several types of difficulties present in vision. The presence of motor problems may also reflect poor organization and inadequate interpretation of visual stimuli, interpretational abilities that may be relatively independent of simple vision (clear sight).

This general principle frequently is made clear to me and to members of my staff when working with awkward children. Some youngsters, although possessing adequate sight, apparently need to cling to their instructors during their lessons. They seem to have difficulty determining precisely where their instructor is, in relation to themselves, because of visual-perceptual difficulties. It is likely that these problems in organizing space also prevent them from adequately perceiving appropriate actions emanating from their peers which, if copied well, would result in better coordination.

Measures of visual perception reveal that this general quality is complex and mult-dimensional. It has been found, for example, that there are at least five different independent visual perceptual qualities measurable in children as young as five years of age. Among these are static as well as dynamic acuity, two qualities discussed in the previous paragraphs. Also included in the list is the ability to fragment space (to decide what is half way between an observer and an object), the ability to determine the relative distance of two objects from an observer, as well as measures of both static and dynamic depth perception. Thus to label a child as evidencing perceptual-disabilities is not very helpful or precise. Instead it should be attempted to determine just what kinds of perceptual problem(s) are present, and in precisely what these problems (or problems) may be interfering with attempts to execute complex motor tasks (Smith and Smith 1966)

The assessment and interpretation of perceptual problems in youngsters has been made difficult in the past because of the presence of large numbers of drawing tasks, within batteries of tasks purporting to assess visual perception in maturing in children. (Frostig 1956). Thus for several decades measures of motor coordination contaminated and modified scores that purportedly evaluated developing visual-perceptual abilities. More recent developmental measures of perception, however, are "motor-free", and consist of measures that evaluate 'pure' visual perceptual organization, rather than hand-eye coordination (Colarusso & Hammill 1972).

The available research indicates that several principles should be followed when dealing with awkward children suspected of having perceptual-visual problems.

(1) Awkward children should also be evaluated by visual-health professionals (Opthamologists, or Optometrists) if any problem is suspected, or before pronouncements are made relative to visual and perceptual deficiencies by motor development specialists, physical or occupational therapists, or by adapted physical educators.

(2) Carefully designed perceptual training may usefully accompany the motor training of such children. For example, the youngster having difficulty with ball skills may at first be encouraged simply to watch balls swung on strings, or rolled across the ground, before being required to position the body and hands for interception.

(3) It should not be assumed that any kind of visual and or perceptual training is likely to aid reading, as reading involves relatively rapid jumps (saccades) that occur too fast for conscious control, together with subtle cognitive qualities whose development are best left to reading tutors.

BODY AGNOSIAS AND DYSGNOSIAS

The word 'agnosia' refers to a lack of awareness that may appear in various sensory modalities. The term dysgnosia has also been used to denote disruptions of sensory awareness. (Lesny 1980) Visual agnosias thus refer to the poor visual perception of various stimuli, including word-blindness, and reading problems. Auditory agnosias, in contrast, denote auditory perceptual problems.

There are also a number of 'body agnosias'. These deficits may involve sensory-perceptual difficulties that children have when attempting to locate their bodies in space. Tactile deficits in the limbs and the fingers, and also poor kinesthetic awareness of limb location and movement are also contained within this general group of symptoms.

These deficiencies have sometimes been referred to as problems poor formation of the body schema, of the body concept, or of the body image. Often the best way to reduce such confusions of terminology is to employ such words in conjunction with specific measurement tools, to operationalize the labels.

In the 1980's researchers began to link these sensory deficits occurring in children to neural abnormalities. In one study, for example, it was found that 50% of the youngsters, who evidenced dysgnosias, also had abnormalities in various components of their central nervous system. These structural differences included including ventricular enlargement (Knuckey et al 1983).

There are two general sources purportedly causing these sensory deficits. One kind is present from birth, and often plagues youngsters from early childhood through adolescence. These may be termed 'developmental agnosias'. Low birth weight is sometimes cited as an instigating factor (Lesny 1980). A second type reflects problems resulting from of some type of cerebral incident, including accidents or stroke occurring later in life. This second type might be labeled 'stroke-related agnosias' (or dysgnosias). At times these sub-divisions are difficult to separate. For example, an accident or cerebral incident may occur as the nervous system is developing, early in life. The resulting difficulties thus appear to be congenital, but actually are due to traumas occurring after birth.

Both in stroke victims, and in young children, various types of agnosias, and the sub-symptoms, accompanying them are hypothetically caused by similar types of neurological damage to the same sensory-mediating components within the central nervous system. Although in the case of developmentally delayed children with bodily agnosias, it has usually been more difficult to confirm the presence of even subtle neurological deficits.

The symptoms reflecting body agnosias may be inseparable from behaviors seen in youngsters diagnosed as evidencing dyspraxias of various types. Thus confusions occurring when moving in space, and when sequencing task movements, may be attributed both to the presence of dyspraxia, and also to the presence of dysgnosias. For example, if a child has difficulties dressing himself/herself one observing clinician may identify the problem as a dressing apraxia, while another will state that the problem reflects a body-agnosia. (a type of somatoagnosia). Thus the same, or a similar, behavioral deficit is likely to reflect the interaction of both an agnosia and also of a specific type of apraxia.

The available research on the topic makes it apparent that body agnosias are composed of various statistically independent sub-components. For example if one asks children to verbally identify their body parts, it will be found that the scores obtained will not be correlated to measures of the sensory-tactile awareness of the body and/or its parts, but to test scores reflecting vocabulary and verbal intelligence. A lack of correlations between scores reflecting sensory and some motor deficiencies, and scores from verbal IQ tests, obtained from children referred to our clinic from schools for the gifted is also strong evidence for the independence of verbal intelligence, various bodily agnosias and some measures of poor motor coordination.

There are measurable sub-components to various types of body agnosias. For example, digital agnosia, reflecting a lack of sensory-awareness of the fingers and/or the hands, is composed of several sub-components, including:

(a) deficits in the ability of the fingers to 'record' sensations and obtain tactile information when objects (placed out of view) are touched or stroked. This quality has been termed 'stereognosis' or, if deficit, astereognosis

(b) the ability of the child to identify fingers when they are named verbally and

(c) the ability to determine where tactile stimuli are applied on one hand, when viewing the other hand (Gerstmann 1940).

Thus digital agnosia should be considered in specific ways, and with reference to the test employed to evaluate different sub-types.

For over one-hundred years descriptions of deficits in the body image may be found in the neurological literature. Initially the only descriptions of agnosias available were those made among stroke patients (Obsersteiner 1881) (Luria 1966). During recent decades, however, agnosias have been studied among maturing youngsters evidencing various developmental sensory and motor problems. Initially a few, selected sensory deficits were described among awkward children brought to clinics for evaluation. Gradually the measures increased in number. Even now, however, the majority of measures in examinations designed to assess the presence of neurological problems in awkward children, evaluate motor rather than sensory qualities. (Tupper 1987, Appendix).

Only a few recent studies are available whose authors have attempted to delineate how various measures of body awareness evolve among normal populations of youngsters. The investigation that have been conducted, often suffer from lack of adequate norms. It is often difficult to identify, with validity, deficits in various bodily agnosias (and dysgnosias) observed among groups of 'suspect children' if normal functioning has not been well documented among different age groups.

In the following sections several types of bodily agnosias are discussed. Included are descriptions of behaviors and scores obtained from measurement tools employed both by experimentalists and by clinicians. References are made both to the possible neural mechanisms involved, as well as to potentially useful clinician interventions.

Spatial Agnosias

General spatial agnosias refer to problems youngsters may have when attempting to transport their total bodies through space with accurate sequenced, movements. Difficulties are encountered, by youngsters evidencing this type of problem, when trying to move around the furniture in a room, or when attempting to pass between classmates and school desks. The bumping that may occur among peers may result in awkward children experiencing social problems.

I was once with a group of child psychiatrists who discussed what they termed 'bumping' scores they had obtained when observing a group of clumsy, learning-disabled children within classroom settings. They pointed out that when these children contacted peers, they often perceived as engaging intentionally in aggressive acts, and thus in turn had aggression re-directed toward them. I was recently contacted by a kindergarten teacher who said she was referring a child to our clinic who, when attempting to move around the her classroom room, appeared to be trying to 'walk through' other children. Thus many awkward children, observed both by teachers and psychiatrists, display sign of spatial agnosias while attempting to move around, and between, their classmates at school.

These types of awkward behaviors, reflecting spatial-motor difficulties may be caused by subtle right hemisphere lesions, or by hydrocephalic conditions, creating cerebral pressures, diagnosed at birth. Even if the latter condition is corrected early through surgery (the placement of a shunt to reduce excess pressure in the cerebral spinal fluid, located in the ventricles) pressure to the adjacent motor-control centers, may result in persistent problems reflecting various types of spatial agnosias.

I have been working with a girl for the past twelve years who, although having surgery to correct a hydrocephalic condition near birth, continues to display problems negotiating safe passages around living room furniture, as well as moving through accurate spatial patterns in childhood games. Her parents are worried about what will occur when she will want to drive a car in the years ahead. The apraxic counterpart' to this type of general spatial agnosia is called 'trunkle apraxia' and was discussed in Chapter 6. A test for this type of trunkle dyspraxia will serve identify the presence of general spatial agnosias (Cratty 1989). It involves repeating a series of up to seven movements of the body, into a pattern of eight 1′ x 1′ squares on a mat, after the sequence of positions are first demonstrated. (*See Appendix*).

There are other clinical measures of spatial agnosias one may employ. For example, a child may be asked to first observe a simple map of a room containing a chair and table, around which a figure-eight shaped line (or a simpler pathway) is drawn The child may then be asked to negotiate a similar pathway, moving his or her body around the furniture, duplicating pathway drawn on the map. (DeFonseca 1985) Marked differences in spatial awareness and in accuracy will be demonstrated by various children asked to engage

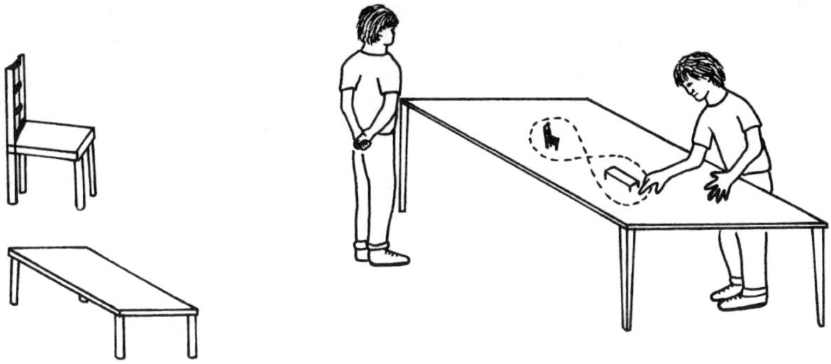

Plate 8-4. Evaluating Spatial Agnosia. In this clinical assessment the child first observes a simple 'map' depicitng a route to be taken around a chair and table in the room. Next, the child attempts to negotiate the route drawn.

in this type of task. The results of these types of assessment should serve to forewarn a clinician, or teacher, so that the real-world management of such youngsters is made easier.

The remediation of, and accommodation, to this type of problem may involve both communicating an understanding of the problem to the child's caretakers, and helping the child understand his or her problem in clear terms. The presence of these spatial confusions should not be interpreted by parents as reflecting their off-spring's ignorance, or lack of willingness to respond correctly to directions. Rather both the child and parents should recognize the presence of the problem and should accommodate to it in various ways.

For example a series of directions, to "go up stairs and to put on a red jacket', should be made shorter and simple. Most of the time partial directions should be given at first. Complex directions to engage in a series of actions, given to such children will often result in an inability to accurately and quickly comply. Rather, these youngsters should be encouraged first to think about such directions, then to repeat them verbally if necessary, and then to ask for their repetition, before attempting to execute them in various real world situations. At times directions to move through a complex sequence may be broken down into parts. At other times maps may be drawn to facilitate a trip to a new store, when moving through a building, or a when learning about the rooms a new home.

Symptoms signalling presence of spatial agnosias of this type, will often puzzle those attempting to administer remedial programs to awkward children. The youngsters will seem to be disobedient when failing to react quickly and accurately to such 'simple' directions as "lie down with your feet nearest me", or to "move sideways to your left".

The inability to react quickly and accurately with an appropriate body movement may also cause safety problems. Such youngsters should be carefully guided across streets, even in middle childhood, as they may be unable to position their bodies accurately and safely in the presence of oncoming cars. These youngsters often have problems when attempting to move accurately in fast-moving team sports. Not only must spatially confused children move their own bodies accurately to prearranged spots in athletic contests, but they must also accommodate to fast moving balls, teammates, and opponents. Difficulties are also likely to be encountered, when trying to learn complex drills during team sport practices, and when exposed to routines in dance classes. Thus, modified and simple drills, and games must be constructed in order to insure the continued participation in desirable physical activities by these spatially confused youngsters.

Right Hemisphere Syndrome

At times spatial agnosias will be accompanied by other symptoms that reflect poor right-hemispheric function. Difficulties may be encountered when the child tries to arrange words and letters appropriately on a page. This general kind of 'right hemispheric syndrome' may also be evidenced in a flat-metallic like quality when speaking. Tonality is believed to be mediated by the right hemisphere, and thus problems in this area produce atonal speech.

Tactile Agnosias of the Body

In addition to deficits in the neurological mechanisms mediating the mental-spatial maps needed to move the total body through space, are problems reflected in the poor tactile awareness of the body's surfaces. Tests to ascertaining the sensitivity of the various surfaces of the body often constitute parts of neurological evaluations. For example, a sub-test assessing of two-point discrimination is often employed. This involves determining how closely two points may be placed together and touched to various body surfaces, before they are perceived by the child as single touch-point. At times the clinician-physician may simultaneously stroke both sides of the body in order to determine possible difference in tactile sensitivity. If differences are found they have important diagnostic significance, including the possible presence of tumors, and thus should interpretable by those with appropriate medical backgrounds.

It is probable that the neurological mechanisms underlying this problem involve pathways and structures mediating light touch. Poor tactile sensitivity on different parts of the body's surface may result in practical and social problems. Often these problems are accompanied by motor incoordination and by inappropriate social behaviors. For example, it is not unusual to find that such youngsters finish their meals with food still on their faces, indicating that they simply cannot feel the food remaining there. Similarly such youngsters are often described as sloppy dressers. When shirts are not tucked in their pants, they are probably unaware of the problem due to a lack of sensitivity to the location of the clothes that are next to their relatively insensitive bodies. These deficits are sometimes grouped under the more general label of *somatoagnosias*.

Remedial methods may consist of both giving the child additional tactile input as part of their therapy program, and also of substituting visual information for the sensory information they may be missing. For example, children who leave food on their face after eating, may be encouraged to inspect their faces in the mirror after meals. The children whose clothing may be poorly arranged may also observe themselves in a mirror during and after dressing.

These problems, like the other agnosias described, are subtle, rather than obvious. Their presence, however, can trigger social problems, whose causes are not always apparent either to the youngster, or to caretakers-teachers. The youngster with various agnosias may not look pleasing to peers, and to parents. The presence of these problems are often judged harshly by those within the social environment, because their presence appears the results of poor character, or due to laziness, rather than to neurological deficits that are beyond the control of the youngster.

Limb Agnosias

In clinical practices, dealing with awkward children, it is common to encounter young clients who evidence the inability to locate their limbs in static positions. Furthermore they also have difficulties when attempting to kinesthetically monitor the movements of their arms and legs. Poor kinesthetic acuity measured in limb positioning, and in movement tasks among awkward children has been verified in data from studies by Hulme and his colleagues (Hulme et al 1984), by Smythe and Glencross (1986) and by Judith Laszlo and her colleagues (Laszlo et al 1980) (Laszlo 1985) (Laszlo 1988).

Motorically inept youngsters apparently obtain late and/or inaccurate kinesthetic information about limb location, speed, tension and/or movement. When throwing a ball, for example, such youngsters may keep their throwing arms in front of their bodies. They do this because they are likely to lose the awareness of their arm's location when they draw it back behind their shoulder and thus out of their field of vision, as they prepare to throw.

When asked to execute a front roll (summersault) youngsters with this problem may incur neck strain. They will likely lose an awareness of their arms' locations when their heads are placed down and through their arms when beginning to roll. Thus they may incur neck injuries because their arms and hands cannot, and do not, support their body weight during the course of the movement.

The most dramatic case of a limb agnosia, I have evaluated, involved a seven year old girl who had just suffered a head injury. The main symptom was a startling one. When seated at a table and attempting to write, for example, one arm would suddenly start to float away out of control. Apparently of its own volition the wayward limb would inscribe a snake-like movement, and would terminate over her head and out of her visual field! Upon discovering the arm's absence, she would suddenly stop what she was doing, and begin searching for the lost arm, surprised at its unmonitored journey. After visually locating it, she would grasp it's wrist with the other hand, and bring it back to the table. This scenario would be repeated several times within a half-hour period and each time visibly upset her. After about six months, however, this unusual symptom somehow terminated.

The apraxic counter-part to limb agnosia, is termed limb kinetic apraxia (*See Chapter 6*), and involves the disruption of demonstrated sub-sequences of a complex movement, involving the hands as well as the arms (Cratty and Samoy 1984). This problem may also be reflected in the inability of a child to integrate the arms and legs in various tasks, as well as the inability to coordinate movements of the limbs in both sides of the body in complex tasks. Difficulties in moving the feet properly, and shifting body weight, when throwing a ball reflect this problem. It is also seen when youngsters try to correctly move their arms, in concert with their legs, when jumping vigorously. Limb agnosias may also be seen when a child attempts to repeat a series of rhythmic movements. This can involve difficulties experienced when attempting to alternately and successively jump from one foot to the other. Thus the presence of a limb agnosia may make learning to skip difficult.

When attempting to remediate this kind of problem it is often necessary to augment kinesthetic input, with tactile stimulation, and with visual information. For example, when teaching a child to throw a mirror placed to the side may prove a helpful teaching aid. The throwing arm may thus be viewed as it is drawn behind the thrower's line of vision. If the problem is severe, tactile input may be helpful. The arms may be gently stroked or rubbed in order to afford more information as to their location and volume. Children whose movement problems include cerebral palsy have traditionally been exposed to this type of tactile intervention. Foot placement when attempting various locomotor tasks, such as skipping and hopping, may be assisted if templates are placed on the ground, into which the feet may be placed.

Digital Agnosias

Digital agnosia is the poor awareness of the location and tactile proprieties of the hands and fingers. There has been a long history of interest in this problem. Digital agnosias include several subtypes. These include problems reflected in tasks assessing sensitivity to touches received by the hand. Difficulties in determining the shape, texture and shape when touching or handling objects reflects another type of digital agnosia, sometimes termed asterognosis. It has been found in several studies that awkward children, when compared to normals, exhibit less tactile sensitivity in the hands (Kinnealey 1989), and also receive less accurate information when both touching and handling objects with their hands. (Haron & Henderson 1985).

Gerstmann identified digital agnosia as one of three problems, within a triad of symptoms. (Gerstmann 1927). The other two symptoms are difficulties in math (acalculia) and body image deficits. Difficulties in carrying out simple mathematical operations is associated with digital agnosia, some have suggested, because these youngsters have problems using their fingers as counting implements when gaining initial quantitative concepts.(Strauss and Werner 1938).

In a recent study my students and I found significant positive correlations between measures of hand sequencing and mathematics abilities, confirming the possibility of a sub-group of children evidencing Gerstmann's syndrome, within learning disabled population evaluated. (Miyahara, Cratty and Goldman 1990). In other studies by Lord & Hulme (1987) and by Hulme and his colleagues (1982) it has been found that clumsy children as a group are likely to be measurably deficient in their ability to obtain accurate tactile-kinesthetic information about the lengths and shapes of various objects when they are inspected manually.

The type of dyspraxia, corresponding to digital agnosia, may be reflected in the inability to engage in pre-conceived motor plans involving the sequential use of the fingers. Finger opposition, touching each finger in order to the thumb of the same hand, has often used to evaluate motor planning abilities of the hands and fingers. The effective execution of this task may also reflect the tactile kinesthetic proprieties of the digits. In one study by one of my students, using ten subjects, a perfect positive correlation was found between a measure of digital agnosia and finger opposition. (Amuchie 1978). These and other data suggest the close association between sensory and motor qualities exhibited by the hands.

Benton (1969) and others have formulated direct measures of finger, or digital agnosia. Essentially these usually consist of asking a child to identify which fingers are touched or stroked by a examiner, on a hand that is kept out of view of the child. At times the identification of the finger touched is made verbally and at other times the child is asked to move the finger, or fingers, involved. In the second case, a movement quality probably influences the scores obtained. In a factor analysis containing a variety of tests including one of 'tactile' finger recognition, digital agnosia appeared to be independent of motor 'soft' signs, and of measures of tactile sensitivity to object shape (asterognosis) (Nichols 1987). Thus the available data seemed to indicate that there may be several, and relatively independent, sensory qualities measurable in tasks using the hands and fingers. (Haron & Henderson 1985) (Kinnealy 1989).

In real life situations a child afflicted with this kind of finger insensitivity may experience a number of difficulties. I recently tested a six-year old girl, who while scoring high on tests of intelligence, was eating with her hands, rather than with table utensils, due to the presence of a severe case of digital agnosia. Often children with digital agnosias, use a fisted grip on their pencils while writing, as they can gain so little tactile information from their pencils when they is held in a the usual way . Attaching four fingers to the pencil thus affords them more tactile-sensory information, than is gained if the pencil or pen is be held in the traditional way. (*See Chapter 7*)

Youngsters with digital agnosias are often fearful of climbing playground apparatus, and may fall if forced to do so. Their fear apparently stems from the fact that they may be unaware of when their hands are clasping the bars upon which they are climbing. Thus they seem to fear, with some reason, suddenly letting go with disastrous consequences. When trying to gain climbing skills, an alert adult should be stationed directly behind young awkward children suspected of exhibiting digital agnosia, to insure their safety.

Children with signs of various types of digital agnosia often avoid making small models. They also find tying their shoes difficult or impossible. They may fumble when attempting to use zippers, or buttons on their clothing. Catching balls may also prove difficult as they obtain late and inaccurate information from the missiles as their hands contact incoming balls.

The hands of youngsters with digital agnosia may not produce accurate information about the shape of objects they cannot see. Tests of 'stereognosis' (or of asterognosis) are contained in some neurological 'schedules. Such a measure was applied to several thousand children in a comprehensive study carried out on a small island off the coast of Great Britain. In this investigation, and in similar studies in which this kind of measure has been employed, it was found that children afflicted with the poor tactile perception of object-shape, were also found to be more likely to evidence other unusual neural soft-signs reflecting developmental lags, including general incoordination (Nichols 1987) (Haron and Henderson 1985).

Signs of agnosias may be seen in both the hands and feet. The child displaying poor sensitivity in the feet, for example may have difficulty properly breaking the shock of descent by quickly bending the knees when landing from a jump. Instead the youngster may display a spastic like extension of the foot (a clonic reaction) upon contacting the ground. The youngster evidencing poor tactile sensitivity in the feet, thus may receive late or inaccurate information from the ground as it is contacted, thus preventing accurate and appropriate motor responses to the landing (a quick knee bend). Abrupt stops at the termination of a jump may thus provide jolting punishments for attempting to leave the ground. Thus some of these youngsters may be discouraged from attempts at this and other vigorous motor tasks.

Summary

This second part of the chapter contains descriptions and explanations of various agnosias involving the poor awareness of the body surfaces its position space, and of the limbs, and hands. Sometimes the behavioral manifestations of the agnosias (and dysgnosias) described, it was postulated, are inseparable from motor counterparts including various forms of dyspraxia. These dysgnosias and agnosias, present obvious and subtle problems to professionals, to parents, and to awkward youngsters themselves, as they collectively attempt to understand and accommodate to the presence of these subtle sensory-perceptual difficulties.

These various perceptual-sensory deficits cannot be seen. Only the behavioral disturbances and consequences that such problems cause are apparent. The existence of these sensory-perceptual deficits should suggest to those conducting programs for awkward children, however, that provisions should be made for the reduction or remediation of perceptual-sensory problems, just as strategies are devised to deal with the more obvious motor problems that are encountered. Among the methods suggested was to enrich tactile input. Attaching additional verbal and visual cues to actions that might be disrupted by poor sensory awareness, was another type of strategy suggested.

It is usually found that the agnosias discussed are statistically independent from scores reflecting academic, intellectual competencies, and verbal abilities. However, these sensory-perceptual problems constitute one of several types of 'hidden problems' that plague neurologically impaired children. Thus it is important to measure and identify these deficits, and if present, to follow such assessments with useful remedial strategies.

OVERVIEW

In this chapter efforts were made to illuminate both obvious and subtle sensory and perceptual problems that potentially influence motor difficulties encountered by awkward children. The problems discussed included those mediated by visual and visual-perceptual mechanisms. These consisted of deficits due to structure anomalies including tumors, and also problems that may be occur within pathways and neural centers that negatively influence both vision and coordinated motion.

Dynamic visual acuity was defined as the ability to perceptually halt, and select out visual information from moving objects. This quality was explained together with the mechanisms involved. Individual differences in this quality among atypical and typical youngsters were also reviewed. It was also explained that there were youngsters who were adequate to superior in the ability to visually intercept and interpret fast moving visual stimuli, and others who were inadequate in this complex ability. Furthermore, it was cautioned that medical specialists conversant with visual pathologies should often be consulted when children evidence problems in visual tracking behaviors.

Various agnosias involving the body and its parts were also discussed. These, it was pointed out, constitute a multi-dimensional problem. Thus these conditions may reflect a lack-of awareness of the body's position in space, and also various anomalies based upon inadequate tactile, and kinesthetic information emanating from the location, and movements of the limbs, hands, and fingers.

Among the agnosias and dysgnosias reviewed included digital agnosia, limb agnosias, and tactile agnosias involving the body. It was pointed out that there is typically a close correspondence between measures of agnosias and the various dyspraxias surveyed in Chapter 6. A important principle thus emphasized in this chapter, and throughout the text, is that there are usually parallel losses in sensory functions, in corresponding bodily locations, when motor incoordination is encountered in its various forms. This section of the chapter also contained explanation of potentially useful evaluative tools. The chapter advanced recommendations of how program content might be augmented to deal with some of the sensory-perceptual problems encountered among groups of awkward youngsters.

QUESTIONS FOR DISCUSSION

1. What is the general meaning of the terms 'agnosia and dysgnosias"? In what sensory modalities is this likely to occur?
2. Can you cite evidence from the chapter that body-sensory and movement qualities are closely linked?
3. How as it suggested that a clinician might test for signs of spatial agnosias?

4. How is digital agnosia evaluated, and how does this deficiency impact upon play and academic tasks of various kinds? Why might a child with this problem have poor upper-back strength?
5. What does dynamic visual acuity mean? How is it measured?
6. What are velocity susceptible and velocity resistant youngsters?
7. What neurological information and confirmation exists for the close association between sensation and motion?
8. How might a child with figure-ground perceptual problems react in ball games? Can you make the case for the placement of such a child in 'closed skills'' rather than 'open skills'?
9. How do visual-perceptual problems, social modeling and imitation, and motor awkwardness interact?
10. What sub-types were described under the general heading of digital agnosia?

Chapter 9
Learning Disabilities and Physical Coordination

INTRODUCTION

Learning disabled children and adolescents, pose difficult assessment and labeling problems. The measurement of both their learning characteristics and motor abilities has not always been made easier by researchers. Most continue to identify sub-types within learning disabled populations by using memory tests (Speece 1987) or information processing measures as guidelines (Swanson et al 1990). Few investigators have employed batteries of tests containing measures of both motor and academic tests. (Cratty, et al 1991).

Clinicians, however, are continually faced with the problem of testing learning disabled youngsters, some of whom appear awkward, and others whose problems are mainly are confined to memory retrieval and reading. Child psychologists, whose evaluation tools include the collection of samples of printing and of figure drawing, may correctly identify a graphic problem, but may then fail to label a child as learning disabled if no academic deficiencies are noted. Some educational psychologists may mistakenly assume that, because the child prints slowly or poorly, academic-cognitive difficulties must also be present. Both awkward and learning disabled youngsters reside in 'grey areas' diagnostically and therefore often present management and educational problems to both parents and teachers.

The significance of motor difficulties among groups of learning disabled and dyslexic populations has been interpreted in various ways throughout the years by scholars interested in these populations. On one hand, Critchley & Critchley (1978) proposed that developmental dyslexia is due to cognitive disabilities which are "requently of constitutional origin" (page 7). Moreover these same authors suggest that the incidence of motor disabilities within dyslexic populations is "entirely coincidental", and thus (poor coordination) is 'apart from dyslexia' (page 89). They concluded that "dyslexic boys are proficient at ball games, while girls may be able in needle work" (Critchley & Critchley 1978, p 92).

Contemporary data indicate that the incidence of motor disabilities within dyslexic populations is usually greater than is expected within academically average groups. Brying & Michelsson found that 18% of a learning disabled group they surveyed evidenced motor problems (1984). Bruininks discovered a similar percentage of poorly coordinated youngsters among a group of learning disabled children. (1978). Klasen places the percentage even higher, finding that 49.2% of the dyslexic group she surveyed evidenced visual-motor difficulties (1972). Jaklewicz after measuring a population of Polish children with dyslexia, in ten-year longitudinal study, also stated that disorders of motor functions coexist with dyslexia in a rather constant manner. Thus she suggested that not only are motor problems pervasive in dyslexic populations, but also that coordination problems persist in individual youngsters over an extensive period of time. (Jaklewicz (1980).

In a study by Sudgen and Wann (1987) it was also found that higher incidence of motor problems existed within a population of children with 'moderate learning difficulties' than is expected among children without learning problems. They discovered that from 29-33% of the learning disabled children they tested evidenced coordination difficulties, as contrasted to the 5% of children with motor problems who are expected within academically normal populations. (Sudgen and Wann 1987). In a recent cluster analysis by Miyahara (1992) it was found that among a learning disabled population numbering one hundred and sixteen boys and girls, Over 60% evidenced either several motor problems or a specific coordination difficulty.

Qualitative differences have also been found when contrasting the motor characteristics of learning disabled, dyslexic youngsters to populations who are academically intact. For example, in series of studies Peter Wolff and his colleagues identified deficits in timing tasks (finger tapping and the like) among academically deficient populations. Wolff et al 1984). They attributed these differences to neurological problems among the learning disabled including either impaired hemispheric communication, or functional difficulties within the left hemisphere. (Wolff et al 1990). They assumed that these differences reflected timing problems common both to reading and to executing relatively simple, rhythmic motor tasks.

During the past four decades well-meaning educators, however, sometimes confused correlation with causation. They incorrectly assumed that since there is a greater incidence of motor problems within learning disabled groups, one simply has to modify movement capacities to elicit positive changes in academic learning. Following the Second World War, numerous writings appeared strongly advocating this position. The titles of books written by these proponents of motor training as a form of academic training reflected these promise. And thus the content and promises made within such books as "How to Develop Your Child's Intelligence" (Getman 1952) and "he Slow Learner in the Classroom" (Kephart 1955) achieved widespread popularity.

However the naive strategy of attempting to rectify learning disabilities by simply improving motor coordination has been laid to rest in recent data surveys. Most illuminating was insightful meta-analysis of the data obtained in numerous studies dealing with this question by Kavale and Mattson (1983). The results of this critical survey suggested that,

(1) not only did well publicized programs of motor remediation not significantly modify learning efforts, including reading, but that
(2) better classroom progress would have been obtained through traditional applications of academic tutoring and that
(3) the motor programs applied did nothing to improve measures of motor coordination.

Other reviews of the literature have also concluded that simply trying to remediate dyslexia through the application of motor program will not succeed in modifying reading or other academic qualities. (Critchley & Critchley 1978) (Hynd and Cohen 1983) (Myers & Hammill 1989).

In summary the best available evidence is that clumsy children are over-represented within groups of learning disabled youngsters. And while some learning disabled children are free of motor coordination problems, the data thus strongly suggest that programs of remedial motor development should constitute an important component of the overall educational program available to many of learning disabled children and youth.

Predicting the presence of learning disabilities in a given child or in a group of youngsters, by evaluating motor coordination, does not seem to be a fruitful undertaking. Rie recently reviewed the literature relating learning disabilities to soft neurological signs, including symptoms of incoordination. She concluded that the mere number of these soft signs present is not predictive of academic problems (1987). Furthermore, as the result of a factor analysis she and her colleagues conducted, it was pointed out that some motor tasks of above-average complexity were moderately correlated to academic abilities (1978).

Denckla and her colleagues (1985), exploring possible relationships between dyslexia, attention and motor proficiency, concluded that there were various sub-groups within learning disabled populations, including those with and without attentional and motor problems. In this same study it was also found that the tests of motor qualities they employed, including measures of synkinesia (overflow), and of rapid-repetitive rhythmic movements, were more likely to predict hyperactivity in children than were measures of specific learning disabilities they obtained. Most important, their data suggested to them that treatment outcomes may be different for the various sub-groups. Outcomes seemed to depend upon the presence of various combinations of learning disabilities, hyperactivity and of types of motor incoordination measured within each sub-division.

In two other factor analyses by Nichols (1978) and by Ayres (1968) it was found that motor coordination and sensory-qualities 'loaded' in factors separate from those containing motor coordination items. It is interesting to note however, that Ayres then proceeded to formulate and promote a program of sensory-integration in which motor-sensory experiences were advanced as producing change in a variety of academic and sensory-perceptual processes. The most reasonable contemporary viewpoint thus seems to be that motor development programs should be one, of several parts, of curricula for learning disabled youngsters. However, simply exposing a youngster with learning disabilities to sensory-motor experiences will do little to modify academic competencies.

In the following diagram of the brain (Figure 9-1) separate functional components are shown. It should be noted that these apparently discrete areas are actually interdependent, mutually influential, and joined by vast networks of complex neural connections. It is thus to be expected that

(1) each child with either learning disabilities or coordination problems may display a highly unique set of behavioral strengths and weaknesses. and that

(2) There are identifiable sub-groups within populations of both learning disabled and the awkward youngsters (Hoare & Larkin 1991) (Miyahara 1992).

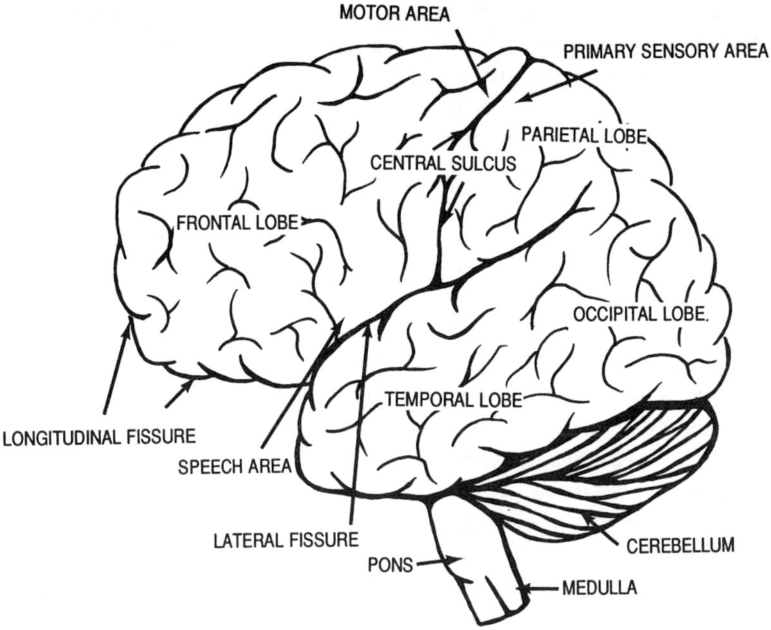

Figure 9-1. The Brain's Functional Areas

Researchers dealing both with populations of the learning disabled, and of awkward children usually are searching for the presence of these sub-groups within both populations. Recent studies by me and my colleagues represent this quest. The data from two of these investigations are summarized and interpreted in the following section. (Cratty, et al 1991) (Miyahara, et al 1992).

PERCEPTUAL-MOTOR PERFORMANCE AND MOTOR PLANNING IN LEARNING DISABLED CHILDREN: TWO INVESTIGATIONS

Study#1: Motor Performance, Fitness, Body-Build, Attitudes & Posture

Introduction

In the first of two studies (Cratty et al 1991) ninety-three boys and twenty-three girls were evaluated, ranging from eight, to sixteen years of age, attending a private school. The school's program focused upon children who evidenced delays in reading (dyslexia) but who did not present marked problems in social-emotional development, or other obviously handicapping conditions.

Motor ability tests were selected primarily from two batteries (1) The Bruinink's revision of the Oseretsky (1978), with some updated norms, and from two versions of the Stott-Henderson (1972, 1984). Several skill-ability components were assessed including tests of muscular power, balance, ball skills, agility, and arm-leg coordination. A posture screening was conducted based upon a scoring system devised by The New York State Education Department (1966).

"Ideal" body-weights were computed based upon norms obtained by Helen Pryor (1946) using measures of body-build, height, and sex. Questionnaire data was obtained (see appendix) to determine attitudes about physical activity, self-concepts about skill and body build, and activities disliked and disliked. In additional selected academic scores were obtained, and contrasted (correlated) to the motor ability scores obtained.

These included age-level scores posted in the Gray, the Slosson, and in components of the Stanford Achievement Tests, evaluating Mathematical Abilities. These tests scores were expressed in developmental-academic ages. Two other academic scores were computed, one reflecting a difference between the children's chronological age, and their overall reading-age, and a second reflecting differences between their chronological ages, and mathematics score. The tests were administered individually by three trained testers. The tests were selected, and in some cases modified to,

(1) cover the entire spectrum of ages tested, and

(2) to result in data expressed in developmental ages, rather than in standard scores.

Motor Tests Employed

Static Balance: The static balance assessment included sub-tests from clinical data, from the Stott-Henderson, and from the Bruinink's Oseretsky. For example, posturing with feet in a heel-to-toe position (the Stott Henderson) resulted in a developmental age scores of from 4. to 4.5 years; a two foot stand on the balls of the feet resulted in a score of 5 years (developmental age) (obtained from the Stott Henderson). A one-foot stand from 6-10 seconds resulted in developmental age scores of from 5.4-5.9 years. One foot stands, from 8-10 seconds on a 1.4″ side balance beam (The Bruinink's Oseretsky) result in developmental balance age scores of from 6.9-7.1 years. At this point, if children achieved a 10 second stand on a 1.5″ wide balance beam they were given a score equalling their chronological age, as static balance tends to plateau at about 7+ years, and thus it was believed that application of a more difficult would not have produced valid, age-related results.

Dynamic Balance: The test of dynamic balance was obtained from the Bruinink's-Oseretsky. It requires a child to walk on a 1.4″ wide balance beam (8″ long), in a heel-to-toe manner, while keeping the hands on the hips. The scores (based upon steps walked, 1-6) result in developmental ages of from −4 to 9+ years. If a child was able to walk 6 steps he/she was given a developmental age score that equalled their chronological age, as dynamic balance plateaus at about the age of nine years. In addition an overall balance score was computed, based upon the scores obtained from both tests of static and dynamic balance.

Arm-Leg Integration: The jump clap test from the Bruinink's-Oseretsky was employed, which requires children to clap their hands together as many times possible during a single jump in the air. The scores ranging from 0-5 claps, results in developmental-age scores of from −4.6 to 17+ years.

General Speed-Agility of the Total Body: A sub-test test from the Bruinink's-Oseretsky battery was employed, requiring a child to run 45′ pick up a small block and return with it 45′ to the starting line. The run, requiring a change of direction was scored in seconds, and tenths, and results in developmental ages of from 4.3 to 18+.

Ball Skills: Catching. Catching was first evaluated using a 8″ (in diameter) playground ball, bounced from 15′ away to the child, five times. Intercepting this from 1-5 times resulted in developmental ages of from 1-5 years, Next two ball interception components of the Bruininks-Oseretsky were administered. The first required a child to bounce a tennis ball at his/her feet, and catch it 1-5 times (developmental ages of from 5-6.9 years). If successful in five attempts in this first test a second was administered requiring a child to catch a tennis ball thrown from 10′ away from 1-5 times (developmental ages of from 5.6 years to 8.3 years). If a child was successful in five attempts in this last test, the age score recorded corresponded to their chronological age.

Ball Skills: Throwing: A target-throwing task was employed from the Bruininks-Oseretsky battery, requiring a child to throw a tennis ball five times at a 10″ diameter target 5 feet away. Scores or from 1-5 resulted in developmental ages of from 4.6 to 11.9 years. If a youngster was successful at all five throws, a developmental age equaling their chronological age was awarded. In addition a combined ball score was computed, combining this test and the previous one.

Power Tests: Arm Power. A test of arm-power was employed from the Bruininks-Oseretsky involving either of two types of pushups (from the knees for girls, and boys eight and younger, and from the feet, with the body straight, for boys nine and older. Scores were based upon number completed in twenty seconds, and ranged from developmental ages of 5 years (1-2 knee pushups for girls) through 17 + years (20 knee pushups for girls, and 20 regular pushups for boys).

Power Tests: Abdominal Power. Abdominal power was evaluated using a curl-up, while lying on the back with knees straight (from the Bruininks-Oseretsky). The score, based upon the number accomplished in 20 seconds, ranged from 1-2 which equaled a developmental age of 6.3 years to 20 which resulted in a developmental age score of 18 + years.

Power Tests: Leg Power. The standing long jump test from the Bruininks-Oseretsky was employed (with updated norms obtained from the test's author in 1989). It was scored in inches, ranging from scores reflecting a developmental age of -3 years (10″) to 19 years (85″-89″. In addition an overall power score (developmental age) was computed combining the three power scores.

Posture Screening: A posture screen was employed in order to selected components of body alignment, viewed from the side, and from the rear. Charts were employed was prepared by the New York State Department of Education (1966) enabling scores to be attached to postural divergences, including kyphosis, sciolosis, and lordosis. Postural divergences were not scored, but were used as clinical data upon which to base later program recommendations.

Pryor Weight-Width Index: Ideal Body Weight. Using Pryor's Weight-Width Index (1946) measures of the children's weight, height, and widths (in centimeters) of their chest, and hips were obtained. Based upon these an ideal body weight was computed. The difference from the 'ideal' and their actual body weight was also obtained.

Attitude, Self-Concepts. Three types of responses were obtained from the youngsters, and the responses scored on a 1-5 basis. These scores reflected attitudes about personal skill (I think I am superior, ok, or inferior in skill), body-build, (I think I am too heavy, ok, or too thin), and attitudes about playing vigorous games (when I am asked to play I am, happy, ok, or unhappy) (See Appendix).

In addition to scores obtained in the ways described, an overall developmental "motor-age" was obtained, by averaging the scores in sub-tests. The mean developmental motor-age by test, was subtracted from the chronological age, to obtain mean differences.

This information was used for individual counseling purposes and for recommendations for program implementation. Differences, between average chronological ages and average developmental motor-ages were also employed to reflect whether the total population (and males vs females), were behind or ahead of the age norms employed.

Findings

Overview. 116 youngsters were tested, ranging in age from 8-17 years. The age of the total population was 12.78 (SD 2.18). The average age of the ninety-three boys evaluated was 12.65 years, and the average age of twenty-three the girls was 10.70. The average grade placement for the overall population was 7.5: and was 7.2 grade for the boys, and 8.04 for the girls. Thus even though the girls were younger, on the average, their mean grade placements were higher than that of the boys. Overall the group motor performance mean (average motor-age) was – 1.8 years less than their chronological ages.

The following Figure (9-2) indicates the average score (in developmental years), by sex in the total test battery of motor test items, contrasted to delays in mean scores representing delays academic achievement.

Delays in Academic Scores, and in Overall Physical Performance Scores of 117 Learning Disabled Youngsters, ages 8–16, Tested during 1989–90 School Year.

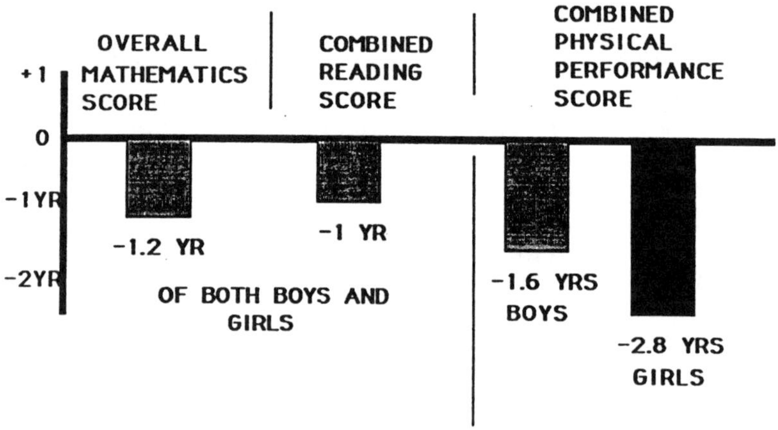

Chart 9-2. Average Delay in Developmental Age, by Sex and By Task, in 117 Learning Disabled Youngsters

A significant difference was obtained upon computing the differences between the delay recorded by males (-1.6 years) and the females (-2.8 years) (t = +2.55 significant at the 1% level), as shown in Chart 9-2. When "motor-age" scores of the individual tests were contrasted, by sex the following results were obtained (chart 9-3).

As shown in (Chart 9-3) significant sex differences were noted when tests evaluating arm-shoulder power (pushups), as well as leg power, overall power, and agility were contrasted. Although the males were developmentally delayed in overall motor ability, the females were delayed more so. Thus provisions in programming should be made to improve these qualities among both the boys and girls within this group, and within similar populations.

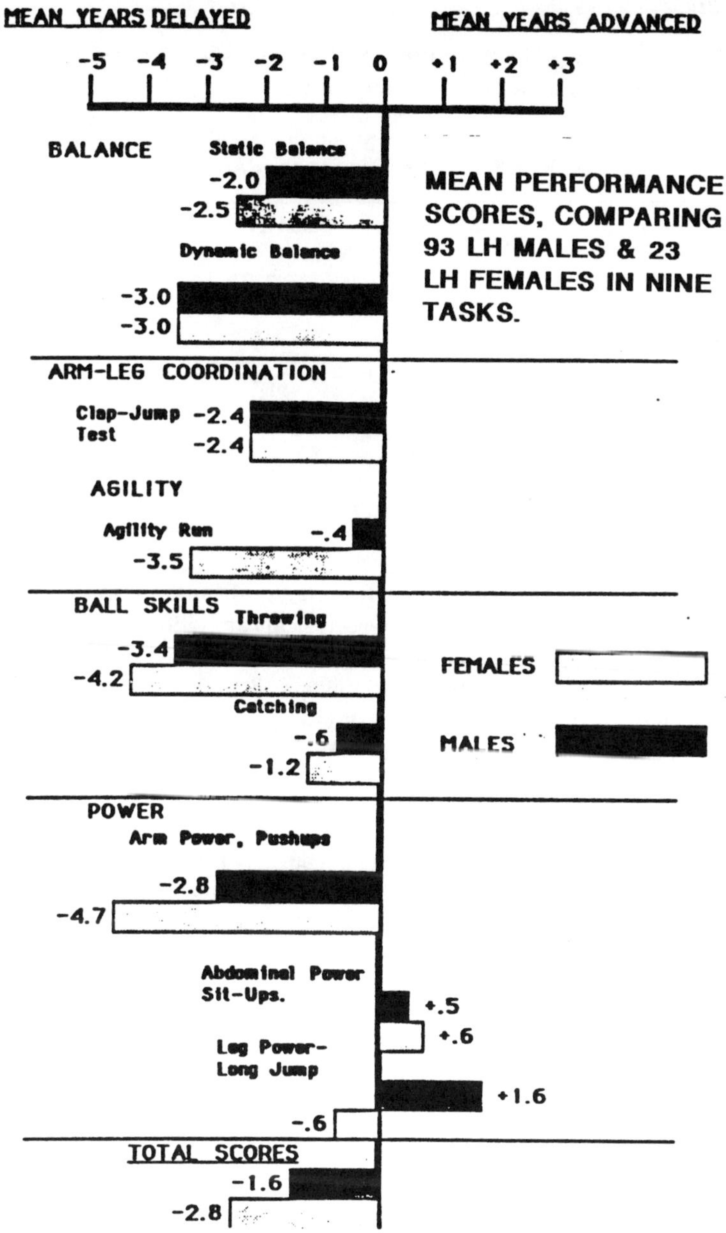

Chart 9-3. Sex Differences in Motor Abilities

Attitude Scores

Scores reflecting self-perceptions and attitudes were contrasted, and the results were as follows.

Chart 9-4. Sex Differences in Attitudes

	Males		Females			
	Mean	SD	Mean	SD	t	Significance
Percept. of Game Skill (5 points)	3.8	1.2	3.3	1.1	1.7	NS
Body Image Deviation from Optimum (5 points)	4.0	1.4	4.0	1.5	.03	NS
Attitude About Playing, 5 Points optimum liked	3.9	1.3	3.3	1.3	t = 2.0	5%

As these data point out, the males felt significantly more positively about participation in vigorous physical activities than did the females. Otherwise feelings about their body-builds and skills were similar, when responses of the females and males were contrasted.

Selected correlations were computed, contrasting selected motor performance scores (based upon developmental ages), of the total 116 subjects. The results of this computation is shown below.

Chart 9-5. Selected intercorrelations, 116 subjects. (Developmental Ages in Selected Motor Performance Measures)

	Balance	Ball	Power	Performance
Overall Balance				
Overall Ball Age	.57**			
Overall Power	.54**	.53**		
Overall Performance	.74**	.78**	.80**	

**Significant at the 1% Level

As can be seen there were significant correlations between some performance parameters. In general the most predictive of the overall performance score were scores in the power tests (combined ages averaged). Moreover the combined scores in the two ball tests were almost as predictive of overall motor abilities, as were scores (ages) from the three power tests.

To determine relationships between the children's feelings about their body-builds, their performance capacities, and their actual body weight (over or under) and performance scores, the following correlations were computed, based upon the scores of the total 116 subjects.

Chart 9-6. Attitude scores, motor performance, and weight: Differences from norms (116 subjects)

	Skill	Body At.	Play At.	Perform.	Wt. Diff.
Peercept of Game Skill					
Body Attitude	.10				
Play Attitude	.61**	−.02			
Overall Performance	.24**	.19	.23*		
Weight Diff.	.01	.10	.03	.22*	

* = 5% Leel of Significance, ** = 1% level of significance

As shown in the above chart (chart 9-6), significant positive correlations were obtained between the youngster's perceptions of their overall levels of performance, and attitudes about playing and their feelings about their skill level (r's = +.61 and 24+). Overall performance and their feelings about their skill were also positively correlated as were their attitudes about playing and their actual performance.

However, the youngsters seemed to evidence inaccurate perceptions of their body builds. Their judgements about whether they believed themselves to be over or under-weight did not correlate to how much these measures actually reflected apparent obesity or an underweight condition.

A one-way Analysis of Variance was computed to determine whether the children scoring differently 1 through 5 on the test of arm-leg integration (the jump-and-clap test) resulted in significant differences in their overall performance scores (performance age, minus chronological age). An F Score of 22.5 suggests that the differences (between the groups scoring, 1, 2, 3, 4, and 5, in this test) were highly significant. The data thus suggests that this test alone would be a useful classification instrument, reflecting overall motor abilities as measured by the total test battery.

Reading and Motor Performance

Selected motor test scores and reading scores were compared, with the following results.

Chart 9-7. Reading and Motor (Age) Scores

	St Bal	Dyn Bal	Clp Jmp	Ball age	Reading
Static Balance					
Dynamic Balance	.54**				
Clap Jump	.40**	.34**			
Avg. Ball (age)	.48**	.58**	.39**		
Reading	.16	.32**	.25*	.44**	
(Grade(s) behind expected grade)					

It was thus found that the best predictors of reading level mean number of years behind their mean chronological age) were a combination of three motor tests, including throwing age, catching age, and dynamic balance (r = .48** (RR = .23). It is thus indicated that 23% (r squared) of the variance of reading scores, may be predicted by combining scores on the three motor tests indicated.

These correlations, however, should not imply that there are casual relationships between the qualities contrasted. That is one cannot be expected to improve reading by heightening balance and ball skills, nor will improving reading likely modify balance!

Rather it is probable that among about 20% of the subjects evaluated, neurological problems are reflected both in academic-reading scores , as well as in the control of postural balance and hand-eye coordinations needed in ball skills. Follow-up studies have begun to identify various sub-types of learning disabled children and adolescents. This work is making it increasing clear that some display academic deficiencies and specific motor difficulties, while others are beset with academic difficulties independent of other signs of neurological impairment including dysfunctional physical coordination (Miyahara 1992)

Overview. Study #1: One hundred and twenty-three youngsters, from eight to sixteen years of age, in a private school for the learning disabled were evaluated in five types of motor abilities, as well as in posture, in attitudes about physical activity, their perceived skill and their feelings about their body builds. Height weight, and body build measures were also obtained. Overall the population displayed deficiencies in upper limb power, as well as in balance and ball skills.

In general upper body weakness was reflected in poor posture scores, as 42% were found to be kyphotic (evidenced round shoulders). There were few significant differences when males and females were contrasted, however differences were found when tests of power, overall performance, and attitudes about participation were contrasted, with the males posting scores higher than did the females. However, as the previous tables have illustrated, the mean scores of most tests administered to both sexes were delayed, when contrasted to norms.

The youngsters seemed more sensitive to their actual physical skill levels, when asked about their attitudes about participation. However they seem somewhat oblivious to their actual body builds, when asked to rate their physiques as "thin", "ok", or "too heavy" (using a 5 point Likert-type scale).

Most predictive of the overall performance scores were scores derived from balance tests, ball skills, and power. A clap-jump test (number of times a child could clap during one jump in the air) was most predictive of various skill-performance categories, ranging from the unskilled, to the highly skilled.

Significant positive correlations between balance scores, ball scores, and academic scores including reading, indicated that perhaps about 20% of the subjects may evidence neurological symptoms that include both gross motor control, and precise eye movements (saccades) needed in reading. Further studies also reflect this possibility (Miyahara 1991).

The deficiencies in balance and in other motor abilities appearing in this data were expected in a learning disabled population. The same finding is typical among similar populations when using measures of motor coordination (Byring & Michelsson 1984) (Jaklewicz 1980), (Sugden and Wann 1987).

Deficiencies in upper body strength found in this study may be associated with skill deficiencies. It could be postulated, for example, that the poorly skilled learning disabled children tested were less likely to play vigorously, and thus evidence average fitness levels, than is true among those without academic and coordination difficulties. Some of the children within this LD group reported that they did not always have opportunities to participate in vigorous activities (gymnastics weight-lifting and the like) that would have stressed the muscles in their upper bodies. The content in programs instituted as the result of this data, included a conditioning facility designed to improve strength, fitness and posture.

STUDY #2: APRAXIA IN THE LEARNING DISABLED

In a follow-up study 72 youngsters (10 girls and 62 boys), from the same population used in the previous study, were evaluated using three tests of motor planning

Tests of Praxic Behaviors. Three sub-tests of praxic behavior were selected from the battery developed by Cratty and Gong (1989). In previous studies these tests were found to be reliable (Cratty and Samoy 1985), and useful as clinical tools (Cratty and Gibson (1986). The praxic sub-tests consisted of a figure-drawing test, containing a diagram-drawing task of seven parts

(a) a test of the replication of up to seven hand positions, modified and expanded from a test suggested by Luria (1966) and later used by Orpet (1972)

(b) a test of the ability to observe, and

(c) an assessment of the replication of up to seven limb positions. (Cratty 1989) (Cratty and Gong (1989).

The Appendix contains the three measures employed in this study. The findings are as follows.

Distribution of Scores

As indicated in chart 9-4 the scores distributed in a bi-modal configuration, demonstrating that were apparently at least two sub-populations within the group studied. One sub-group in possession of adequate motor planning abilities, and a second group who evidenced measurable symptoms reflecting dyspraxia.

Age Trends. As can be seen below (chart 9-95), there were no obvious age trends in each of the three motor planning tests.

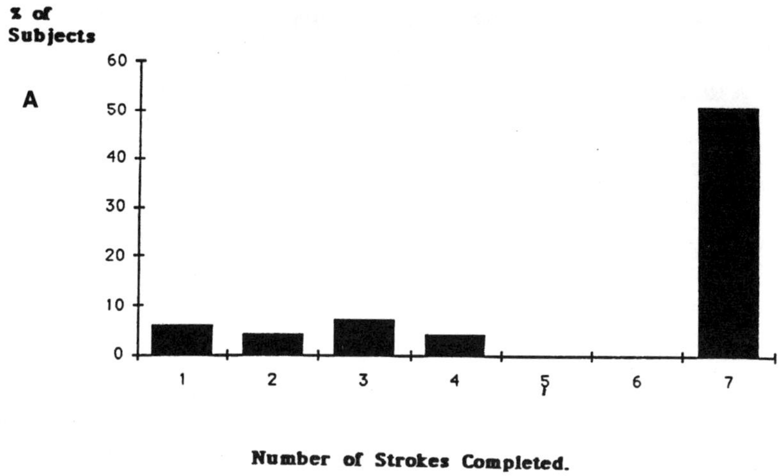

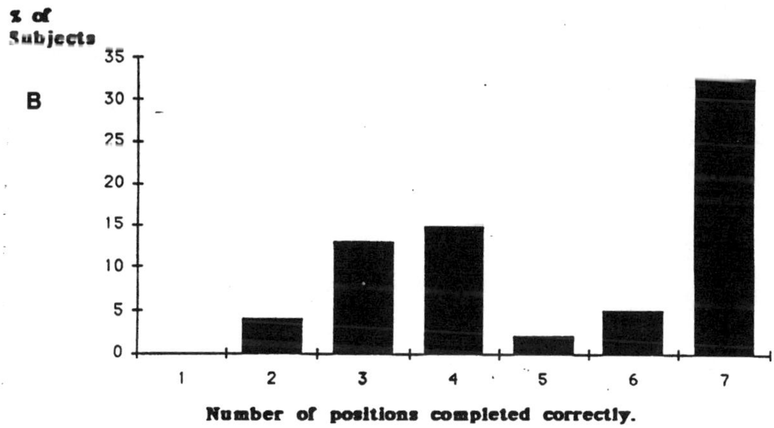

Chart 9-8. Distributions of scores on two tests of motor planning, 342–343
(A) Distribution of Scores obtained when 72 Learning Disabled Children were exposed to a drawing a geometric figure, containing up to 7 strokes.
(B) Distribution of Scores obtained when 72 Learning Disabled Children were exposed to a task involving the replication of up to 7 arm positions

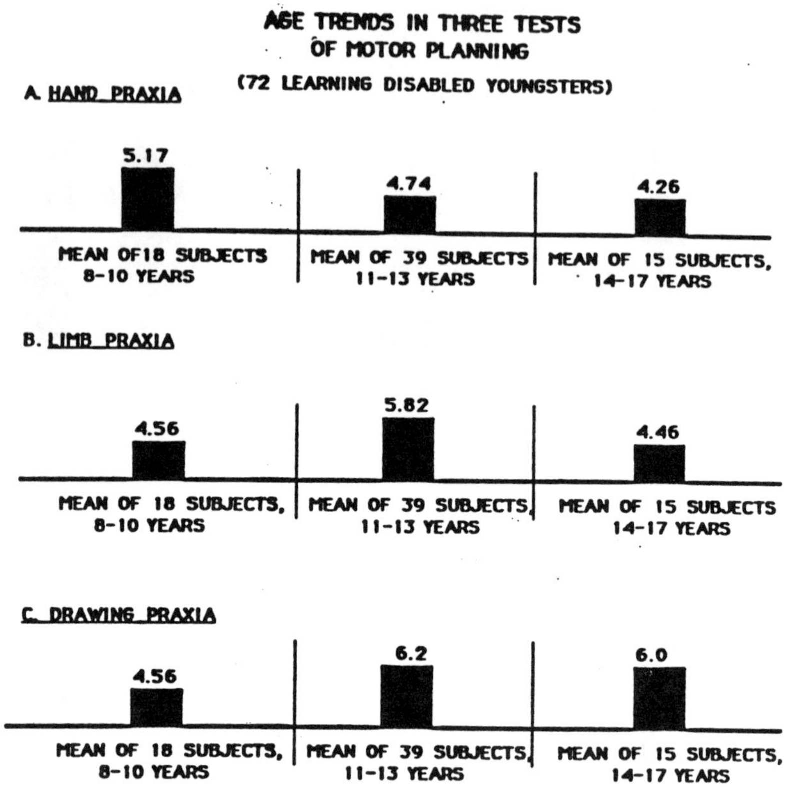

Chart 9-9. Age trends in three tests of Motor Planning, 344

Inter-correlations of Selected Scores

The Chart (9-10) which follows reveals moderate, to low a correlations, between the three sub-tests of motor planning employed.

As can be seen in Chart 9-10, No significant correlations, other than those expected by chance, were found between the tests of motor planning when contrasted to more traditional tests of motor performance also employed in the study. However there were significant positive correlations between the scores obtained on the test of hand praxia and the scores reflecting mathematical ability. The data was not analyzed further (using cluster analyses) due to the few number of subjects tested.

Chart 9-10. Inter-correlations of Scores From Three Motor Planning Tests. To Each Other, and to Selected Motor and Academic Performance Measures (Based Upon Data from 72 LD Youngsters)

Praxic Tests	Drawing	Hand	Limb
Hand			
Limb	.380**		
Drawing	.267*	.483**	
Static Balance	–.014	.068	.057
Dynamic Balance	–.099	–.016	.131
Clap Jump	–.028	.170	.127
Agility Run	–.051	.261*	.240*
Throwing	–.161	–.024	–.100
Catching	–.008	.082	.084
Broad Jump	.114	.133	.076
Push-up	–.188	.034	.015
Sit-up	.167	.281*	.092
(N = 69)			
Gray	.076	.104	.026
Slosson	.155	.162	.001
Read. Compreh.	.075	.265*	.027
Reading Average	.215	.220 +	.170
(N = 50)			
Math Concepts	.092	.364**	.152
Computation	.039	.339**	.062
Application	.109	.410**	.174
Math Average	.088	.407**	.142

**p<.001, * p<.05, + p = .007

Discussion of Findings in Study #2

These data contain several important findings, and implications. The lack of age trends, within the tests of praxia employed, are believed important to consider. Improvement with age was noted in previous studies in which the tests were applied to non-learning disabled children. It thus could be concluded that dyspraxia may persist within learning disabled populations of the type evaluated in this study. It appears therefore as if some learning disabled adolescents are as likely to become confused when presented with sequential information to be expressed in serial-motor tasks, as are younger learning disabled children. Similar age-persistent trends, reflecting poor information processing, have been noted in the data of other investigators exploring abilities among learning disabled youngsters of various ages. (Bruck 1989).

It thus believed important that many learning disabled adolescents must continue to be taught sequential motor skills, including writing and sports skills, with the same patience as is required when working with younger learning disabled children. Furthermore it appears that perhaps the sequenced tasks that *are* acquired by the older population involve the acquisition of specific "splinter" skills, whose learning is not likely to transfer positively to other complex serial order skills to which they also may be exposed. It is probable that this kind of improvement in specific skills is only obtainable with intensive practice, reflecting overlearning. Whether or not a general motor serial memory quality, may be improved with remediation, should be the subject of further investigations. New research strategies intended to do this have been formulated by several workers whose suggestions are reviewed in Chapter 12.

The data from this 2nd study resulted in a bi-modal picture of motor planning abilities. There were probably several 'sub-types' of subjects contained within this population. One group contained those youngsters whose academic-learning problems were accompanied by dyspraxias, and who thus function at low levels in motor serial memory tasks (and perhaps in serial memory tasks involving other kinds of stimuli including auditory-verbal information).

The data also reflect the existence of a second sub-population, within the group evaluated. This second group's learning difficulties were not accompanied by marked signs of motor dyspraxia. A third sub-group seemed to consist of learning disabled youngsters whose motor planning skills are intact but who evidence other coordination problems including balance and fitness deficiencies.

The lack of significant correlations between scores on motor planning tests, when compared to other standardized tests of motor performance are also important to consider. These non-significant correlations indicate that the motor planning tests are independent of scores obtained from other, more traditional, tests of motor ability. Thus the ability to *acquire* a complex movement demonstration is apparently independent of the eventual ability to *perform* both simple and perhaps complex motor tasks. Age trends reflecting improvement with age, were seen in previous studies of general motor performance scores (Cratty et al 1990), obtained by testing similar populations. Thus the lack of age trends in these tests of motor planning further reflect the independence of performance between the two types of tests. The low, moderate inter-correlations obtained between the three tests of motor planning tests further indicated that these tests sampled relatively independent, but related qualities.

Finally the moderate, significant correlations between the test of hand praxia, and mathematical tests suggests the possible presence of Gerstmann's syndrome was evidenced by a number of youngsters within the population studied. Gerstmann's Syndrome is a collection of several problems combining body image deficits, finger agnosia, acalculia, and sometimes includes dyslexia. (Gerstmann 1927)

SUMMARY AND OVERVIEW

The data from these two investigations corroborate information from previous studies of learning disabled children. As a group the youngsters in this study displayed motor coordination qualities inferior to current developmental averages. These two investigations also produced several findings useful to those planning school programs. For this type of population. For example it appears that learning disabled girls may present special problems when confronted with physical activity and physical education. They may lack both motor activity capacities, and also harbor extremely negative feelings about how they both look and function in motor skill situations. The data revealed that the females were even further behind norms, than were their male classmates, when measures of coordination, fitness-strength, and self-concept were averaged. It appears that special attention should thus be paid to special needs of learning disabled girls when programming for physical improvement.

The marked delays in fitness recorded in the studies could be explained in several ways. The most probable supposition is that poorly coordinated learning disabled youngsters tend to avoid physical activity in general and thus evidence the results of this avoidance in scores reflecting poor fitness levels (reflecting what has been termed a 'dis-use' syndrome). The attitude scores obtained from this population and low performance scores indicate that special program content should be instituted for learning disabled populations. When working with such groups close attention to motivational factors and to strategies designed to enhance their self-esteem. Most of the data we and others have obtained related strongly suggest that many learning disabled youngsters are not happy with their body's appearance and with the sports skills they are able to exhibit.

The data also suggests that important sub-groups are present both within populations of awkward children and also groups of the learning disabled (Lubs et al 1991). On the basis of this data it appears that learning disabled children may be divided into at least four sub-groups, relative to physical competencies. These include one group who is relatively free of motor problems, and indeed may be able to compensate for academic deficiencies through vigorous and sustained participation in recreational sports, and in related activities.

A second sub-group seems to consist of individuals who evidence motor planning problems along with academic difficulties. There is recent evidence that this sub-type may be pervasive within family complexes (Regehr & Kaplan 1988). A third group may evidence adequate skills and fitness, but require a longer period of time to acquire complex skills because of the presence of dyspraxias of various kinds.

Still another sub-group of the learning disabled may be able to learn skills reasonably well, but lack the muscular and cardiovascular fitness and the coordination needed to fully and vigorously participate in sports and games. This fourth group seems to possess physical capacities that remain under developed, because they apparently lack the motivation to participate in vigorous physical activities. Other more precise data reflecting sub-divisions among groups of awkward children has been reviewed in chapters 5 and 7.

Data from this study indicated that motor planning problems in the learning disabled are pervasive. Rie also refers to the problems learning disabled children have executing complex serial skills. (1987). Important to consider in this data, in addition, is the lack of age-trends in the scores obtained. This finding suggests that basic problems in sequencing may persist in learning disabled populations. If this is true, older learning disabled children and adolescents should also be patiently taught new and complex skills, as is true when dealing with younger children within this type of population. Further longitudinal studies of motor planning abilities and disabilities among this population are currently underway. Longitudinal studies, reviewed in Chapter 13, also substantiate the persistence of motor problems, and neuro-motor soft signs, among groups of clumsy children for as long as ten years.

Overall this and similar data suggest that motor coordination problems are an additional difficulty with which many learning disabled children must contend. Thus helping the learning disabled to improve physically is an important goal to be pursued along with strategies intended to elicit academic competencies. Low and positive correlations between academic scores and motor functions in this investigation, do not indicate that simply modifying motor coordination will magically improve academic competencies.

However, *not attending* to the coordination, fitness, and participation needs of learning disabled children, displaying deficiencies in these task areas, is likely to blunt the self-esteem of youngsters who do not need additional evidence of their incompetencies. The elevation of motor-skill and fitness capacities may have some 'overflow' effect into academic work. However, further research is needed to determine the manner in which the intervening variable, self-esteem, is likely to be positively influenced by the acquisition of increased physical competencies, and then in turn to find out if elevation of the self-concept will positively influence classroom effort and performance. Studies employing path-analyses could be used to illuminate possible chains of causal relationships.

QUESTIONS FOR DISCUSSION

1. How might members of the various sub-groups found within the data of the study on dyspraxia behave, both in classrooms and on the playground?
2. Discuss implications reflected by lack of significant correlations revealed in the studies listed, between tests of motor planning (praxic behavior) and scores reflecting scores from more traditional tests of balance, ball skills, coordination and motor performance capacities.
3. Discuss the lack of correlations between the learning disabled children perceptions of their body size, and their actual body sizes as measured.
5. Why do correlations between reading scores and measures of motor ability not necessarily imply causation? What variables might cause both reading scores and scores reflecting motor abilities to vary slightly in the same directions, as current data indicates?
6. Do meta-analyses of studies demonstrate the validity of the assumption that exposure to a few perceptual-motor tasks will positively change reading and other academic competencies?
7. What does information, and the data, contained in the chapter imply for those attempting to formulate ideal programs of motor development, physical education and athletics, for large and learning disabled populations, containing youngsters with diverse motor, emotional, and intellectual competencies?
8. What does a bi-modal distribution of scores from tests of motor planning, discussed in the chapter, suggest when devising both an ideal academic program and a good physical education program for learning disabled youngsters?

9. What did the apparent lack of age trends in motor planning data presented in the chapter, suggest for helping youngsters to acquire essential and complex academic and self-care skills throughout the life of a learning disabled person?
10. What sex differences were found in the data presented, relative to fitness, self-concept and motor capacities? Might these differences be reflected when devising an ideal physical education and motor development-fitness program?

Chapter 10
Social and Emotional Accompaniments to Poor Motor Coordination

INTRODUCTION

Those studying and chronicling the characteristics and habits of awkward children have been virtually unanimous in the observation that various emotional problems accompany physical ineptitude. It seems logical to assume that negative social feedback and poor self-assessments resulting from the inability to write well in a classroom, coupled with poor play skills, will likely result in lowering awkward children's self-esteem. Much of the available evidence from contemporary, data-based studies is beginning to confirm this hypothesis.

Self-esteem is believed by many to be an important cornerstone of good mental health. Thus it seems reasonable to hypothesize that incoordination accompanies emotional states that are less than adequate. Furthermore, poor feelings about the self often results in undesirable social behaviors, reflecting attempts at over-compensation.

The logical relationships between motor incoordination and poor self-esteem, have inspired several recent studies whose data seems to substantiate this assumption. Data from the studies available, together with field observations, seem to support the conclusion that motor incoordination undermines the formation of an adequate self-concept resulting in immature and insecure social functioning.

DATA-BASED EVIDENCE

The empirical studies available, reflect several approaches to the exploration of possible relationships between mental health and physical coordination. In one type of study comparisons have been made between the self-concept of children labeled clumsy, in contrast to how physically average children report feeling about themselves. In an investigation of this type conducted by me and post-doctoral students several years ago, a questionnaire-type self-concept test was used containing questions reflecting children's' feeling about their appearance and physical ability. The test was originally constructed by Dale Harris and Ellen Piers (1964). (*See Appendix*).

In four of the twenty questions tendered to the 222 male subjects, differences were found between the two populations contrasted (Cratty et al 1972). The awkward boys reported, more often than did the physically adequate boys, that they were sad most of the time, that they did not believe themselves, strong, and that they would rather watch than play games. A significantly larger percent of the awkward boys also reported that reading was not easy for them. This final finding perhaps reflects the presence of a significant percent of boys with learning difficulties often found within populations of awkward children.

It is interesting to note that, in the same study, contrasting the responses of awkward girls, to those with average physical coordination, no significant differences were found between the percentages offering 'low self-concept responses' to the various questions. This lack of difference may have occurred because at the time the study was conducted (1972) the self-concept of females was not as predicated upon physical prowess as was true among young boys.

A student and I recently followed up this 1972 investigation with another, using a highly similar questionnaire. (Dalrahim & Cratty 1990). Eighty-three awkward boys, averaging 6.3 years of age, were polled relative to the feelings they had about themselves, and how they felt about their physical appearance and ability. These were children, whom we had evaluated during the past thirty-six months at our clinic and averaged delays of from 1 to 1.5 years in physical coordination. The scores of 17 awkward girls were used in the same study, using the same questionnaire. They averaged 6.5 years of age, and also were delayed physically from one to two years.

Of the twenty questions there were marked differences in the percent of low-self-concept responses on the questions indicated in Figure10-1 below. Contrasted are responses of normal subjects in the 1972 study (Cratty et al) to the responses of awkward populations polled in the 1990 study.

In this second study, the questionnaire contained a query about whether they tired easily in games. It was interesting to note that 41% of the awkward boys and 65% of the awkward girls reported that they experienced high levels of fatigue when confronted with vigorous physical activity. (Dalrahim & Cratty 1990).

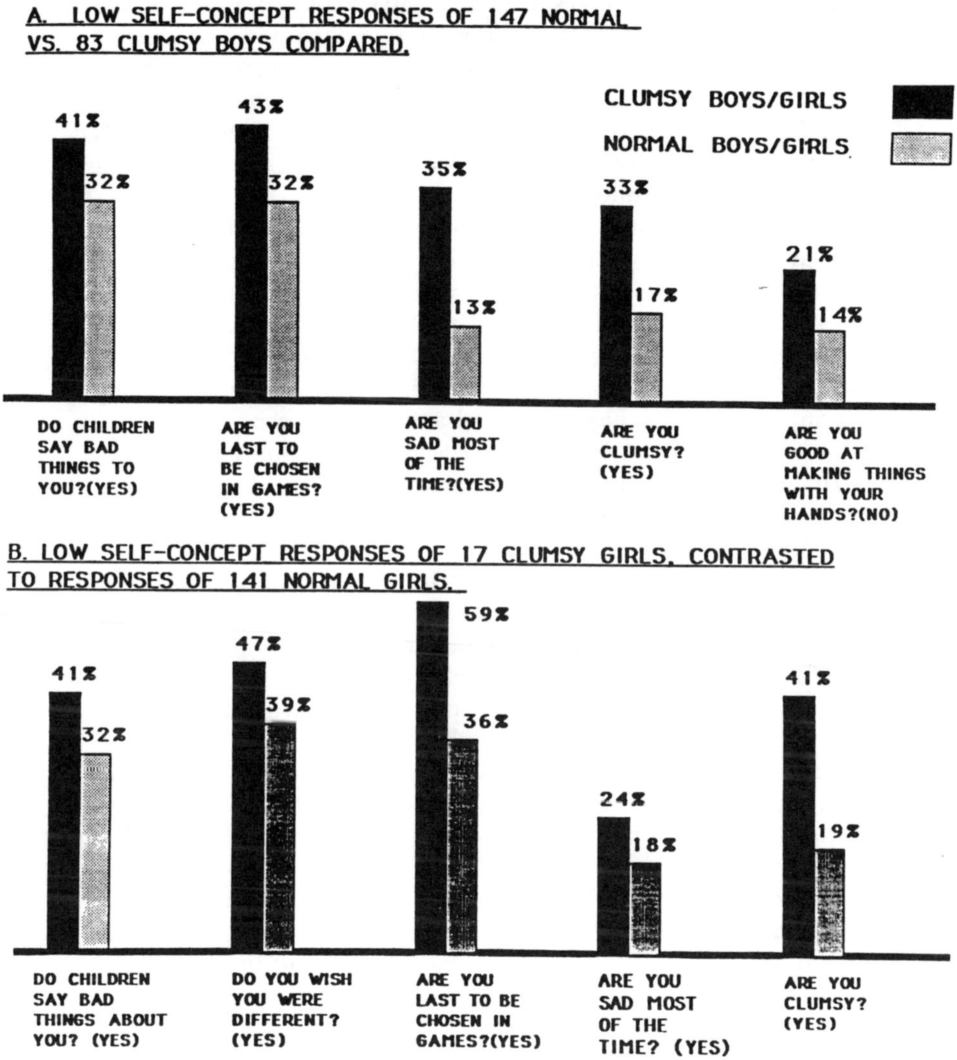

Table 10-1. Comparisons of selected responses on a self-concept test, administered to clumsy children (1990 study) and to normal controls (1972 study)

In second type of investigation, comparisons are made of the motor competencies of children within various atypical groups. Including in these have been groups of children labeled learning disabled, the mildly and moderately retarded, and the emotionally disturbed. Two of these studies are located in administrative manuals accompanying tests for physical awkwardness in children. (Bruininks 1978) (Stott and Henderson 1972).

Data D.H. Stott and his colleagues obtained data from children labeled "emotionally unstable" (1972). One of the purposes Stott stated for his motor test battery, was to provide an "independent means of measuring subtle neurological impairments such as could affect behavioral adjustment". To determine if his battery accomplished this goal, comparisons were made of children evidencing varying degrees of emotional mal-adjustment based upon their scores from *The Bristol Social Adjustment Guide* (Stott and Marston 1971). The criteria for mal-adjustment in this study (Stott and Marston 1971), were those scoring in the lower 10%, within six categories of disturbances.

Stott found that emotionally disturbed population identified was over represented among awkward children. Hostility score were found to be closely associated with motor impairment, as were scores reflecting the tendencies to both over-react to the environment, and to under-react and behave in overly passive ways in social situations. Stott found that 'inconsequence' (failure to inhibit impulses) was the quality most highly associated with motor impairment. The scores Stott obtained from the Bristol Social Adjustment Guide also correlated with mean scores from the tests of motor impairment administered.

Summarizing this work, Stott pointed out that three times as many mal-adjusted children, compared to well adjusted youngsters, were motorically impaired: and likewise three and a half times as many motorically impaired youngster, as compared to motorically normal children, were maladjusted. (Stott et al 1976).

The data from other, more contemporary, studies by Hulme and his colleagues (Hulme et al 1982) (Abbie et al 1978) and Henderson and Hall (1982) also indicate motor ability tests can statistically discriminate between groups of emotionally normal youngsters and groups of youngsters evidencing various psychiatric syndromes. Data from additional investigations, including those by van Rossum and Vermeer (1990) and Kalvergboer and his colleagues (199) and others (Henderson et al (1989) also indicate that there are strong links between physical awkwardness, low self-esteem, and social problems.

Factor analyses have also been conducted containing tests reflecting both emotional qualities and movement qualities, including tests of coordination and motor 'soft signs.' The data from these also point to associations between social-psychological stability and movement competencies. For example in a study by Nichols (1987) tests of hyperactivity, emotional stability, and attention span loaded in a factor containing scores from two drawing tests. Thus the overall picture from this and similar studies is that motor ineptitude likely causes various symptoms reflecting emotional upset.

The relationships between emotional instability and motor impairment may be circular. Stott, for example, suggested that the inter-active relationships he found were due to the presence of general types of neurological impairments that may influenced *both* motor and emotional qualities in the youngsters he evaluated. The correlations found in the studies that have been reviewed, thus require close scrutiny in order to determine possible causal relationships present, and the direction of the causation.

Some believe, therefore, that valid data demonstrating possible causal relationships between motor ineptitude and emotional health is lacking (Duele & Robinson 1987). For example, general neurological problems and emotional instability may, in some children underlie both hyperactivity (usually viewed as a sign of poor emotional health) and motor incoordination. Hyperactivity, coupled with a tendency not to remain long at various motor tasks, may result simply because a child does not wish to be exposed to the sustained scorn and ridicule of teachers and peers in situations requiring physical performance. Finally hyperactivity and inattention, qualities common both to groups of emotionally disturbed and motorically inept children, also may impede the execution of motor skills when they are presented in a test battery requiring prolonged periods of time to complete. For example, both Henderson and Hall (1982) Hulme and his colleagues (1982) pointed out that emotionally disturbed children they assessed often took longer, than did normal children, to accomplish most tasks. This tendency is typically found among emotionally disturbed youngsters whether confronting physical challenges classrooms, or in competitive and recreational sports.

Data from a few studies are now beginning to illuminate the possibility of modifying emotional states by exposing awkward children to remedial program. In recent work by Laszlo and her colleagues, for example direct evidence was obtained of 'dramatic' changes in social-emotional behaviors occurring among children exposed to a program, that also produced parallel and positive changes in their physical skills. (Laszlo et al 1988).

Most encouraging, however, are the recent appearance of longitudinal studies. Investigators are beginning to survey, not only motor characteristics, but also the emotional states of youngsters assessed during several testing sessions taking place throughout the formative years of life. These studies are obtaining evidence obtained during significant time periods within the lives of the young subjects studied. In one of the first of these it was found that, while some awkward children improve over time, many continue to have difficulties, of several types, well into their teens (Gillberg & Gillberg 1989).

A comprehensive, longitudinal study was published recently by Anne Losse and her colleagues. They compared measures of emotional health and physical coordination, obtained from thirty-two youngsters at both their sixth and sixteenth years of life. They found strong evidence that the youngsters surveyed continued to have motor problems, attracting the attention of those attempting to teach them motor skills during this entire decade of their lives. During the several testing sessions necessary to complete this study, it was also observed that many displayed 'intense personal feelings of failure' throughout this ten year period.

It was concluded by Losse and her helpers, that clumsiness is not a benign disorder confined to childhood, but rather awkwardness continues into the teens. Their data also made it clear that persistent and measurable evidence of motor ineptitude during the years the study took place, was accompanied by feelings of social inadequacy among mos t of the youngsters taking part in the study. However they also observed that among some subjects who had been extended continuous and effective parental support, symptoms of poor emotional health were significantly reduced, and in some cases apparently eliminated (Losse et al 1991).

The available data from both correlative and longitudinal investigations thus strongly suggest that motor ineptitude both causes, and is accompanied by, low self-esteem and associated social adjustment problems in many children and adolescents for significant time periods during their formative years. Motor task performances constitute concrete, and observable, measures of competency, or of incompetency. A youngster who cannot perform well thus sees vivid evidence of his or her failings, and concurrently receives negative social feedback from observing peers, parents, and teachers. Thus both self-perceptions and the social judgements of others combine to lower the self-esteem of many awkward children and adolescents.

The values in various school-play settings, and at home, likely influence the amount of social punishment incurred by awkward children. In a home setting in which physical competence is highly valued, for example, the awkward child's self-concept is likely to suffer more than if he or she is being reared in a home environment in which physical prowess is not as important as performance in other arenas. However it is becoming increasingly clear that continued and sustained negative reinforcement from those surrounding the child, will likely result in the youngster's poor emotional health coupled with symptoms reflecting a low self-concept. Moreover the youngster will likely engage in various compensations and avoidance behaviors that are likely to be viewed as signs of less-than-adequate emotional health. In the following section the nature and meaning of some of these compensations are explored.

CLINICAL OBSERVATIONS OF COMPENSATION AND AVOIDANCE STRATEGIES

A number of compensatory behaviors reflecting inadequate social-emotional adjustment are likely to be exhibited by awkward children. Parents, professions in clinics, and teachers are among those whose best efforts are often thwarted by these, often abrasive, ways in which awkward children act. These compensations and avoidance strategies are at times subtle, and at other times obvious. In either case, how these behaviors are expressed, and the forms they take are both important to consider, when assessing and providing programs for children with coordination problems.

Engaging in these strategies serve several important needs on the part of a clumsy youngster:

(1) A compensation sometimes reflects the child's attempts to totally avoid situations in which physical performance will be required;

(2) A another group of behaviors that are seen within performance situations the child has not been successful in avoiding. Thus while on the playground the child finds ways of not actually participating.

(3) Still a third type involves ways clumsy children have of modifying both their own performance and performance demands so that they have a chance to succeed, but on their own terms.

Often an awkward child will engage in several of these avoidances-compensations, in quick succession, or at different times throughout a single day. A compensation or compensations may be selectively used when an awkward child is confronted with specific demands made by adults, children and by various situations encountered. That is many youngsters will learn to carefully match a specific compensations to various demands and stresses. It is typically found that each child favors one or more of these compensations, and consistently relies upon them. Some of the more common of these compensations are discussed in the following paragraphs.

School Phobias and Similar Problems

Some poorly coordinated children may attempt to avoid school attendance completely. They may do this for various reasons, including the knowledge that they must take a fitness test in their physical education class that day. Upon arising in the morning their effort to avoid school may range from claiming illness, to 'throwing' temper tantrums. Their protestations may even be accompanied by measurable medical symptoms. They may become nauseous when contemplating their school day, and accompany these feelings with pleas to remain at home. These, and other symptoms may be exhibited by poorly coordinated children who believe that their school day will reveal physical incompetence, either in unstructured play situations, or when confronting specific tasks within structured physical education settings.

School phobic reactions may occur intermittently, or be seen every morning, or be expressed in anxious talk at the end of a school day. Their causes may transcend needs to avoid physical activity, and may include important medical and/or psychological symptoms that should not be ignored. The frequent occurrence of these avoidance symptoms are often indications that something is indeed wrong, and that an emotional health specialist should be consulted. School personnel also should be contacted, to determine what components of the school program may be triggering the phobic reactions displayed.

Similar avoidance reactions may be displayed in other settings. For example, when an awkward child returns home from school and believes that it is likely play with neighborhood children may be required, he or she may plead illness, fatigue, and spend the afternoon by the television set or at the computer. Birthday parties, when games are about to be engaged in, may constitute another place in which avoidance compensations are exhibited. In this setting, poorly coordinated children may cling to their parents, to avoid game participation.

The classroom ares still another setting in which avoidance reactions may be displayed. At school the awkward child often voices the wish to remain in the classroom at recess, and help the teacher. Thus many seemingly amenable "teacher's' helpers" are, in reality, poorly coordinated youngsters, evidencing the avoidance of physical activities at recess.

Avoidance reactions, reflected in anxious talk by an awkward, have been reported to us by some parents as occurring just prior to entering our clinic program. During the program, the child may often function well and participate fully. Afterward, however, these parents also report that their offspring's avoidance reactions quickly resume. Thus avoidance reactions and phobias, including negative feelings about both clinic and school situations, may be heard and observed both prior to or after potentially stressful performance situations are likely to be encountered.

Learned Helplessness and Infantilization

One of the most pervasive, and potentially harmful, compensations involves the display of learned helplessness. Infantilization may be partly the reflection of inappropriate caretaker behaviors, including the tendency of some mothers and father to unknowingly reward "babyish" behaviors. Infantile behaviors arise from the fact that developmentally delayed children often are subtly rewarded for their incompetence and inabilities to perform physical tasks well.

The problem can also stem from an attitude, adopted by the clumsy child, that most of what he or she attempts will likely be unsuccessful. Thus they give up trying when confronted with physical performance situations. If not encouraged by caretakers to try to accomplish various motor tasks, over time helpless feelings become more pronounced.

Symptoms within this general pattern of helpless include displaying immature play patterns, and a disinclination to attempt or to persist at motor tasks. These symptoms may even include delays of speech and language. Infantile speech patterns are common among children who have learned to be physically helpless. Signs of social and emotional immaturity displayed by an infantilized child may include frequent temper tantrums, thumb sucking and similar behaviors that are not age appropriate.

The three year old who simply points and yells for objects, rather than asking for them, is displaying another type of infantile behavior. The six year old who requires the maid to dress him/her every morning is also exhibiting a sign of learned helplessness. This syndrome also may be exhibited by a child of eight or nine years, who remains in a sandbox playing in isolation or with one playmate, rather than participating in group games with complex rules and requirements that are expected of youngsters in middle childhood.

This pattern of behavior, if continually reinforced, will persist into adolescence. Parents who continue to refuse to demand mature behavior and performance will likely produce psychologically and physically helpless teenagers. It is striking to observe these symptoms evidenced by some adolescent learning disabled adolescents, for example.

This pattern of behavior is often seen when evaluating children in our clinical program. For example, when asked to draw a simple geometric figure the child evidencing infantile helplessness may make light marks that are barely discernable on paper, while failing to form the diagram correctly. The pencil marks made may consist of light swipings, that are difficult to see, executed as the pencil is held in a limp-fisted grip. The helpless syndrome is also discussed within the chapter 7 dealing with Dysgraphia.

Other signs may appear when a helpless child is confronted with motor tasks. For example, a ball may be passively dropped at his or her feet when a child, who has learned to be helpless, is asked to "throw the ball as hard as you can." If these symptoms of learned helplessness persist during the application of a remedial program, clinicians' best efforts are likely to be sabotaged. On the other hand if the youngster is made to feel adequate and effective during initial remedial sessions, progress in skill acquisition is often the result. Thus often we have such children learn to tackle a dummy, and in other ways engage in vigorous and sometimes aggressive behaviors, so that they learn that they can have an effect on something (knocking down the dummy) rather than being a passive and helpless person.

Learned helpless is likely to be engendered by parent reactions, and also by the responses of others with whom the child comes in contact. Some caretakers may have needs to keep their child dependent on them, and to exercise their parenting and caretakers roles in distorted and exaggerated ways. Essentially often caretakers reward their offspring for signs of incompetence, and for immature babyish behaviors.

These rewards may be extended to the child in a variety of subtle ways. For example, increased parental concern is engendered when the child evidences delays, a concern which the child observes, and may enjoy. Thus if possible, parents should correct infantile behaviors they observe, in a non-judgmental and unemotional manner. Frequent parental arguments about how to 'handle' the child's problems are often rewarding to the observing offspring. Thus parents should try to set goals for mature behavior that both are able to agree upon, while their child is not in attendance.

Visits to numerous professionals in efforts to evaluate and to remediate the problem may also serve to sustain infantile and inappropriate behaviors. Thus care should be taken not to over-evaluate such children. Observing the often dramatic effects upon powerful adults with which they are surrounded, motorically delayed children may persist and evidence less-than-mature performance delays in a variety of tasks required of them in both social and in educational situations.

Perhaps most vexing to clinicians are some parents who have somehow send their awkward children the message that it is cute or otherwise desirable that they are clumsy. This type of parental reaction at times accompanies reluctance to enter their child in a remedial program. This same parent may suddenly withdraw their immature offspring from such interventions when it is seen that progress is being made! This remarkable behavior is engaged in when the helplessness that both child and parent somehow value, and the latter has nurtured, seems to be in danger of being overcome by the appearance of positive changes!

It has been our experience over the past thirty years, that the appearance of symptoms signaling learned helplessness are more the rule than the exception among young, motorically delayed children. Typically a five-year-old, will display the motor development of a four year old, and then may be further delayed socially, emotionally, and linguistically, still another year by social forces promoting infantilization.

Generally the caretakers of these youngsters are observed to 'operate' at two levels when approaching those who purportedly may help their child. At the conscious level, they seek out professional advice, evaluation and remedial programs; while at a second level, of which they may not be aware, they undermine the professional advice, and the best efforts of clinicians in remedial programs. For decades the appearance of this kind of helpless behavior by young children has proved highly frustrating to both teachers and to clinicians who come in contact with developmentally delayed children, including the physically awkward.

The answer to this problem is usually intensive family therapy, so that the mother and other caretakers are provided a mirror in which they may view the ways they are rewarding, and thus maintaining, their offspring's helpless and ineffectual behaviors. After gaining an awareness of how their parenting practices influence their children, attempts should then be made to modify these behaviors. However, often 'selling' the need for such therapy is a task that professionals contacting parents are not always able to accomplish.

Comedic Behaviors and Other Types of Compensatory Verbalization

Within play situations, the awkward child runs the risk of not been noticed. Being overlooked may appear to such children to be a form of punishment worse than receiving ridicule. Thus the uncoordinated youngster often makes an effort to make the other children know they exist. One strategy is to use an excess of verbal behaviors at play, and in other situations. These verbal behaviors may include:

(1) A constant attempt to be funny, by engaging in excess comedic behaviors.

(2) Compensatory bravado, consisting of statements that express an overly self-confident demeanor, "I can make the Olympic Team!".

(3) Constantly voicing statements that have nothing to do with a play situation.

(4) Verbal pre-occupation with the rules, acting like a 'playground attorney'.

At times this excess verbiage ('hyperverbalization') may become abrasive to the uncoordinated children's playmates. However, this hyperverbal behavior may persist, serving several purposes including:

(1) Excess words assisting the awkward child to be noticed, despite the fact that this attention is often accompanied by negative social evaluations,

(2) Excess barrages of words may help the awkward child stave off the need for performing, to 'wall off' others who attempt to interact with them physically. This second purpose often surfaces in our clinic program both when the child is evaluated, and later during initial remedial sessions. We have found that the chatter of the poorly coordinated youngster can be shrill, voluminous and constant. Usually suppressing this extraneous verbiage is usually necessary before significant improvements occur in physical skill within remedial and educational settings.

The content of hyperverbalizations varies. This excess chatter may consist of persistent attempts to joke and be funny, including making fun of the play situation and of other children. At other times this hyperverbal behavior consists of intellectualizations, about the skills required or about other aspects of the games. Still another focus of this chatter may be upon rules and their interpretation. In this latter case the awkward child may sound like a youthful attorney, while engaging in sophisticated arguments about scores, rules and the like. This type of verbal behavior thus may also effectively block requirements to exhibit physical skills in the games confronting the youngster

When working with awkward children emitting these excessively verbal compensations, several strategies may be pursued. At times the effusive statements may be ignored. At other times it may be pointed out that too many words interfere with good play. In our clinic we have had success with the initiation of rewards systems For example we often give a colorful sticker if, the child is able to suppress excess verbal activity for increased periods of time. If these kinds of compensatory verbiage are carried to excess, the child must be directly confronted with the need to stop talking and to perform. At the same time the chattering youngster may be informed as to the reasons he or she is behaving in these ways, and that the verbiage is neither socially attractive nor performance enhancing Often the reduction of these verbal compensations is a valid clue that real skill improvement is taking place and is often accompanied by positive changes in the child's self-confidence.

Aggression

Lacking adequate play skills, awkward children sometimes engage in excess physical and/or psychological aggression against others. Sometimes this aggression appears in the form of verbal abuse, or even of obscenities directed toward peers. At other times aggression may consist of simply chasing weaker or younger children around the playground. At still other times, direct physical aggression is engaged in. Case studies of young adults who have evidenced marked sociopathic behaviors often contain scenarios of how, as children, they lacked adequate play skills, and thus began to take out their frustrations in the form of aggressive vengeance against others.

One theory about the formation of aggressive feelings rests upon the triggering role of frustration. Most competitive sports and rules are formulated so that one person, or team wins and another loses (what social psychologists term a sum-zero condition). Losing is usually frustrating, so that it may be postulated that the frequent losing experienced by awkward children (or the potential to do so) is likely to raise levels of both frustration and thus heighten aggression.

Within a clinical setting we often encounter overly aggressive children who lack adequate play skills. Care has to be taken to introduce them to skills in which they have a chance to succeed. At the same time we have to avoid any hint of competitiveness in the situation, except with themselves, as they attempt to improve in various tasks. Furthermore, cooperative games may be played, in which two children cooperate to, for example, keep a ball in play in volleyball or handball. (Orlick 1978).

This frustration-aggression chain may be seen as awkward children attempt to place their thoughts on paper, and fail badly to adequately execute writing skills. It is critical, when working with awkward children, to first limit and then eliminate excess aggression that many emit in social-play situations. Various forms of anger may be directed at teachers, parents and/or at peers. Aggression may also be reduced by the institution of psycho-therapy, for both the child and to the parents. Helping parents to understand what is likely to reward and punish these unwanted aggressive behaviors can also prove useful.

Retreat to Academia (Into the Computer!)

As is true of all of us, awkward children do not persist in tasks in which they lack skills, but instead veer toward achievement areas in which they believe success is likely. Negative self criticism and punitive social criticism, as well as positive evaluations from others, mold the performance routes we all take in life. It is thus not unexpected, to find poorly coordinated children finding other ways to express their personalities than by participation in physically demanding games. Among the detours uncoordinated youngsters take is to engage in academic activity, and also to explore the fascinating worlds offered by their computers. Either of these two routes may be taken compulsively, or be entered into in more relaxed ways.

Awkward children thus may become super memorizers of facts. They may become avid collectors of various kinds of objects, and/or become 'experts' at early ages within a narrow or broad scientific subject-area.

It be could be argued that the faculties of many major universities consist of an inordinate number of individuals who, as children, were less than adequate in play situations. Instead these future academicians began, in sensible ways, to devote their energies to expanding their intellectual strengths rather than remaining on playgrounds and athletic fields to encounter the ridicule of their peers. Youngsters growing up do not always 'buy' the concept of becoming "well-rounded", by acquiring a balance of both physical and intellectual skills. Rather they will typically enter performance realms in which they are likely to be rewarded and avoid arenas in which they are likely to encounter failure.

This type of intellectual compensation is thus one of the more socially desirable strategies a clumsy child make employ when frustrations are encountered, as they attempt to master physical skills. Proper guidance, as this type of compensation is seen, becomes easier if the child is given a complete battery of tests including those measuring academic potential and ability. In this way the intellectual pressures that may be 'handled' by the child within academic contexts may be measured and educational plans may be gauged accordingly. Practical educational judgements have to be made about just how much physical activity and what kinds of physical activities in which a highly intellectual, but awkward, child should be encouraged to engage. Often it is appropriate to interest a youngster evidencing this type of compensation in the physiological underpinnings of physical activity. They may therefore sometimes focus their intellect upon the mechanisms within their body that are activated during exercise and begin to engage in sports and exercises. These youngsters sometimes find that individual sports, and endurance activities are more attractive than those which requiring them to confront the prowess of physically more adequate peers. Creative and intelligent, but awkward, children may also participate in the formation of their own developmental programs and games, a subject that has been discussed elsewhere. (Cratty 1988) and in books (Cratty 1974, 1986)

OVERVIEW

Acquiring adequate emotional development by awkward children is made difficult for various reasons. They are likely to experience constant negative social evaluations from their playmates, and siblings. Their parents may react to them in ways that often confuse them. Their fathers and mothers can exhibit behaviors that may include, denial that their problem exists. Caretakers may unknowingly extend rewards for passive delayed behaviors. Parents may become angry, and/or express too much concern about imperfections their youngsters may exhibit. Moreover those in positions to help poorly coordinated youngsters, including classroom and physical education teachers, may display continual irritation at their clumsiness, and/or less-then-adequate teaching skills. (Losse et al 1991).

Family values about the importance of physical prowess differ markedly, ranging from a high emphasis upon sporting activities, to values among family members who other forms of success, including artistic and/or academic attainment. These and other differences in family values interact with at least three components of the youngsters self-concept, components that include feelings about physical ability, social competence, and intellectual attainment. (Harter 1981).

It could be hypothesized, therefore, that the most marked feelings of inferiority are engendered in physically inept children whose family members place high values upon physical prowess and skills. In contrast, less negative feelings may be engendered by families whose members are not as enthusiastic about sports, but reward success other types of endeavors. It also may be true that in family complexes in which physical skill is highly valued, the most marked changes will occur in the child's self-concept when their children's physical abilities undergo improvement.

However it is difficult to find American families whose members do not value academic achievement. Thus when physical awkwardness involves exhibiting inaccurate printing and writing, most parents members take quickly heed, and begin to evidence marked concern. The dysgraphic child thus may encounter more social pressure in many homes, than does the youngster who cannot play games well.

The simple axiom that an improvement in physical skill will result in a heightened self-concept needs careful examination. Continued negative social feedback from family members directed toward an awkward child, whose skills may be improving, can serve to maintain a persistent low self-concept. Improvement of physical skill within a remedial setting needs to be accompanied by change in family members' perceptions of the awkward child, in order to produce real changes in how the awkward youngster perceives himself or herself. Losse and her colleagues emphasize the importance of good parent understanding and support, in the production of emotional health among awkward children, in her recent longitudinal study. (1991). I know of one program in which the youngster's skill changes are carefully explained and illustrated to family members, in order to stimulate positive social feedback from them. (Morris 1985).

The compensations that awkward children evidence, while irritating unusual and bizarre, constitute what could be construed as the only rational ways to behave in situations that to them are irrational and perceived as unfair. It may be useful to first evaluate the physical coordination of various children in a large school by visiting the playground and observing avoidance behaviors. After this initial screening the children identified might be exposed to formal motor testing. For decades a principal in an elementary school year UCLA, referred children to my program, based upon her the compensations she observed among youngsters on her school's playground. The objective evidence we then obtained, after assessing these childrens' physical skills, invariably confirmed this principal's insightful observations.

Most important, upon consideration of the social-emotional accompaniments to physical awkwardness, are the following principles:

(1) Those conducting program intending to improve physical skill should become aware of how the children in their charge will attempt to avoid direct tutoring efforts, and should adjust teaching behaviors program accordingly. The compensations discussed reveal the real threat that physical activities pose for physically uncoordinated children.

(2) Program content should be carefully devised so that the difficulty level permit measures of personal success, rather than producing failure and frustration.

(3) Children brought to a program of motor remediation may require extensive psychological or psychiatric evaluation intervention. Thus often youngsters should be referred to mental health specialists, rather than only focusing upon motor skill enhancement.

As has been pointed out earlier, there are both obvious and subtle interactions between perceived success in physical tasks, and good mental health. However, the contention that skill improvement will inevitably result in better mental health is simplistic. Enhancing physical skills may, however, make a significant contribution to the mental health of many awkward youngsters. The evidence collected by Losse and her colleagues (1991) strongly suggests that unless both good parental support is extended, and effective educational interventions are obtained, emotional stress is likely to be a persistent accompaniment of motor ineptitude for a good part of the lives of many awkward children.

QUESTIONS FOR DISCUSSION

1. What chain of events results in both acting out compensations and evidence of low self-esteem among learning disabled youngsters? Can you diagram these relationships?
2. What kinds of compensations are seen on the playground, and in other contexts by youngsters seeking to avoid physical activity in which they are likely to incur failure? Which of these seem useful, and which are not?
3. What might you do to re-direct a negative social compensation expressed by a clumsy child, into a positive behavior or attitude? Be specific, just what would you do?
4. What forms might hyper-verbalization take? As an instructor In a remedial program, how might you reduce the amount of extraneous verbiage engaged in by a poorly coordinated child?
5. What kinds of tests are explained in the chapter, with which to obtain self-concept data from youngsters? Do you know of other types used? Can you locate other kinds of assessment instruments within the literature?
6. What forms might 'school phobia' take? How and when would evidence of school

phobia appear? What might be done to reduce or eliminate school phobias due to the need of the child to avoid physical activity or physical ability testing?

7. What forms might pseudo-play, as an avoidance behavior, take when an awkward child is faced with various sports situations?
8. A child's self-esteem may be differentiated into at least three components: including the social self-esteem, academic self-perceptions, and feelings about physical ability and appearance. Discuss the interaction of differing family values and these three components of the self-esteem seen among various groups of children.
9. How might reasonable goal setting help to bolster the self-esteem of an awkward child? How might re-location of an awkward child to another playground, school, or neighborhood either hinder or help his or her self-esteem.
10. Might there be sex differences in the manner in which awkward children react emotionally to limitations in their physical-coordination? What would you hypothesize these differences might consists of?
11. Discuss the possible dynamics of parent-child interactions that result in a child feeling and acting helpless in physical performance situation.

Chapter 11
Evaluation and Assessment

INTRODUCTION

Historical Perspectives

Effective evaluation of the numerous medical and psycho-social facets of human beings is both an art and a science. Meaningful assessment requires a philosophy that reflects a healthy combination both of mature sensitivity and the scrutiny of data emanating from available scientific tools. Attempting to 'get a handle' on the complex behaviors emanating from an awkward child thus requires not only the collection of test scores and observations, but a penetrating interpretation of the evidence within the social and cultural ecology unique to each youngster.

Over three thousand years ago administrators of some oriental cities gave intelligence tests to ferret out potentially useful civil servants. The scientific awakening of Western Europe in the 16th century, encouraged scholars to measure various dimensions of the physical and biological world. The first physical measures of humans including height and weight. For example, in 1830 Quentelet a Belgium astronomer and statistician, measured the sizes of soldiers in Napoleon's army. He found that the scores arranged themselves in a "normal curve" with the majority of the measures clustering around the average, with fewer scores at the extremes. He then conducted a longitudinal study of children's heights. (Scammon 1927).

Throughout the remainder of the 1800s other testing programs began to focus upon other human abilities. In the 1880's directors of the first experimental psychology laboratories in Europe and in the United States devoted a large part of their energies to measuring motor qualities, such as reaction time and movement speed. The measurement of coordination represented the first attempts to survey intelligence of both adults and children. These early psychologists based these efforts upon a "faculty theory of intelligence". They postulated that the possession of good physical qualities, such as a fast reaction time, were signs of well-functioning nervous systems, that also enable people to think effectively. The extensive use of movement tests resulted in these early efforts becoming labeled 'motor psychology'. Thus during the last century the assessment of physical abilities formed an important part of efforts expended by the first experimental psychologists.

In the late 1870s Alfred Binet formulated the first intelligence tests for children developed in Western Society. He felt the need for more precise measures of mental retardation, after observing the then common practice of assigning children to schools for the retarded, following a brief interview by a medical doctor. Prominent components of Binet's test included printing and drawing tasks. These same motor tasks are presently found in contemporary versions of Binet's efforts (The Stanford-Binet), as well as in other modern tests of children's cognitive functions, including the Weschler Intelligence Test for Children. Currently a thorough evaluation of intelligence thus results in scores reflecting both verbal intelligence, and performance intelligence. The latter sub-score reflects the extent to which youngsters' perceptual and motor characteristics met expected age norms.

At the beginning of the second decade of the present century, at the Neurological Institute in Moscow, the first tests were formulated whose purposes were to assess motor coordination in children. In 1920 Nicholas Oseretsky constructed a battery of tests to evaluate what he labeled 'motor idiocy'. During the following decades Oseretsky's test stimulated the development of similar instruments in numerous countries of the world, (Sloan 1955) (Bailer, Doll & Winsberg 1973). In the 1970's, and the 1980's modifications of Oseretsky's battery, in the United States have resulted in tests formulated for use with populations of awkward children. (Stott and Henderson 1984) (Bruinink 1976).

Several scholars have factor analyzed various versions of Oseretsky's original test, in order to determine the basic qualities that groups of the sub-tests are actually assessing. (Thams 1955). Others have formulated useful shorter versions of Oseretsky's original instrument (Beitel & Mead 1980). Data from several contemporary versions of the Oseretsky have been used to illuminate the assessment strategies, discussed later in this chapter.

The formulation of precise criteria for the identification of clumsy children from within normal populations however, presents several problems measurement problems. In the 1979 study by Keogh and his students, for example, it was found, that there was a lack of agreement when comparisons were made between information gained from a movement test battery, and observational data from a teacher-administered checklist, after both measures were applied to the same first grade children (Keogh et al 1979). Laszlo and Bairstow have also alluded to the difficulties when trying to locate effective evaluative instruments to assess the movement characteristics of children (Lazslo & Bairstow 1986).

Several factor analyses of motor ability traits conducted from the 1940s to the present are helpful in the identification of basic motor qualities, in both children and adults. The most prominent and useful of these programs of research was an extensive series of studies conducted by Edwin Fleishman and his colleagues, stemming from work during World War II, among air-force pilot trainees. Toward this program's latter stages, Fleishman and helpers began to focus on skill-families that depended upon the adequate functioning of both larger and smaller muscle groups. In 1965 Fleishman published an evaluation instrument, based upon test scores obtained upon 20,000 youthful subjects. The resulting assessment battery was 'factor pure', that is each sub-test was designed to evaluate a separate and independent motor quality. (Fleishman 1965).

Other scholars during the 1970s focused upon the basic motor qualities found among different groups of children. G. Lawrence Rarick at the University of California at Berkeley completed a comprehensive factor analytic study in 1976 to identify motor ability sub-groups among both retarded and normal children. The youngsters were divided into two age classifications. The first ranged from six to nine years. An older group was from ten through thirteen years of age. (Rarick et al 1976). Forty six tests were given. Measures of physical size, body composition as well as of muscular flexibility, strength, and motor coordination were employed. Manual abilities were also tested for. After the scores were factor analyzed, several ability groupings were identified.

Rarick identified six factors common to the various sub-groups, and also that were similar in analyses of both boys and girls. These factors were identified as:

(a) *Strength and body size:* containing tests of biking against resistance, and also height and weight.

(b) *Gross limb–eye coordination:* including target softball throwing.

(c) *Fine visual motor coordination:* included tests of peg manipulation, and tapping.

(d) *Fat or Dead Weight:* including measures of skin fold thickness, and of trunk width.

(e) *Balance:* including both moving and static balancing tasks.

(f) *Leg-power and Coordination:* the inter-correlated tests making-up this factor included running speed in a 35 yard dash, and the height of a vertical jump.

Data from these types of analyses are essential when formulating valid test batteries. Components of remedial programs for awkward children have also been identified through the application of factor analytic techniques.

During the past two decades a number of neurological evaluations have been formulated with which to assess the presence of movement related 'neurological soft-signs'. These subtle signs of neurological dysfunction were first observed and written about at the end of the last century. It has only been within the last twenty years, however, that attempts have been made to objectively evaluate, classify and draw meaning from their presence. These minor signs reflect dysfunction of the nervous system, and are not usually accompanied by easily diagnosable lesions, tumors and other.

The content of these specially designed neurological evaluations include tests of synkinesia (associated movements), dyspraxia, sensory awareness, variations in muscle tonus, gait characteristics, balance, and various measures of motor coordination. Most of the research conducted with these instruments has been descriptive, rather than experimental. (*See Tupper 1987 for a survey*) A comprehensive factor analysis by Nichols (1987) and an investigation involving several thousand children, conducted within an island community, by Rutter (Rutter et al 1970) are among the most useful studies of these subtle indicators of neuromotor dysfunction.

The interpreting the results obtained from these special neurological 'schedules' often proves vexing and presents both practical and theoretical problems. For example, the signs observed are often transitory, thus making their reliable measurement tenuous. (Hertzig & Shapiro 1987). Further, arguments have arisen as to how these symptoms should be grouped and classified. Finally, and perhaps most important, the presence of these 'soft' motor signs have often proved difficult to interpret within an acceptable neurological model.

It is usually found, however, that a one or more of these soft-signs are over-represented in sub-groups of atypical children including the hyperactive, among the learning disabled, and when assessing psychiatrically unstable groups. The ways in which these relationships should be interpreted, both when assessing neurological functions and planning programs, remain elusive, however. There are controversies as to just what measures should be included within a list of 'soft-signs'. Reviews of these data and the issues involved may be found in the book by Tupper (1987); while definitional issues may be examined in the book by Small 1982) and in an article by Tupper (1986).

CONTEMPORARY GUIDELINES

Professionals from various disciplines may evaluate movement behaviors of children. These include pediatricians, neurologists, orthopedists, psychologists, educational therapists, occupational therapists, physical therapists, and physical educators. Members of these diverse groups, as might be expected, often display various purposes for sampling these qualities in youngsters. These numerous professionals also take one, or a combination of, several avenues when evaluating motor coordination.

For example the usual reasons for a medical-neurological evaluation is to determine the presence of possible pathologies within the central or peripheral nervous system. Professionals in the psychiatric and psychological communities may observe movement behaviors in order to gain additional insights into the mental and emotional health of young clients. Educators of various persuasions may assess motor abilities in order to derive motor (developmental) age levels, that reside within various ability groups. This information then is often used to formulate useful remedial programs.

Types of Evaluation Tools

There are several other dimensions to evaluation and diagnostic programs that should be considered. These include operational and scientific concerns, as well as philosophical considerations. For example potentially useful assessment instruments may range from general checklists on which the presence or absence of the execution a motor act is noted, to more precise tools. Some may contain tasks that may appear within several type of numerical ratings. These scoring systems may range from 1–100, from 1–7, include a score of pass or fail, or consist of developmental age rankings that proceed from birth to adolescence.

A test may be based upon normative data, obtained directly by those constructing the test. Some, on the other hand, rest upon general age appropriate averages, obtained by others, and that have been surveyed by the test formulator with reference to the available literature. These latter instruments are often termed criteria-referenced tests. Another important dimension of motor evaluations to consider consists of whether or not the instrument is "age appropriate". For example, some evaluation tests are useful only in infancy. Still others are appropriate to employ in childhood, while others are useful only in late childhood and/or in early adolescence. Testing protocols, and tests, appropriate for infancy and childhood are explored in a section which the follows.

The specific motor abilities contained a test battery are also important to consider. An evaluation tool may focus upon only a limited portion of the overall motor abilities profile of a child. On the a test battery may contain numerous measures, resulting in a broad and comprehensive picture of how both the larger and smaller muscle groups function. Often in a psychological evaluation, for example, only tests sampling printing, and drawing behavior are employed. In contrast a physical therapist may be interested in assessing only motor qualities that reflect functioning of the larger muscle groups that sub-serve walking. Some professionals, wishing an even broader picture of variables related to motor functioning, may employ instruments evaluating various components of the child's self-concept, and measures of activity level, in addition to using tests of coordination and physical capacities. Selected items from various neurological schedules may also be added to enhance information obtained from standard tests of motor performance.

There are essentially two general types of motor test batteries available. One type is based upon 'hard-data' and norms obtained by the test's author. These vary markedly in quality, and may or may not be based upon scores obtained from adequate numbers of children of various ages, and/or of both sexes. (Fleishman 1965). An important way in which these tests may be judged is to determine whether they have been based upon data which has been well factor-analyzed. This step is critical in test construction to determine whether each sub-test evaluates an independent motor quality. A test battery whose components are found to actually measure separate and independent qualities, as identified by a factor (or cluster) analysis, is said to evidence good 'construct validity.' This means that the battery is evaluating the individual components of motor behavior that it purports to measure.

A second type of assessment tool is termed a criteria-referenced test. These instrument are based upon criteria obtained by the authors' surveys of the literature. No norms have been obtained by the author when constituting a criteria-referenced test. Rather the test maker has consulted developmental literature and formulated levels, or criteria, from this library survey. One must, therefore, rely upon the test maker's interpretation of information that has been obtained indirectly.

Care must be taken when using this latter type of evaluation tool, however, in so far as many authors of such "tests" have not consulted 'hard' data themselves, but have in turn rested their criteria upon *other* criteria-referenced tests. It is possible, therefore, to obtain criteria-referenced tests that are second, or third "generations" removed from actual data collection. Thus the validity of some of these instruments is suspect and their usefulness is limited. Among the useful criteria referenced tests available, is that by Koontz (1974) in which a precise survey of motor abilities among young children is presented. The instrument also contains precise remedial strategies appropriate within several ability areas, on a month-by-month basis.

The space in this chapter does not permit a complete review of all the available tests, and test batteries which may be employed assess motor functioning, and dysfunctions in infants, children and youth. A reference by Cratty (1989a), and a review chapter in the the book by Lazslo and Baristow (1986) also contain discussions of available assessment devices. A chapter by Goldstein and Tupper (1987) contains a useful discussion of the nature of test reliability and validity, pertaining to the measurement of neurological soft signs.

In the following two sections it has been attempted first to present what are believed to be the most useful evaluation instruments available to assess infants suspected of motor dysfunctions. The final part of the chapter contains appropriate screening criteria with which to identify clumsy children within populations of typical youngsters.

ASSESSMENT IN INFANCY

Many tests of motor abilities in childhood emerged from the efforts of child development specialists who formulated comprehensive behavioral scales in the 1920's and 1930's. These pioneers included Nancy Bayley at the University of California at Berkeley (1935),

Arnold Gesell and his colleagues at Yale (Gesell 1925), and other scholars at the Universities of Nebraska and Iowa.

The influence of these early efforts are apparent in more contemporary scales, which closely resemble these early tools, both in content, and intent. (Battelle 1986). The data resulting from application of these recent tools are often influenced by cultural variables including playmates, parental stimulation, race, ethnic sub-group, as well as by toys and play equipment that have been available to the infants. The scores obtained from some are vague and subjective, such as trying to determine just when a child is able to 'walk with assistance'. Thus even contemporary versions of these earlier tools, lack precision. The scales designed for assessing development in early infancy thus must be carefully administered, and their results judiciously interpreted. Furthermore it is important to consider the temporary emotional states of the infants assessed, and the cultural and social contexts in which the data are obtained.

More sophisticated, evaluation tools were constructed after World War II. These devices began to focus upon more basic motor abilities, than was true in earlier instruments. They also assessed patterns of movements and interactions not captured by the earlier tests of motor development. Some, including the Denver Developmental Survey (Frankenburg & Dodds 1967) began to point to an age *range* within which a given motor 'milestone' should appear, rather than arbitrarily selecting a specific time in the life of a 'average' child at which a developmental task should appear. This Survey and others began to contain norms, taking into consideration developmental differences found within various ethnic and raial sub-groups.

Infant reflexes and basic responses

Just before, and shortly after birth, infants engage in a variety of writhings and squirmings. For centuries these actions appeared random and without significance. Within the past several decades, however, reflexes and other early patterns of movement have been closely scrutinized, classified, named, and inspected for meaning. Albrecht Piper in a classic book published in the 1960's (1965) clearly described these actions, accompanied by interpretations. In research that followed Piper's efforts, it became clear that some infant reflexes have useful survival value, others are important beginnings of voluntary movements, while still other reflexes, if they persist, delay the appearance of imperative voluntary actions.

In the late 1960s the interactions of reflexes and voluntary movements were incorporated into assessment instruments. Among the first to do this were two Italian pediatricians Milani-Comparetti and Gidioni, (1967). They formulated a model and test assessing the intricate inter-weaving of reflexes and the assumption of various components of voluntary motor activity. An updated version of this useful tool appeared in the 1980s (Milani-Comparetti Gidioni 1987).

Using their test, one may graph the manner in which reflexes and such voluntary actions as standing, turning, and sitting are interwoven. To give two examples, their model illustrates how the persistence of the asymmetrical tonic-neck reflex (which occurs when one arm is extended to the side, and the head also turns toward the same side) will impede the infant's efforts to turn over by acting as a brake; and conversely how when this reflex phases out, voluntary turning is able to be accomplished.

Another example is how the persistence of the plantar flexion reflex in the feet (the feet curling, and grasping the ground) will delay the appearance of the stable support needed for normal standing and walking; and conversely how a stable standing support position is able to be achieved when the plantar reflex becomes subordinated by maturing higher centers. The ways in which infant reflexes contribute to, and detract from, the acquisition of normal positions and actions preceding walking (turning, kneeling, sitting, and standing) has been discussed in a previous publication by the author (Cratty 1989c).

In the 1970s and 1980s other workers began to expand on the assessment ideas initiated by Milani-Comparetti-Gidoni (Hoskins and Squires 1972). These later workers devised more expansive scoring systems, so that signs of early motor delays could be more precisely assessed. For example, the test developed by Ellison and her colleagues in the 1980s (1983) further objectified how unusual patterns of movement and motor delays, assessed during the neonatal period, and during the first two years of life, predict the appearance of later coordination problems. Using their system, its authors claim, will illuminate abnormal motor behaviors, by attaching numerical scores to the behavioral interactions observed.

In addition to reflexes, infants display a plethora of rhythmic behaviors that appear in the limbs, and in the trunk, while sitting, standing and kneeling. These were not accorded much developmental importance until Esther Thelen and her co-workers in the late 1970s began both to count and measure what they termed 'stereotypies'. They also attempted to determine the relationships of these normal rhythmic actions to the assumption of normal voluntary activities and postures. (Thelen 1979, 1981, 1987)

Thelen concluded that the appearance, and vigor of these actions have developmental significance. Their appearance do not occur in a random manner, she postulated, but are seen just prior to, or accompanying, related voluntary actions and postures. It is not entirely clear, upon considering Thelen's suppositions, which comes first, a given stereotypy, or the position in which the rhythmic behavior occurs. However, it is possible that further careful assessments of these rhythmic movements, will also aid in the early prediction of children who may later become dyspraxic, or who might evidence other movement atypicalities including hypertonia or hypotonia.

Scales by Ellison and her colleagues (1983), by Cratty and DeOliveira (1989) and by Eichel (1986), have also been developed which purport to evaluate the inter-dependency of reflexes, of voluntary movements, and of these rythmic-stereotypies. (*See Appendix*). These have been found useful for the precise evaluation of infants stressed with maternal drug use (Cratty 1990). With further research these instruments may also predict the later appearance of coordination and tonus problems, in a variety of 'suspect' infants, including those with low birth weights.

Thus contemporary assessment instruments, designed for application to infants during their first months of life, have focused with increased precision upon a variety of qualities. In addition to those reviewed are other tests designed to assess psycho-social behaviors among infants (Brazelton 1972). The scale recently formulated by Case Smith also appears to have promise in the evaluation of fine motor abilities and object manipulation among young children. (Case-Smith 1989).

MOTOR EVALUATION IN CHILDHOOD

Good tests with which to assess motor abilities in early childhood are not plentiful. Reluctance on the part of the United States Government to fund normative studies has contributed to this problem. One comprehensive research program involving 20,000 youngsters by Fleishman (1965) included averages for children from 10–15. However, similar well normed instruments designed to test the motor abilities of younger children are largely lacking. Despite the dearth of evaluative instruments, there remains a great need to assess children from two to five years of age, in order to predict school readiness, and to expose those evidencing developmental delays to programs of remediation and enrichment.

There have been several approaches to the assessment of motor abilities in childhood. One avenue was based a medical model in which "suspect" children are exposed to a neurological evaluation composed of tasks intended to expose minor neurological dysfunctions. This approach was pioneered by Touwen and Prechtl (1970). Portions of the neurological "schedule" they formulated are sometimes used by insightful doctors in order to assess subtle motor dysfunctions that might otherwise might remain undetected. This type of tool evaluates muscular strengths and weakness, subtle variations of reflex functioning, excess neuromotor overflow, (discussed in Chapter 6), as well as the presence of other subtle problems.

The backgrounds of some professionals, however, do not permit them to administer and to precisely interpret a neurologic test of the kind devised by Touwen and Prechtl (1970) and others (Tupper 1987). Thus educators, and therapists may employ various testing tools that have not been well formulated. Some of these are 'in-house' instruments' composed within a specific settings, and consisting of checklists indicating whether various motor tasks are passed or failed, based often upon vague criteria. Others are developed by consulting the available the literature, and consist of general age-related averages for various tasks based upon the data collection efforts of others.

Still others that are available are normed tests based upon averages obtained by the test's authors. Sometimes this type offers some promise, but they have usually been 'normed' with reference to limited samples, both in number and in ethnic make-up. The more promising of those, include a recent revision of the Stott-Henderson (1984) and the Bruinink's Oseretsky (1978).

A scientifically well-grounded test should have what is termed 'construct validity'. This means that the qualities the tester purports to be testing should be sampled by the test components. Meeting this criteria requires a test based upon data that has been factor analyzed, depicting which sub-tests sample specific and independent abilities. An effective test battery is often based upon an extensive evaluation program. The Fleishman battery is one of the few instruments that meets this criterion (1965). An effective test battery applied to awkward populations might also include components assessing basic motor abilities, graphic-writing skills as well as essential self-care tasks.

Tests of self-care skills are also useful additions to evaluation programs. These instruments are often used with populations who are obviously handicapped. Modifications, however, should result in some becoming useful when evaluating important self-care skills in groups of awkward children. (Jepson et al 1969) (Lynch & Bridle 1989). The skills sampled in this type of test should include not only those involving grooming and dressing, but also essential skills needed when bathing eating. (Gisel & Pollock 1988).

The results of the applications of test batteries should provide afford directions to those constructing remedial programs. The presence of each test, within an evaluation program, implies that if a precise problem is present, the tester will then somehow attempt to fix it! There thus should be a close correspondence between stated program objectives, program content, and the components of accompanying tests. Unfortunately these kinds of relationships are seldom encountered in the real world of education and remediation.

The professional is confronted with several problem when constructing a useful and valid a test battery. The final instrument formulated should be compatible to the situation, and in line with time and financial constraints. Some of its components should be suitably normed with reference to the age and ethnic make-up of the population to be surveyed. Parts of the assessment may be based upon, however, depend upon the collection of information from observations or from a check-list. Most important, the content of the evaluation should lie within the experience and background range of the tester, so that scores are *interpretable* both to the clients, and to their parents and guardians. Giving tests and obtaining scores are undertakings, as is *interpreting* the scores. The latter job requires penetrating insights stemming from a thorough and appropriate professional background.

Moreover the level or depth to which the interpreter-tester probes for and discusses meaning, should be compatible with his or her professional background. Educators should confine their speculations to behavioral data; emotional health professionals should be excepted to add emotional and social dimensions to parent conferences following the assessment of a clumsy child. Interpretations delving into etiologies that refer to vision and visual perception should be engaged in by those whose backgrounds include either medical or optometric schools. Neurological-medical interpretations should be the purview of those with appropriate medical degrees.

DEVELOPMENTAL SIGN-POSTS

In the following section a selection of testing criteria are presented. These criteria have been obtained from test items in useful (normed) tests, and from the author's clinical and experimental experience. The tests and criteria for pass and fail, are based upon the assumption that the test will differentiate between the motor abilities of children in the upper 80–80% and those within the lower 10–15% in a populations of pre-school and of school-age children, from which those evidencing obvious sensory and motor handicaps have previously been removed. The tasks have been placed within several ability sub-divisions, including locomotion, both static and dynamic balance, ball skills including throwing and catching, agility and arm-leg integration, manipulative abilities including self-care skills, and printing-drawing capacities. References are also made to measures of leg, abdominal and shoulder-girdle strength and power.

Pre-Locomotion and Early Locomotion

Pre-locomotion skills are imperative in establishing a normal base for later locomotion. During the first year of life these first consist of head control, and proceed through the abilities to turn over from front-to-back, and from back-to-front, usually occurring between the fourth and sixth month of age.

By the sixth and seventh month, the infant can sit, unaided. By the eight month most infants creep, first crudely and later using a cross extension pattern (in which the left knee proceeds forward in concert with the right hand) By around the first year of life infants usually pull themselves to their feet, and within a month or two attempt to walk without assistance. Generally these latter stages occur earlier in thin, muscular children, and in girls before being accomplished by boys. These important development milestones are pictured next page.

Walking usually is seen first with the hands held high, in what is termed a high-guard position. During the second year of life the arms gradually lower, and will begin to swing at the sides in rhythm while walking. The child's gait becomes narrower and more rhythmic in nature during this same time.

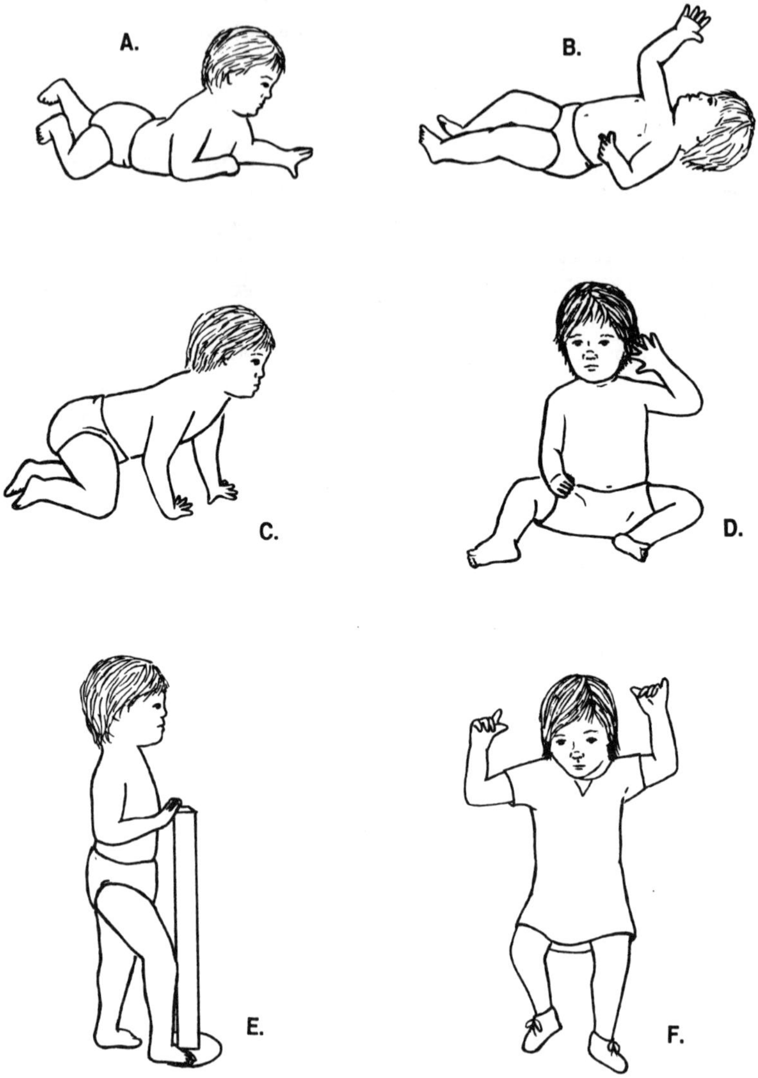

Plate 11-1. Stages in Pre-Locomotion
The infant begins to exhibit head control, a support response (A) from the first to third month, by the third to fourth month will turn over (B) and assume a hand-knee position (C) used in creeping by the sixth month. Unassisted sitting (D) is seen by the sixth to eighth month, while between the tenth and twelfth month the child will usually pull to a upright stand. (E) Unassisted walking (F) usually is accomplished from the 11th to 14th month.

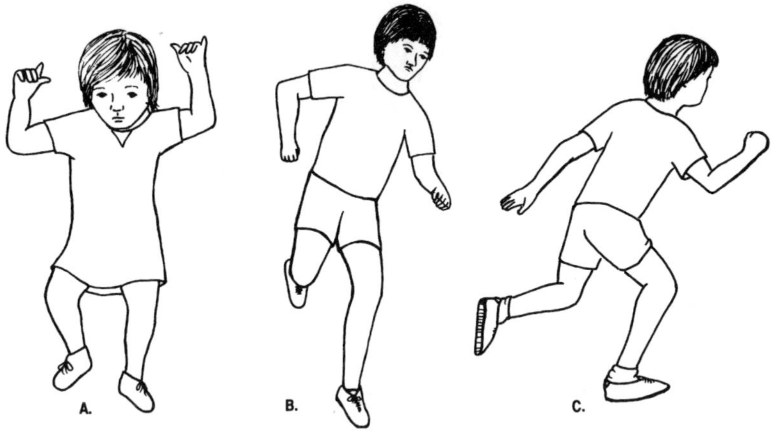

Plate 11-2. Stages in walking
(A) The first walking efforts are marked by the arms held high in a "high guard" position, locomotion is later accompanied by a rhythmic arm swing (B) by the third to fourth year, and later a cross-extension pattern when running (C) by the fifth year.

During the second and third year of life additional locomotor skills are seen, that first include a 'hurry' which is a fast walk-like run, during which the feet never leave the ground. The first rudimentary 'jumps' also are accompanied by a vigorous thrust upward of the arm, and downward with the legs, but the child usually does not leave the ground. The first true jumps occur only when the ratio of limb strength to body-build becomes favorable, often not until the middle, or at end of the fourth year of life. As is expected, bulky heavy babies jump and run later than do thin more muscular and 'wiry' infants.

Three year olds, begin to jump; and shortly may exhibit three or four jumps consecutively. A simple shuffle-like gallop is seen at this age, but both feet usually remain on the ground throughout the cycle. Some three year olds can execute an unsupported step, taking off on one foot and landing on the opposite foot. Walking is usually accompanied with a consistent cross-extension pattern (right arm swinging forward with the left leg, etc.) by three-and a half to four years of age. However, when running at this age, the same cross extension pattern is seldom exhibited.

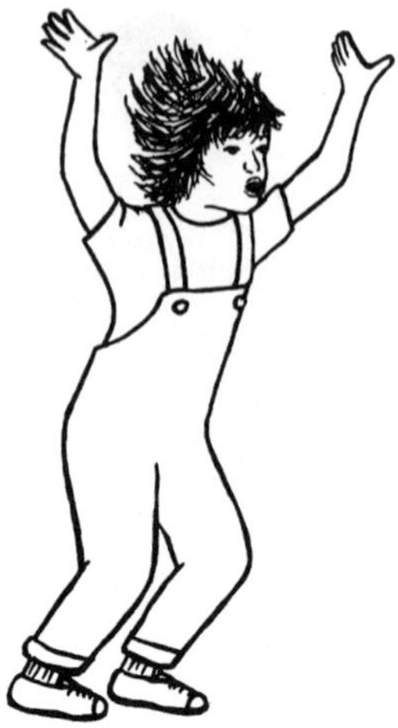

Plate 11-3. A false jump is often seen during the second to third year, as the infant is unable to leave the ground because of a disadvantageous ratio between body weight and leg strength. The arms and legs imitate a regular jump, while the feet do not leave the ground.

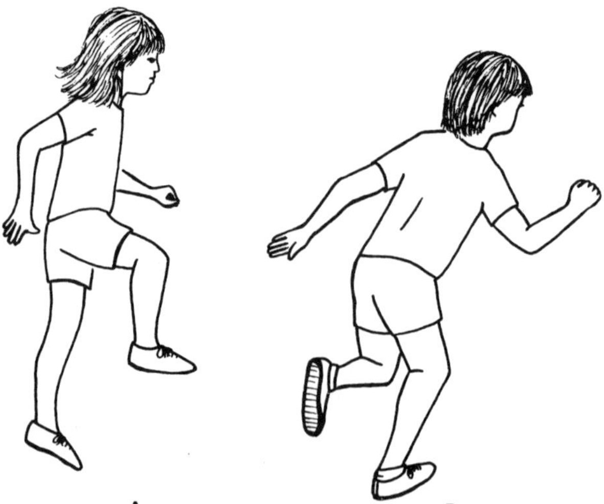

A. B.

Plate 11-4. An unsupported step occurs when a child takes off on one foot, is momentarily unsupported, and lands on the opposite foot (A), as shown below. Hopping involves taking off and landing on the same foot (B), and is seen later.

Three year olds may hop once, but by the beginning of the fourth year most children can hop on a preferred foot, three or four times in succession, taking off and landing on the same foot. By four most children evidence a true run (with both feet off the ground at sometime during the complete cycle). Running is often accompanied with a good cross-extension pattern (the left arm moving forward with the right foot, etc). Also by four, lateral movement is often accomplished, but not with good accuracy and speed. Galloping becomes possible by about four and a half, with both feet leaving the ground at once, during each cycle.

Five year olds may to try to skip, but often only succeed with one foot at a time, while the other takes a simple step. Most Girls at six years, and many boys at the same age, can engage in a true skipping action. While girls at six can usually jump continuously and rhythmically from one foot to the other in a 2-2 rhythm. Moreover hopping is likely to gain precision during these years, and both boys and girls of six and seven can hop with precision into a series of squares that are 1′ x 1′ in size.

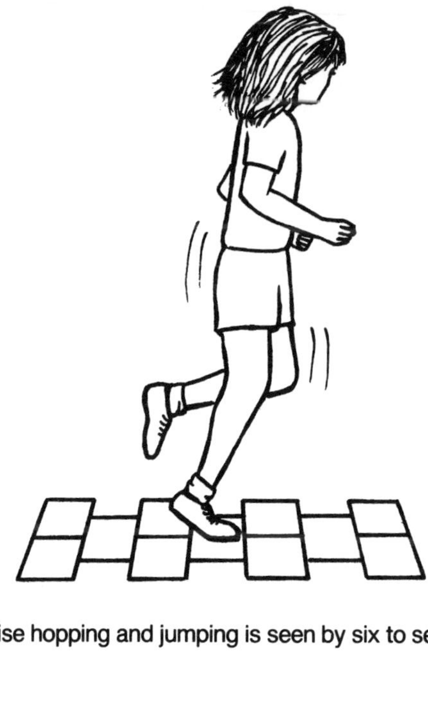

Plate 11-5. Precise hopping and jumping is seen by six to seven years of age.

By seven years most girls, and some boys of eight years can continuously hop in a continuous manner from foot to foot in a 3-2 rhythm. This action consists of hopping three times on one foot, and transferring immediately to two times on the other foot, and continuing in this way through several cycles. Most seven year olds can engage such complicated tasks as rope-jumping, and two-wheel bicycle riding.

Static Balance

Children can statically posture with their feet about shoulder-width apart by the middle of their second year of life. By their fourth birthday they can posture with their feet together, and by five can rise on the balls of both their feet without "wobbling extensively", for from four to six seconds.

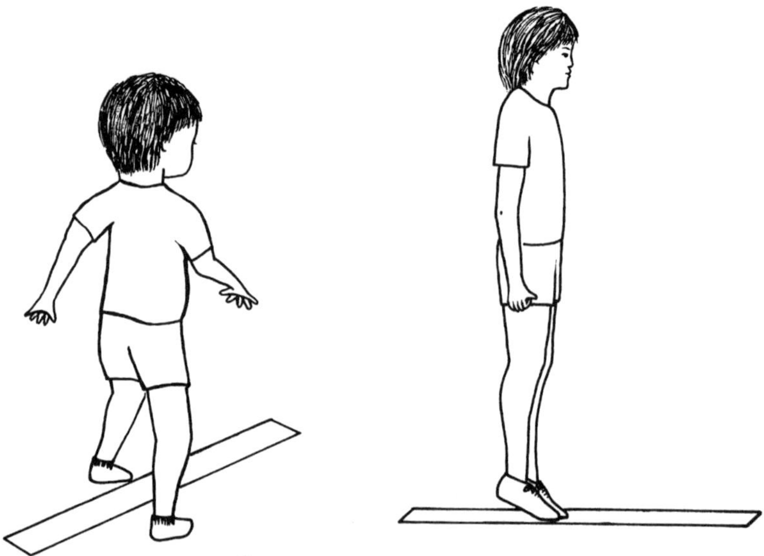

A.

B.

Plate 11-6. A three-year old can balance with feet shoulder-width apart (A), while by five they should be able to posture in a stable position on the balls of the feet as shown (B)

Six year olds may begin to stand on one foot, with the other held up at a right angle, flexed at the knee. A one-foot balance task is enhanced if a target is placed at eye level as shown (Plate 11-7 below), and the child is asked to look at the target while posturing. Control in this type of one-foot stand, for from 6-8 seconds, is usually expected by the age of six in girls, and by seven in boys.

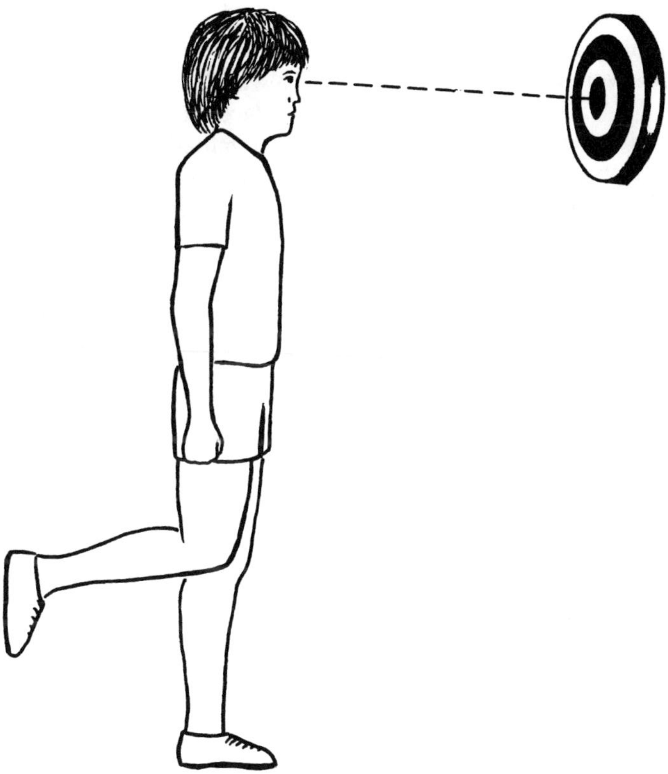

Plate 11-7. Static Balance with a target
Static balance is enhanced, if a visual target is placed at eye level as shown.

Youngsters eight years and older, with adequate static balance, should be able to posture in a one-foot stand, hands on hips, on a 1.5″ wide balance beam for from 6-8 seconds. Tasks more difficult than this do not adequately discriminate between children with, and without, balance problems, as static balance tends to mature by about the eighth or ninth birthday.

Dynamic Balance

Children as young as three can walk a 2″ wide line painted on the floor. By four years youngsters can walk, alternating feet, along a 4″ wide balance beam, if it is placed about 4″ from the ground. By the age of seven, children can successfully walk balance beams that are from 2″–1.5″ in width, if they are placed close to the ground. Females are usually superior in tasks evaluating both static and dynamic balance. Both types of balance tasks are found in the Bruininks Oseretsky, (1978) as well as in other evaluative tools (Stott & Henderson 1974).

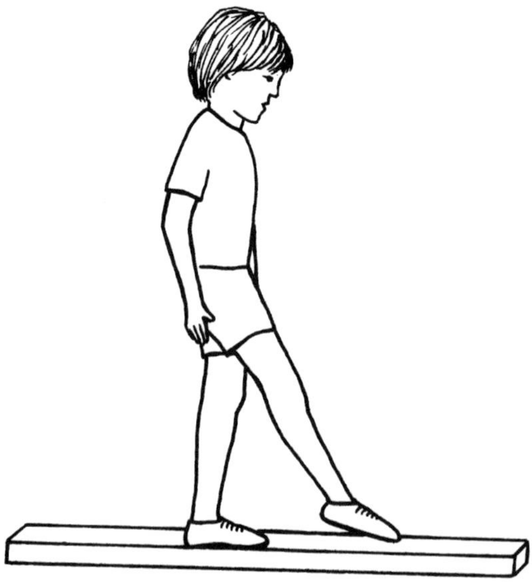

Plate 11-8. Balance beam walking is a common means of testing dynamic balance, and may be scored by counting steps accomplished on a beam of a given length and width. At five, children can usually alternate steps on a beam 4′′ high and 4′′ wide. By eight and nine, children can walk a beam 1.5′′ wide.

Ball Skills: Throwing

Throwing may be evaluating with reference to mechanics, by measuring accuracy, and also by determining the distance of the throw. Biomechanically children pass through several phases when throwing from a stiff armed release of the ball, without any shoulder rotation, nor weight shift of the body, seen during the 2nd and 3rd year of life. Also during these first attempts, the method they select to throw will vary from trial to trial.

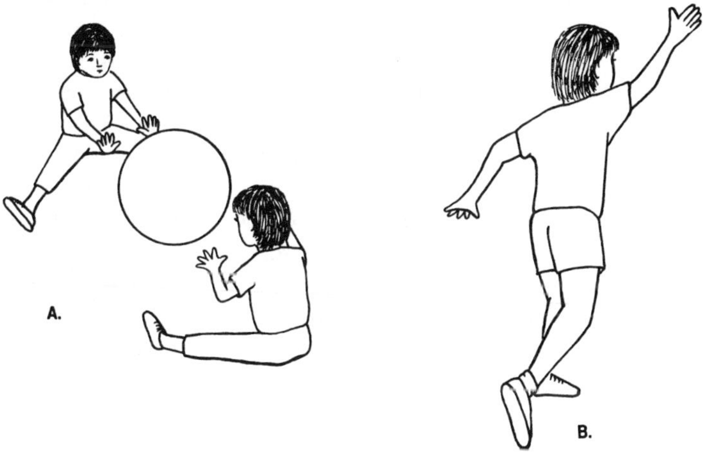

Plate 11-9. First efforts to propel balls will consist of merely pushing a missile as shown (A), while final mature efforts seen between five and seven years consist of the pattern shown (B) in which a vigorous step is taken with the foot opposite to the throwing arm-hand.

Later by about four years releasing the ball, will likely be accompanied by a forward weight shift. But four year olds will not usually execute a long throw by taking a simultaneous step, with the foot opposite the throwing arm. Instead at this age they will usually step with the foot under the throwing arm.

By five years a weight shift will likely occur, and now many youngsters will step forward simultaneously with the leg opposite to the throwing arm. At this age boys are likely to evidence a mechanically more mature throwing pattern than are girls. By six years, and older, children will usually evidence a mature throw, when asked to throw distance, or to throw as 'Hard as you can', with a weight shift accompanied by a step with the foot opposite to the throwing arm. A test assessing throwing accuracy is contained in the Bruininks Oseretsky (1978). Generally, however, well-normed tests of throwing accuracy are difficult to locate in the available assessment instruments.

Ball Skills: Catching

Two and three year olds will be able to intercept a ball rolled to them, if it does not come too rapidly. At three a 'catch' will be made with stiff arms, cradling the ball when it arrives after being bounced to them. By four years a simple catch will be accomplished of a 8″ diameter playground ball, about 3 out of five times, when bounced toward the child from a short distance away (about 10–15′).

By five years youngsters will be successful in its interception of the same size ball five times out of five, bounced carefully to them and arriving chest high. By six years children will be able to bounce a tennis ball, at their feet, and catch it, as shown in Plate 11–10.

Success in this task at six years, will occur from 3-5 times out of five chances. By seven years most children should be able to catch a tennis ball thrown to them ("on the fly"), and arriving chest high, from a distance of about 15 feet, four or five times out of five. In later childhood youngsters are able to catch, or intercept, a tennis ball projected toward them from greater distances, requiring reasonably accurate and rapid adjustments of their bodies, forward, backward, or to the sides.

Kicking

Youngsters in many countries of the world engage in games involving the ability to kick and to guide the ball, as when dribbling in soccer football. Kicking evidences predictable progressions. Initially a child will not involve his total body when kicking, and will merely push the ball. Later the ball will be kicked with mechanics of increased sophistication and reflecting mature mechanics in which the total body is involved.

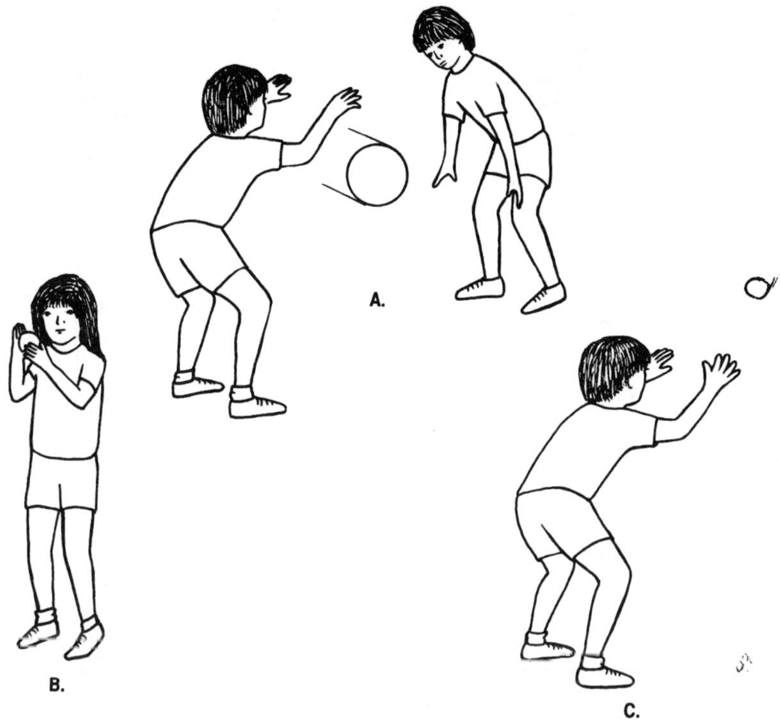

Plate 11-10. At four and five years children may intercept a 8″ diameter playground ball bounced from 10–15″ away, from three to five times out of five (A). By six a tennis ball may be intercepted after being bounced at the feet (C) and by seven the same size ball may be caught when thrown from a short distance away (C)

Agility

Agility tests may sample the accuracy of the body when hopping and jumping and the like, how well the total body can move in a vertical plane, and/or running agility in which the child is required to change directions while running. Test makers have agreed when selecting agility tests, and when defining the term. The Bruinink's Oseretsky (1978) contains an agility run in which an object must run to, grasped, and then returned to a starting point. We have found this task satisfactory in evaluations we have carried out. However, like several other tests in this battery, the complete dimensions of the testing area are not given in the instruction manual.

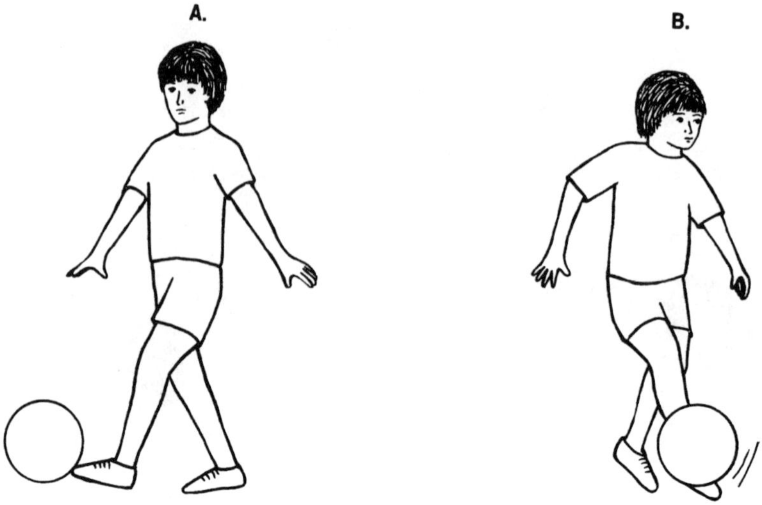

Plate 11-11. Kicking evolves from a simple pushing of the ball with the foot (A), at about the third year, to a vigorous and mature action (B) seen between five and seven years of age.

Moving up and down in a vertical plane may employed to test a child's ability. Asking a youngster to "get up, as fast as you can" from a back lying position will illicit both mature and immature attempts. At three and younger a child will often turn completely to his/ her front before retaining an upright position. By four years and five a child will make a partial turn, before arising. And by six and older the child will arise to a stand without turning over. The quality of the performance in this task depends also upon body build, with thinner stronger children arising more maturely than heavier, weaker youngsters.

Coordination

Measures of coordination are traditionally included in batteries of motor tests. Numerous types of 'coordination' tests have included those sampling qualities of both the larger and smaller muscle groups. Definitions of coordination, as is true of agility, abound in the literature Their diversity is matched by the wide variety of tasks that have been formulated to evaluate this apparently mult-dimensional quality.

A test of arm-leg integration found in the Bruinink's Oseretsky (1978) has been found useful in our research. It is scored by counting how many times a child can clap his/her hands together during a single vertical jump (late 11-13). Age norms are available, and the test appears to separate children well into broad motor performance categories as well as any single test is likely to do. At four years a child may execute a single clap, by five two, and by six years three claps in the air. After the age of six only athletic children and youth are likely to perform four or five claps during a single jump.

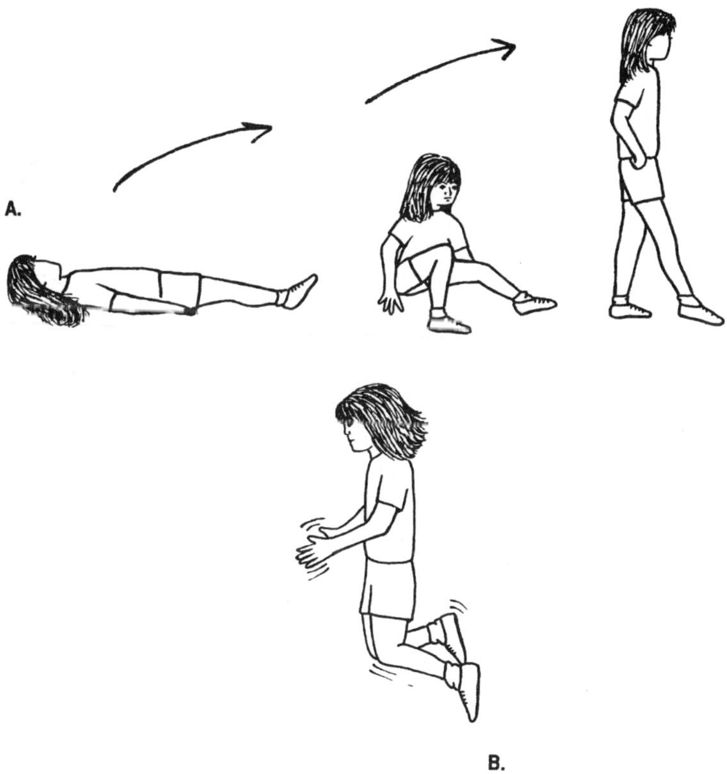

Plate 11-12. Agility Tests
(A) indicates the phases in a 'how fast can you arise?' test, attention is paid to the matuity of the middle phase, in which a mature child may remain in the original direction, while less mature children either partially, or completely, turn to their front, before arising. (B) depicts the useful jump-clap test, scored by counting how many times in the air a child is able to clap, during a single jump.

Manipulation

Often on several infant scales a manipulative tasks often involves grasping an object. The maturity of the grasp is observed. For example, it is noted if the child uses the palm of the hand (fingers together) when grasping. This palmer grasp, as shown in Plate 11-14. This type of grasp is often seen between the second and fourth month of age. Later a more sophisticated grip for handling objects is seen, involving the fingers, opposite the thumb. This 'pincer grip' is usually seen used by infants between the 8th and 12th month of age.

Plate 11-13. (A) depicts a palmer grasp, while (B) shows a more refined pincer grip in which the first and other fingers oppose the thumb.

Cube-stacking is also a task employed infant to evaluate manipulative abilities. It is usually scored by counting the number of one-inch cubes the infant can successfully stack in a tower. Two cubes may be stacked in this manner by the 12th month; while by the 18th month a tower of from 4 to 6 may be built. The available evidences suggests that by the age of five years, among normally functioning children, a stack of twelve 1″ cubes are able to be stacked in a stable tower.

Many self-care skills require manual dexterity. The ages at which each is acquired, is often molded by the culture, and by the teaching efforts of available caretakers. Generally it is assumed that by a year of age the child can begin to use a spoon, a little later clothes may be removed, with some help from the parent-caretaker. Shortly after a year of age, the child can usually hold a cup with both hands and drink from it. However, it is not until about two years later than a knife and fork will begin to be used while eating.

Hands are washed and dried by the middle of the second year of life. Buttoning, using zippers and other skills needed to put on clothing, are not usually seen until the middle of the third year of

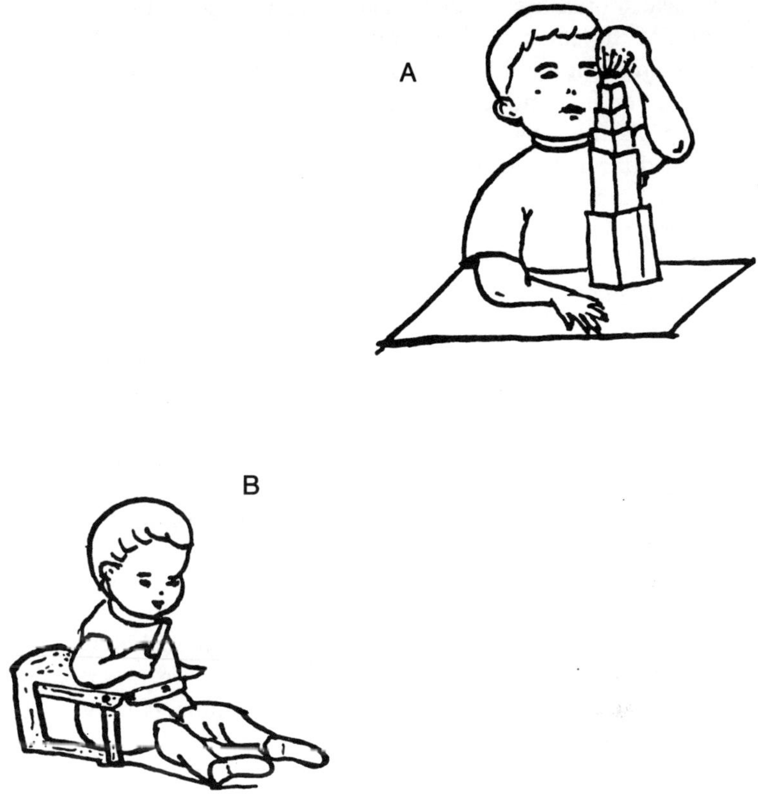

Plate 11-14. Cube stacking (A) is often found on the 'adaptive' sections of infant development scales; while self-care skills (B) are useful criteria to use when evaluating manual skills, but may reflect family values, as well as ethnic and cultural specifics.

life. Unsupervised dressing is not usually accomplished until the middle or latter part of the fifth year of life, after the fourth birthday.

Finger Opposition

An often-employed test of manipulative ability, likely to reflect success at dressing-buttoning, holding table utensils and the like consists of asking a child to touch each finger, in order, to the thumb of the same hand. This task is usually not accomplishable unaided until about the fourth or fifth year.

The task should first be demonstrated, and is scored by timing the duration of the effort, and also by recording errors. (Denckla 1973). At three and younger a child's may accomplish the task, but only if the examiner first moves each finger to the thumb, and then the child repeats the movement with each finger. By late in the fourth year and during the fifth year, a child with adequate manipulative abilities should be able to accomplish this task, slowly, with one or less errors, but must closely watch the fingers and hand.

Older children about the age of seven, should be able to execute finger opposition quickly and accurately, after it is demonstrated. Girls tend to be superior to boys, in this kind of task. Mirror movements, similar movements of the hand not engaged in the task, may also be seen in children when this task is required. These mirror movements (sykinesia) in the non-involved hand, commonly occur in normally functioning children younger than five and younger. Among children with immature neuromotor systems, however, these associated movements may persist after the ages of six and seven.

Printing & Figure Drawing

The ability to execute simple figures evolve from scribbling behaviors, that were seen as early as the second year of life, and that have been depicted in Chapter 7 dealing with dysgraphia. (Cratty 1989b).

A.

B.

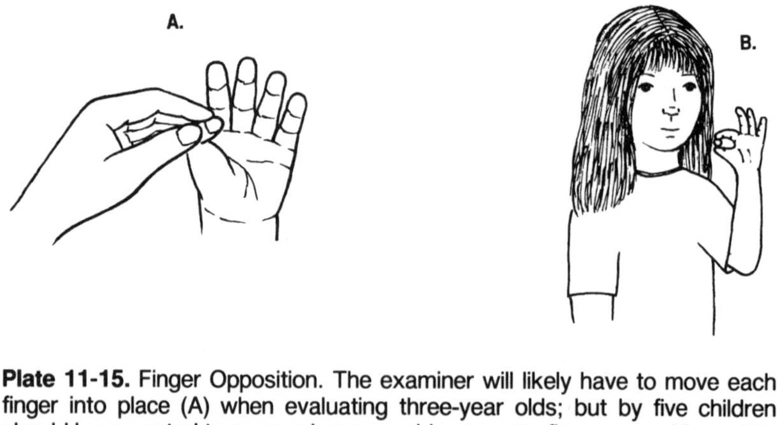

Plate 11-15. Finger Opposition. The examiner will likely have to move each finger into place (A) when evaluating three-year olds; but by five children should be expected to engage in reasonably accurate finger opposition, while carefully watching their progress (B). By the ages of seven most children evidence rapid adult-like abilities, with girls generally more precocious than boys in this taks

The first figure that can successfully copied by children, about the age of three-and-a-half, is a simple line cross.

A Line Cross **B Rambling Circle**

Plate 11-16. First Scribbles and Drawings

By four years children can draw a reasonably good circle, but not a square. But by about the fifth birthday a child should draw squares and circles that are clearly different. By five and a half, many children, if given some encouragement, will copy most block letters about 2″ high, will attempt to print their first names.

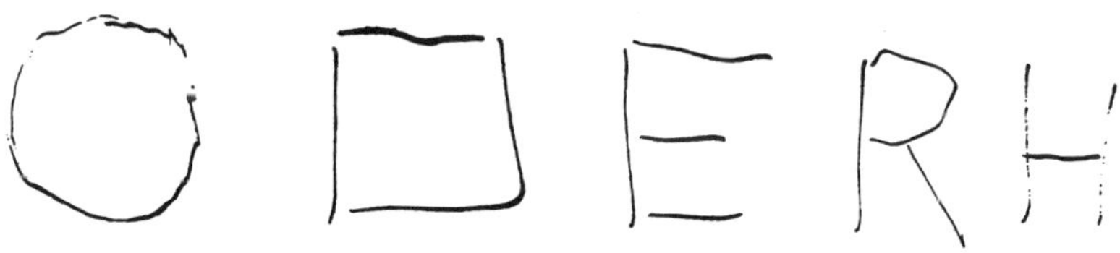

Plate 11-17. Circle, Square, and Block Letters.

During the sixth year the letters will executed with more accuracy, and will replicate letters smaller than was possible a year earlier. Many children this same year are able to draw a triangle, if it is first drawn for their inspection.

By seven and eight reproducing a diamond is possible, and youngster's reproductions of human figures, houses and the like become more mature. People drawn have full limbs, rather than the stick-line arms and legs seen earlier.

Also by this age both upper and lower case manuscript letters are usually able to be printed legibly. By eight most school systems in the United States introduce children to cursive writing. In many drawing tasks at this age, girls will be superior to boys. However boys will often be superior in later childhood when asked to replicate three dimensional figures; a cube, or cylinder for example.

A further discussions of the complex dimensions of children's drawings may be found in Kellogg's exhaustive treatment of the subject (1969). The development of graphic behaviors has also been discussed and illustrated in Chapter 7 dealing with dysgraphia

Additional Qualities

Other qualities that may be assessed within a comprehensive evaluation can include the presence of associated movements, as well as of motor planning behavior. Guidelines for the evaluation of these important qualities are found in Chapter 6 dealing with "movement characteristics". Strength-power items including leg, arm and abdominal strength may be evaluated, in children from about 5 to 16 years, using the tasks contained in the Bruininks Oseretsky (1978). The leg power tests in Bruinink's battery consist of a standing broad jump; arm and abdominal power involves scoring the number of pushups and sit-ups accomplished within twenty-second intervals.

Summary

Caution should be applied when interpreting the results of an evaluation in which the above tasks are employed, or when using any battery made up of simple screening items with which pass-fail scores are obtained. Care should be taken not to commit either of two types of errors. One error involves a *false-positive* assessment. This first error involves falsely stating that the child evidences a motor problem, or problems, when indeed none is (are) really present.

The second type of error is a *'false-negative'*. This error consists of not correctly identifying a motor problem, or problems, when in truth problems may be present. The guidelines described in the second part of this chapter should be used only in general ways. It may be more useful to use some of the standardized testing instruments now available, surveyed within the first part of the chapter. Committing either type of error, the false- negative or false-positive, can be extremely stressful to parents and teachers, and to other professionals contacting the child. Such mis-diagnoses may even result in legal problems for the tester.

Interpretational problems also arise when attempting to correctly evaluate the efforts of children with various body-builds, within various economic and racial-ethnic sub-groups, and of youngsters whose parents have subjected them to varying amounts of exposure to and demands to perform various kinds of motor tasks. Useful efforts at interpreting test results should thus be based upon the tester's knowledge of the total racial-social-ethnic-family context in which the child has developed, or failed to develop, prior to his or her confrontation with the testing instrument and with the evaluator.

OVERVIEW

An historical review of the evaluation of motor abilities of children was first presented. Motor testing was traced from its early beginnings involving the placement of motor tasks in the first measures of intelligence, through the development of the first motor test batteries in the 1920s, and finally to the emergence of contemporary evaluative instruments useful in the identification of clumsy children.

Testing criteria were also presented, by which a'good evaluative instrument' might be scrutinized. Emphasis was placed also upon the importance of the tester's interpretational skills. It was pointed out that any valid assessment should be based, not only based upon 'objective' scores, but also upon interpretations related to the ethnicity and race of the youngster, to the socio-economic conditions and to family environment and values to which the child has been exposed. Moreover the nature and depth of the interpretation should rest upon the professional credentials in possession of the tester. The strengths and weakness of both normed tests, and of those based upon authors' surveys of the literature, were pointed out. The latter are usually labeled criteria-referenced tests.

Selected evaluation tools, useful for the assessment of infants and children within various age groups were surveyed. These included instruments designed for the early identification of motorically 'suspect' infants, including the Milani-Comparetti Gidioni (1987). Others based upon the interweaving of infant reflexes with imperative voluntary motor tasks including sitting, standing, and walking. Others tests reviewed included those appropriate for the identification of motor problems in pre-school children and among those in middle childhood.

The chapter concluded with developmental-task guidelines, upon which a check-list might be based. The movement tasks contained in this check list included balance, locomotor and ball skills, as well as agility, arm-leg coordination, manipulative abilities, and printing-drawing criteria. The ages surveyed relative to performance of these tasks, were from birth to middle childhood. In general the criteria listed, if not met, would likely identify children whose abilities lie within the lower 5–10% of youngsters from 'normal' classroom populations.

In a broad sense the following approach to evaluation might be considered. One first might evaluate a child, both qualitatively as well as quantitatively, and from this data an overall picture of the main sub-syndrome(s) evidenced might then be formulated, together with a profile of precise deficiencies identified in specific ability areas. After this initial motor evaluation is completed, one might further ascertain, via personal observations, or from the indirect reports of others, the general type(s) of social-psychological compensations the child typically exhibits. These might include those described in Chapter 10, and range from various forms of hyperverbalization (the 'lawyer' ... the comedian etc) to aggressive behaviors, and also include infantile withdrawal from age appropriate activities. The final step is to formulate a'plan of attack' within a remedial-clinical setting. This plan should include appropriate instructor behavior, reward system, as well as the length of time and group size to which the child may be exposed. Chapter 12 contains guidelines for program formulation. A schematic of this three-part model for the evaluation and remediation of children with coordination problems follows.

QUESTIONS FOR DISCUSSION

1. What general philosophical criteria should be considered before formulating a testing program?
2. What important practical considerations useful to consider when beginning to test youngsters?
3. What does test reliability mean, how many types of reliability should one consider? May a test be reliable and not valid, valid and not reliable? Explain
4. What is face validity, with reference to a motor test? What does construct validity mean? How is construct validity determined?
5. Discuss what self-care skills might reflected in the scores obtained from a test of finger opposition? What ability stages at what ages are seen in this test?
6. Discuss the principle of closely matching program criteria, with program content, and with components of the program's testing program. What objectives are

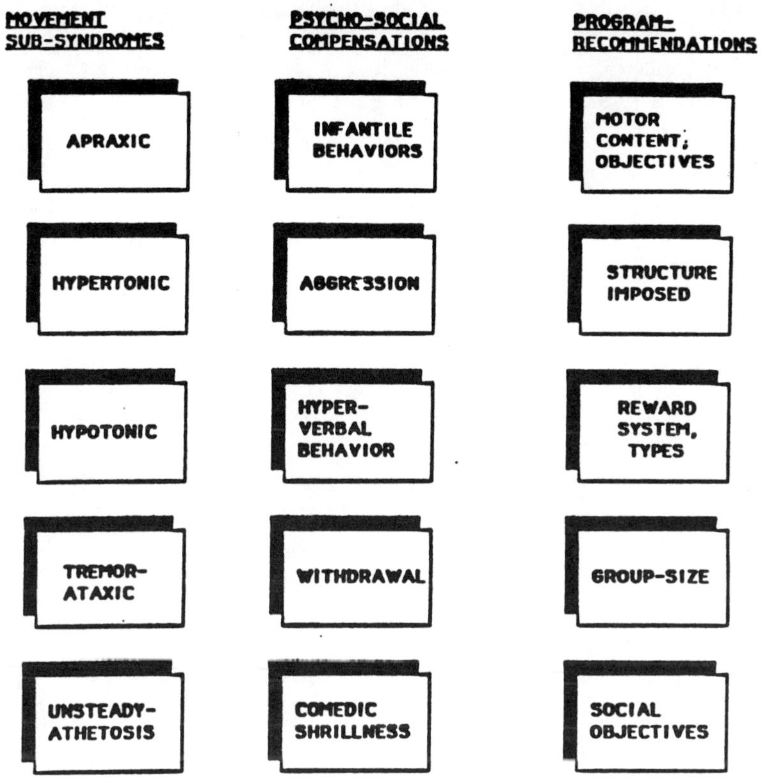

Plate 11-18. Motor sub-syndromes, psycho-social compensations, and program recommendations.

frequently not tested for? What might be the later reactions of a youngster's parents to program outcomes, if tasks intended to remediate qualities, initially assessed, are not placed within the program?

7. Discuss the interactions depicted on Plate 11-19? How might you profile a given child using such a schematic? What is missing from this diagram?
8. Discuss what might constitute a good social setting for evaluating a child. What variables might detract and contribute to from the reliable and valid testing of a child?
9. What are the strengths and weaknesses of a criteria-referenced test? Discuss these qualities with regard to the ability to generalize from the results. What about the usefulness of a criteria-referenced test to works within a specific setting?
10. Bring to class copies of a test designed to evaluate the inter-action of reflexes an voluntary movements seen in infants. Discuss the advantages and problems with using such an instrument. Who seems qualified to apply this kind of measurement tool?

Chapter 12
Formulating Remedial Programs

INTRODUCTION

Remedial programs designed to improve coordination and related qualities in awkward youngsters are of several types. They are also found at various locations. For example, a parent may encourage their child to learn self-care skills at home, and to improve recreational skills in the backyard. Formal programs include those focusing upon the improvement of self-care skills of developmentally delayed adults and children within institutions. Adapted physical education programs may be conducted within school settings. Occupational and physical therapists sometimes work to improve the physical skills and fitness of poorly developed children in both out-patient and inpatient programs found in hospitals. Some departments of special education and physical education in colleges and universities, have provided part-time remedial services for awkward children.

Diversity also becomes apparent upon surveying the titles and backgrounds of those engaged in programs of physical improvement. Administrators and clinicians range from physicians to occupational and physical therapists. The personnel within school settings may include interested teachers and parents, and also adapted physical education specialists. Tutoring in graphic behaviors is often applied by educational therapists and psychologists. Faculty members of special education, psychology and physical education departments sometimes conduct programs within their institutions.

The format and objectives for these programs also have varied. Some are administered by appointment, and the child given individualized tutoring. Others meet tri-weekly, bi-weekly or weekly and consist of small class instruction. The objectives of some of these efforts are limited to the improvement of sports skills and related abilities. Other programs have focused solely upon improvement in fine motor tasks including graphic behaviors, and self-care skills.

Motor activities have been employed in many programs instituted throughout the past decades, in conjunction with programs also designed to improve general academic competencies. Other clinicians offer services intended primarily to improve upon both fine and gross motor skills during a child's visits. Still others believe that simply applied sensory motor experiences will inevitably influence higher centers, that in turn will transfer to and remediate all perceptual and academic difficulties the child may evidence. Thus compounding the problem of selecting services are the variety of the sometimes theoretical orientations of those seeking to give help to children with coordination problems. Often these professionals are not in philosophical agreement about what exposure to physical activities will likely to accomplish

Thus numerous types of programs espousing a variety of objectives, and run by personnel with varied backgrounds, offer potential help for infants, children and youth with problems in physical coordination. Therefore, it often proves difficult for parents, seeking useful assistance for their offspring's problems, to sort out the variety of personnel and services available.

However there appear to be both practical and theoretical principles useful to consider, when assessing and conducting current programs, and when formulating new ones. An overview of helpful management and remedial strategies may be also found in a chapter on this same subject by McKinlay & Gordon (1986). The present discussion focuses upon some important broad guidelines. The principles and operations, discussed in this chapter, are based both upon evidence in the available literature, and upon the author's experiences as a clinician.

PRINCIPLES AND GUIDELINES

General Objectives

There are a number of important general objectives that are applicable for a variety of educational and/ore remedial programs, directed toward youngsters evidencing a variety of atypical behaviors. These principles also are relevant to the modification of movement qualities in children.

(1) *Remedial program should be constructed, and carried out with reference to the social-cultural setting in which the young clients reside.* A program of motor activity should be formulated while keeping in mind parental demands, the social-economic conditions surrounding the youngster, and also taking into consider-

ation the nature of peer pressures to which the child may be subjected. Some of these cultural variables may be modified by the therapist, while others are difficult to change. Parental attitudes may be changed, for example, if the individuals conducting the motor program present clear evidence of their children's improvement. An awkward youngster, upon showing positive skill changes, may benefit by having his or her school setting changed. The presence of abrasive peers who may not credit the child with real improvement that has taken place, project attitudes the clinician is unlikely to alter.

(2) *A comprehensive remedial program should consider three general types of approaches to a child's problem.* These include (A) engaging in direct interventions directed toward specific culturally-imperative skills; practicing letter formation for example. (B) Aiding the child to engage in compensations for skills not easily mastered. Providing special fasteners for shoes, when shoe tying is a problem, is one example. Another compensation is to assist a child to learn to type, when handwriting proves slow and tension producing: and (C) Seeking to lessen cultural pressures for quick and accurate physical performance. Application of this third principle might consist of asking a classroom teacher to reduce the lengthy of written homework , and/or to substitute oral reports for written work.

(3) *The social emotional accompaniments of motor incoordination should be accommodated to when constructing programs.* For example, an objective for such programs is often to reduce excess compensatory verbiage that often issues forth from the mouths of awkward children, so that better attention to the task at hand becomes possible. Poor self-esteem and a background of failure when attempting motor tasks may be overcome by presenting the child tasks, during the first remedial sessions, in which success is likely. The program content should also prove intellectually challenging and provide creative experiences. (Cratty 1988, 1985b).

(4) *The content, and teaching strategies within a remedial program should be based upon a sound and thorough knowledge of normal child development.* Both quantitative and qualitative differences in motor behaviors seen among awkward children should be considered (Chapters 5, & 6). Difficult tasks should be broken down into sub-stages for more effective learning. This is only

possible if the personnel conducting the program are able to analyze carefully when, and how, normal children are likely to acquire imperative motor tasks.

Qualitative differences in developmentally delayed youngsters, should be accommodated to. The clinician should be aware of abnormal movement qualities seen in awkward children. (Chapter 6). When possible these should be modified. Other individual differences to be taken into account include variations in learning strategies adopted by poorly coordinated youngsters, and the possibility of the appearance of unexpected emotional responses occurring during remedial sessions.

(5) *There should be a close correspondence between stated goals, program content, and evaluative instruments used.* It is common to observe programs in which their stated objectives are not reflected in the program content. Likewise it is common to see things done in programs that are not evaluated. In the former case it is unlikely that the stated objectives will be reached; while in the second case real changes may occur, and yet not be recorded. Later in the chapter, a discussion of transfer-width enlarges upon this principle.

I am aware of programs for learning disabilities in which an emphases are placed upon content intended to improve graphic behaviors. Yet in this same program no evaluation instruments are administered to give the administrators an idea of whether gains in writing and writing is forthcoming. Many individuals running programs include statements about enhancing the self-concept as an important goal. In these same programs attempts are seldom made, however, to evaluate components of the self-esteem and related emotional qualities. In these same programs there are often few specific strategies employed that will likely raise a child self-esteem to any significant degree. Program content and components for which no sub-tests are given are likely to result in efforts expended by clinicians that are neither illuminated nor rewarded. Objectives which are stated, and tested for, but for which no specific program provisions are made, are not likely to be achieved.

Program Objectives

The material in Chapter 13 dealing with prognosis for change, makes it clear that positive changes in motor functions are not the inevitable outcomes of movement programs administered to children. The available information suggests that without careful planning and good teaching various motor abilities may, over time, evidence regression, rather than improvement. These measurable set-backs may reflect a 'disuse' syndrome. This means that the motor capacities a younger possesses may be blunted, because he or she desists from engaging in physical activities in which continual failure has been experienced. Chapter 13 contains more information about expected changes due to intervention.

Important principles to guide planners of the operations and content of motor development program have been grouped into strategies intended to enhance of motor learning, principles related to the social-emotional environment, and operational guidelines governing program scheduling and staffing.

Principles of Motor Learning and Skill Acquisition

These principles governing motor learning include strategies involving spacing versus massing practice in time, using effective motivational techniques, whole vs part teaching, principles of transfer of training, and teaching for maximum retention over time.

(A) *Practice periods, containing content intended to improve physical skills, should be of short-duration and spaced over time.* There is vast amount of data pertaining to the way in which motor skills improve because of rest days inserted between days of practice. (Cratty 1975). Too frequent practice sessions of a single skill may result in little improvement. To the contrary the psychological fatigue (response inhibition) produced by excessive practice may result in performance decrements. In contrast if the practice of a given skill takes place in sessions spaced in time, more rapid improvement is likely to take place.

This does not mean that a daily program of physical activity and skill development will not be effective. During daily sessions different skills and fitness activities and games may be practiced on alternate days. For example a child may be educated in sport skills and engage in fitness exercises on Monday-Wednesday and Friday; while crafts, and efforts at improving printing and writing are placed into a Tuesday, Thursday and Saturday schedule.

(B) *The practice of skills should be well-motivated, and appropriate rewards should be constantly available.* Often younger children require various extrinsic rewards (tokens or toys) during their initial exposure to a motor development program. These may be important to administer at frequent intervals, particularly to children whose attention deficits are marked. Recently, for example, we administered colorful sticker rewards every minute to two boys whose attention spans were less than sixty-seconds when first entering our program.

Gradually over a period of two months the sticker rewards were given for more prolonged periods of attention, lasting from five then seven, and finally ten minutes. At last the sticker-reward were withdrawn, and verbal reward-statements reflecting social approval, were substituted. For some youngsters only signs of social approval, and/or the intrinsic knowledge that they improved in a skill, may be enough. For most, however, giving more concrete signs of improvement may initially have a more immediate and useful impact, before the mastery of skills becomes intrinsically rewarding.

Extrinsic material rewards have limitations, however, including the following. They are only effective if the child finds them truly rewarding, and also attaches their appearance to specific performance changes of which he or she is aware. Rewards should be extended not only for obvious performance changes sought, but for improved effort including more prolonged periods of time during which the child attends to the task. Finally such rewards may be attached to the termination of unwanted social compensations, including various types of hyper-verbalization, engaged in by some insecure children when exposed to motor task situations.

Extrinsic, material rewards also may not transfer to life situations, because it is unlikely that the child will receive stickers, toys etc, every few minutes as he or she spends each day. Thus every effort should be made to give the child clear evidence of positive changes in skill levels that may be occurring, and at the same time register social approval for the improvements achieved. Also an excess of intrinsic rewards given randomly and not attached to performance changes contributes to learned helplessness. The child, exposed to these latter conditions begins to believe that engaging in physical activity, when indiscriminately rewarded or over-rewarded, must constitute a noxious form of work for which one should be paid, even though no effort is expended or improvement takes place. (Cratty 1989h).

(C) *Goals should be clearly stated, precise and frequently set.* The data research findings from studies on goal-setting are clear. Admonishments to 'do your best' extended to groups or to individuals, are not likely to produce any measurable positive performance changes. In contrast groups, or individuals have been found to perform significantly better over time, when confronting both mental and physical tasks, when they are faced with precise goals.

Furthermore, goals need to be clearly understood by the learner, formulated with precision, and carefully described and stated by the teacher-clinician. Whether goals are formulated by the learner or the instructor is not as important as whether they are *accepted* as reasonable, and are clearly understood by the learner.

Performance objectives should consist of establishing both short-term and long term goals. Performing youngsters should be shown how short-term goals contribute to long term goals. It should be clearly understood how a short-term goal, to be reached the next day or by the end of a week, contributes to clearly stated and measurable long-term goals, to be attained over longer periods of time. A chapter on goal setting research, related to physical activity, may be found in another text by the author (1989h).

Goals should be precise, easily measurable and understood by the child. It is more important that *improved effort* should be rewarded, either through extending social-reward-approval statements or by giving extrinsic rewards, than it is to reward performance improvement. Rewards for improvements of in individual effort, including more prolonged attention to the task and the reduction of evasive behaviors, will likely have positive effects upon performance and learning.

Improvement-graphs reflecting upward fluctuations of measures of effort or performance, are useful. Youngsters need clear evidence of their improvement, presented to them in terms they understand. Every paper completed during the practice periods intended to improve printing, used by the children in our program, are retained and dated (See The Case Studies in

Chapter 7). Using this evidence a child may, after a few weeks or months of practice, clearly observe performance improvement. Other skills may also be graphed. These may depict age-related changes in gross motor skills, and should be retained for later inspection by the children. Care must be taken to determine that the child both understands the nature and measurability of the goals set, and also understands the nature of the improvement depicted.

(D) *Complex Skills must often be taught using a progressive-part strategy*. It is highly satisfying, both to teacher and learner, if a child can observe and then perform an entire movement that has been demonstrated or explained. However this rapid acquisition of complex actions is often not possible by clumsy youngsters. Thus complex skills must be taught in parts. However seldom is a 'pure' part method useful. This would consist of teaching-demonstrating and learning each part separately and then performing the entire action by putting all the parts together at the same time.

The progressive-part method is usually better. This consists of first demonstrating and learning the first part of an action, and then the second component. These two parts are combined and then performed together, before learning and then adding a third part. The three parts are then practiced as a whole, until acquired. Then a fourth part is learned, before being added to the 'whole' composed of the first three parts. This system is continued until the entire action-sequence or pattern is acquired. This method is appropriate when teaching dyspraxic children to tie their shoes. Seldom can this, and other, multi-part skills be acquired wholes. Many such tasks must be broken down into parts, and then built up into the whole, using the 'progressive-part' way described elsewhere.

(E) *Sound principles of transfer of skill should be followed*. Acquiring skill in one task cannot be counted upon to transfer to improvement in another task. For example, years ago the literature contained data demonstrating a lack of correlation between large and small muscle activity. Similarly in our clinic program we consistently observed that large muscle activities did not improve hand-eye coordinations needed in manipulative tasks, and when printing and writing. It was found that practice in printing letters was needed to improve letter formation, just as specific practice in ball throwing and catching was needed to enhance these important playground skills. Program content should thus reflect in precise ways the specific task-needs of the participants.

The program should be based upon what is termed 'narrow transfer width'. The child should be confronted with relatively specific tasks in which it is hoped to elicit improvement.

In contrast, adherence a 'wide-transfer width' principle suggests that with the practice of a few tasks, improvement will occur in a wide variety of tasks and ability categories. In general this latter hypothesis related to transfer, has proved popular with many over the years. In general, however, motor development program promising too much simply by exposing the child to a few sensory and/or motor experiences are clearly unsound and lacking in scientific veracity. The following diagram contrast the concepts of narrow, in contrast to wide transfer width, relating program content to expected outcomes.

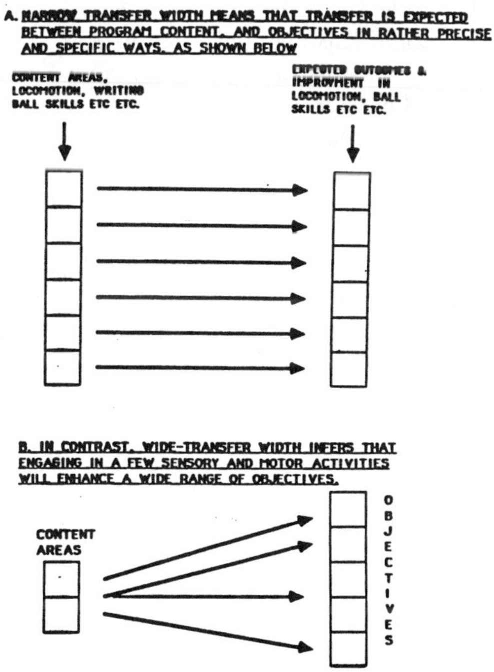

Chart 12-1. Wide and narrow transfer width

An effective program should provide specific content-experiences which specifically address a child's individual competency needs. Unfit children should be exposed to specially designed groups of physical exercise intended to improve weakness in specific muscle groups, children with balance problems should have balance training, while those having trouble with locomotion and agility should contain opportunities to improve tasks within these skill areas. For the most part, since most awkward children evidence three or four types of performance problems, the program content should be similarly varied, and contain opportunities to engage in at least four to five types of activities and skills.

Transfer cannot be left to chance. It is a common supposition, for example, that letter reversals are produced by children who do cannot identify their own left and right hands and body parts. However not only is there not a statistical correlation between left-right discrimination and letter reversal, but simply training youngsters to identify their left or right hands will not modify letter reversal, (or the reversing of letter order in words).

To modify letter reversal *cognitive bridges* must be built from the child's body to the page. This may be accomplished, for example, by having the child first identify their left and right hand, and then touch the corresponding side of the page with each hand. At this point, sides of the pages may be labeled with the words "left" and "right". Then various letters and numbers may be oriented on the page, relative to whether they "face", or open to the left or right hand sides of the page.

The transfer of general principles governing skilled performance may not occur, unless taught for. For example, a useful biomechanical principle, common to more than one motor task, often must be re-taught when confronting each task. The concept of making a forward weight shift of the body when executing a vigorous throwing movement, must often be demonstrated and taught again and again when instructing youngsters to execute other forceful movements in which the same principle is applicable, including hitting and striking. Each of the movements containing this weight-shift principle (or any other principle) should be practiced, and the principle re-explained during each different session. Young awkward clients, without direction, cannot be expected to transfer and apply useful biomechanical principles from one task to another without a great deal assistance by a teachers or therapist.

(G) *The content of a program should include provisions for enhancing basic movement qualities, as well as more specific and complex skills.* When formulating program content the focus should be upon tasks reflecting different levels within a comprehensive classification system. Including should be those designed to enhance qualities ranging from basic movement factors to more complex skills, and skill families. The following Chart (12-2) illustrates such a hierarchy. Thus the content decided upon should reflect both the individual performance needs of the young clients, as well as specific skill demands required in the sub-cultures; competencies that include "skill families" useful at play and in athletic competition, as well as complex groups of self-care skills.

SKILL "FAMILIES"

ALL THE SKILLS IN FOOTBALL, BASKETBALL, SWIMMING STROKES AND STARTS, ETC.

COMPLEX MULTI-PART SKILLS

SERVING A VOLLEBALL, OR SOFTBALL, KICKING A FOOTBALL, SERVING A TENNIS BALL, A JUMP SHOT IN BASKETBALL ETC.

SIMPLE MOVEMENTS AND MOVEMENT SERIES

ONE JUMP FORWARD, SKIPPING, BOUNCING A BALL, RUNNING A ZIG-ZAG AGILITY COURSE

BASIC MOVEMENT AND PERCEPTUAL FACTORS FOUND IN FACTOR ANALYSES OF GROUPS OF MOTOR PERFORMANCE SCORES.

BODY AGILITY, LIMB SPEED, STATIC STRENGTH ENDURANCE, FLEXIBLITY, RUNNING SPEED ETC.

Chart 12-2. Levels of performance

(H) *Special provisions should be made for the perceptual–sensory as well as for the motor aspects of skill.* Precise training in the perceptual as well as the motor components of skills should prove useful. Thus such aspects of skill acquisition as perceptually anticipating the location of incoming balls, as well as kinesthetic awareness of the positions of body parts should be incorporated into efforts as enhancing skill directed toward poorly coordinated youngsters.

(I) *Special strategies are needed to insure retention of skill.* There are clear-cut practical differences between the concepts reflected in the terms *performance, learning and retention.* Performance changes often occur during a brief short-period of time, reflecting momentarily heightened emotional or motivational states. In contrast, learning implies permanent changes in behavior caused by practice. Retention is the ability to re-perform a task after a period of no-practice lasting several weeks, a few months, or even longer.

Simply because a child is observed performing a task, or group of tasks during a single practice session (printing all the letters of the alphabet, to give one example) does not insure that the skill(s) will be retained over time. Extra practice is often necessary, past some established criteria, to produce long-term retention. Over-learning, if well-motivated, will serve to insure the easy re-performance of a skill(s) at a later data.

A four or five year-old, for example, exposed to letter-printing practice may forget how to execute many of the letters of the alphabet after a short-period (7-10 days) during which no practice occurs. It is if some internal 'floppy (memory) disc' has been erased within their personal computer inside their head! Forgetting occurs partly because initial over-learning has not taken place. Because The performance levels observed prior to a lesson-vacation may actually constitute a temporary state reflecting highly motivated effort, rather evidence that true learning has taken place.

Rhythmic motor skills are remarkably resistant to forgetting. An adult will suddenly climb on a bicycle and ride it, even though no practice may have occurred for several decades. However skills containing difficult combinations of sequences, including shoe-tying and dressing. In contrast those lacking coherent relationships are easily forgotten, and require over-learning to produce true retention. For example printing the letter A, upon hearing the sound "ah."., and similar 'illogical' motor tasks and stimulus-response combinations are more difficult to retain, than are the rhythmic order of strokes used when writing capital cursive letters.

Other factors contribute to skill retention. Remembering and re-performing a motor task will be facilitated if, for example, during the learning process, youngsters understood that the task is an important one, a skill requiring retention and one which must later be re-performed. More retention is likely to take place if awkward youngsters are aided to understand that the skills they practice are important over their life time, and are not only of momentary importance. Other principles of skill retention are summarized in a 1975 text (Cratty 1975).

(J) *The age and/or developmental levels of the child-clients will influence the degree to which general movement qualities versus specific skills should be incorporated into the program.* In general more activities intended to enhance general qualities should be contained in programs designed for younger children, or those more developmentally delayed. With age ability profiles tend to fragment, evidencing more specific abilities and disabilities. (Cratty 1989b) In contrast, when working with older youngsters and/or those more advanced, more emphasis should be placed upon the introduction and practice of specific skills, both motor tasks needed for the playground and self-care activities. This relationship between maturational-developmental level, and the specificity of skill training is illustrated below in Chart 12-3.

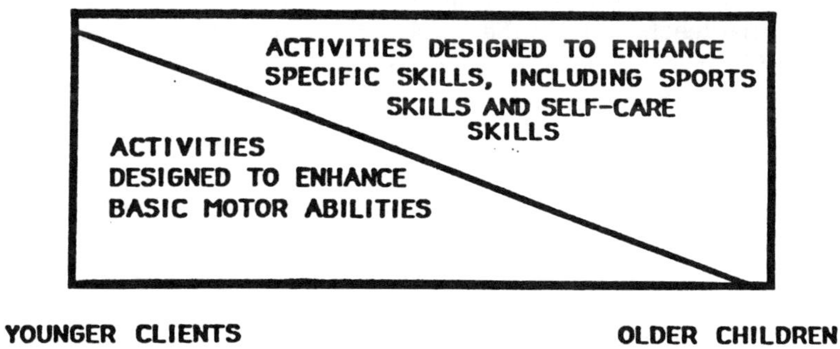

IN INFANCY AND EARLY CHILDHOOD EMPHASIS SHOULD BE PLACED UPON ACTIVITIES DESIGNED, TO ENHANCE GENERAL MOTOR ABILITIES, HOWEVER AS THE AGE OF THE CLIENTS INCREASES, THERE SHOULD BE A SHIFT TOWARD ACTIVITIES DESIGNED TO ENHANCE SPECIFIC SKILLS ENCOUNTERED IN LIFE, INCLUDING SELF-CARE SKILLS

Chart 12-3. Basic vs specific skill content in programs of motor development as a function of age

The Emotional Environment

Adherence to several principles should help to optimize the emotional environment in which remedial efforts take place. These include guidelines applicable to teacher-learner interactions and those governing parental behaviors directed toward an awkward youngster. Efforts to encourage responsible parental responses to their youngster's physical efforts often requires the help of effective family counselors.

(A) *Improvement of self-esteem in physical activities should be a constant goal.* Specific strategies and techniques should be directed toward achieving that objective. How children feel about themselves comes about because of combinations of negative and positive social evaluations. What people say about a youngster's physical performance efforts, including parents, friends, teachers and others, have a marked impact upon how youngsters feel about their body's capacities to move. Thus to change how a child feels about himself or herself there is a need to modify how others react the awkwardness seen among these youngsters.

Parents should be helped to become aware of both the negative or positive impact their statements may make upon their offspring. Most important parents must be given precise and clear evidence reflecting performance improvement evidenced by their child, so that their perceptions of his or her efforts and performance are modified. If parental perceptions are changed, hopefully the child may begin to receive more positive social feedback from them, for both improved effort expanded, and for measurable improvement that has taken place.

Often the negative social feedback from playmates and school 'friends' can emotionally crush the performance of an awkward child, even after measurable improvement is achieved. At times it may be necessary to place an improving youngster in a new school setting. This type of relocation may permit new schoolmates to give him or her chances to enter games, and new teachers who respond more positively to classroom work completed, than was true in the former school setting.

The children's self-perceptions of physical performance and abilities, do not form their entire self-concept. Often separate are feelings about intellectual accomplishments, and social skills and acceptability (Do people like me?). However children's physical performances are one of the most observable behaviors others judge. Thus if negativisms are constantly voiced, this constant social censure may "spill over" into social and intellectual components of youngsters' self-esteem.

It should be emphasized that a child's self-esteem is somewhat compartmentalized. Even by the age of five it has been found that there are specific groups of feelings a child has about himself or herself. These include feelings about social acceptance and abilities, perceptions of academic competencies, as well as what a child thinks about his or her physical appearance and abilities. These self-perceptions continue to fragment and become more specific in older children. In early adolescence, for example the youngster perceives different kinds of social acceptance as arising from a close friend, versus a more global social group in which they function.

Thus movement educators should be aware of the possibility that improving a child's physical 'self' does not always easily transfer into other components of the child's self-perceptions. It is often seen when testing the self-concept among entrants to our clinic, that a child may believe himself or herself adequate socially and intellectually, but feel deficient in physical skills. Thus young clients entering clinic programs in which an objective is to enhance self concept, should have their self-concept evaluated with precision. Following this evaluation, specific means should be taken to enhance the component of the self-concept the clinic personnel is claiming to modify.

(B) *Parents should be encouraged to formulate reasonable expectations for their children's capacities, and for potential skill changes due to educational efforts and programs.* Parents often need to be aided to determine what recreational and self-care skills are able to be accomplished at their child's developmental (not chronological) age. If care-givers impose undue pressures, they may undermine the best efforts put forth by both their children and by clinicians.

Helping parents to formulate ways of aiding a child to acquire important self-care skills is important. For example, laying the child's clothes out in the order they are put on when dressing should assist a dyspraxic child to get ready in the morning. However, most parents should not be pressed into service as home-teachers. It is enough for the parent to concentrate upon the overall happiness and mental health of their child, rather than impose additional stresses upon the child-parent dyad that are likely to be experienced if the parent is asked to teach the child at home.. Unreasonable pressures from parents to succeed in motor tasks can sabotage the best efforts of competent clinicians and teachers. Finally parents are not likely to be effective home-teachers because they have already used up the rewards and punishments available to them as they get their off-spring through the day's activities. Adding the stress of tutoring to the social pressures already born by the mother-child paid, will often break down effective communication and interaction between the two.

It may be useful to impart counseling about the kinds of sports in which awkward children may expect better performance outcomes. Generally children whose perceptual problems preclude their participation in often-confusing team sports may be encouraged to participate in individual sports in which the perceptual demands are not too great. The concepts of "open" and closed skills may be useful to explain during this type of conference.

Generally more success is achievable in closed skills, by awkward children, than when confronted with open skills. An closed skill is one in which the performer has control all of (or most of) the task"s components. Closed skills include jogging, golf, swimming, practiced dance movements, and body-building. On the other hand open skills are those containing unexpected components to which the child must suddenly adjust. Open skills include those in which the performer must react to the unpredictable actions of others. Open skills include volleying in tennis, playing outfield in baseball, hitting a pitched softball, defensive actions in volleyball and most skills used when playing both ice and field hockey.

Finally parents should be aided to place emphasize upon a clumsy child's abilities, rather than upon their disabilities. Constant reminders directed toward a youngster of what he or she cannot do, is likely to be psychologically crushing. On the other hand an emphasis upon both improvement, and what a child *can do well* are likely to have positive emotional outcomes.

(C) *Teacher-clinician behaviors should encourage effort, and reflect positive expectations.* Data from studies such as that by Martinek and Johnson (1979) have indicated over the years that teacher expectations are important molder's of children's efforts and improvement in educational programs. Negativism, or even passivity, on the part of an instructor-clinician in a remedial program will likely have negative consequences. Instructor behaviors reflecting optimism will likely elicit positive change.

(D) *The program's task content should be designed to insure initial success.* Prior to the institution of tasks which may prove difficult and threatening the awkward child should be exposed to easily accomplishable activities in which initial success is guaranteed. The awkward child is usually insecure in a physical-activity environment. These insecurities, unless overcome with success, will likely produce various kinds of avoidance behaviors early in the remedial process. Avoidance strategies appearing may include hyperverbalization, and/or aggression, and even include tearful withdrawal from the task situation.

After success is achieved, then moderately stressful skill levels may be gradually introduced. The awkward child typically has a very narrow range of acceptability of task difficulty, with regard to physical tasks. Skilled activities which are perceived as too easy may prove immediately insulting and avoidance reactions are likely to occur. In contrast, tasks believed by the child-client to be too easy, quickly prove insulting, and again the youngster will likely display withdrawal and avoidance strategies.

Adjusting task difficulty is often difficult. The task of the effective clinician, however, is to constantly identify tasks within the child's narrow range of acceptability, in order to reduce or eliminate avoidance behaviors and "distractible" reactions. Making the accommodation of task difficulty even harder, is that the child-client"s range of acceptability may change from session to session!

Operational Principles

(A) *Personnel should be selected with reference both to having good technical-professional skills and also possess superior personal-social competencies.* Both sensitivity to individual needs, as well as a knowledge of motor skill acquisition and child development are important to consider when staffing programs of motor development. Having a high level of technical skill and knowledge, without the ability to elicit good personal-social interactions will blunt the best efforts of those possessing several university degrees. While simply liking children and being able to relate to them will not insure that a program of effective physical activities are presented in a manner that is technically sound, educational useful, and safe.

Personnel may be obtained from those graduating from schools of physical and occupational therapy with good backgrounds in normal motor development, and some experience with moderately awkward children. However the training of many emerging from these institutions have prepared them primarily for working with the aged, post-operative cases, and/or with obviously handicapped youngsters. Adapted physical educators are often useful, but lack the background to enhance graphic skills.

Students with backgrounds in psychology as well as physical activity are often helpful, as are physical education and classroom teachers with additional work in motor development. Some experience with learning disabled children can help, because of the prevalence of motor ineptitude among this population. Often a program is well staffed if a several individuals reflecting a variety of backgrounds render service.

(B) *Programs should be available to children from 2–5 times a week, in sessions lasting from 40 minutes to more than an hour.*

Once-a-week sessions do little but document the maintenance, or the steady decline, of abilities the child may possess. While too frequent exposure to the pressures of learning skills may similarly blunt progress. Often best is a program, of from two to three sessions spaced throughout the week.

The length of the session depends upon the ages of the children served. Younger children should be exposed to shorter sessions of formal instruction. The length of a single session should will often depend upon the variety of motivating and varied experiences available. In general the more varied the offerings, including crafts, recreational skills, and graphic-drawing content, the more motivating and varied the components of session are likely to be, and thus the child should be able to sustain his or her interest for longer periods of time.

One-hour, or a forty-five minute remedial period, should be divided into several *task sessions*,. Each task session may last for from two to three minutes, to from ten to fifteen minutes. A task session is a relatively short period of time during which a single task, group of highly similar tasks or a single game, is engaged in.

Usually task sessions are longer when the youngsters are older, and/or their attention is reasonably good. Sometimes task sessions last only 3-5 minutes when a 'busy' five year old is being dealt with. A task session should generally last as long as a child is engaging in motivated work.

When working with a hyperactive-distractible child the session should be prolonged slightly longer than the child is willing to work. Thus if avoidance behaviors (either physical or verbal) are encountered during the 4th minute of a task session, the session should be prolonged, perhaps 2 minutes more. A task session may be made to last longer with (a) the help of verbal contracts made with the child ("Work a few more minutes and we will go to the computer next") or (b) with the aid of extrinsic rewards ("Two more minutes of work with the ball will earn you a pretty sticker").

The duration of task-sessions in which same task is continually practiced, may vary from session, when working with the same child over a week or months. The length of task sessions will depend upon the temporary mood state of the child, fatigue encountered as well as other variables evaluated by a sensitive clinician. A single clinical-session, lasting from thirty minutes to over an hour, may thus consist of from 4-10 task sessions each of which may be from 3-10 minutes in duration.

(C) *Semi-structured play may produce remedial benefits.* Structured sessions containing formal instructions, are not the only way to elicit improvement in youngsters' movement capacities. Well conceived play, molded to varying degrees by clever developmentalists, will often produce hoped for changes in movement capacities. This approach may be particularly effective with groups of infants from 1–4 years of age. This molding may be accomplished by (a) the use verbal suggestions (b) by the provision of selected play materials, (c) by using obstacle courses requiring various motor abilities to traverse, and/or (d) arranging the size of children's play groups. Socialization goals may also be achieved within such sessions, particularly of games and apparatus requiring cooperative-sharing efforts are employed. I once observed several kinds of paired activities usefully applied in a motor development program designed for blind and low vision pre-schoolers. The activities forced cooperation and social interactions by the nature of their requirements.

SUMMARY AND OVERVIEW

Development program need to be carefully constructed and contain content specific to the individual needs of children they are designed to serve. Both programs containing both formal instructed task-sessions, and programs consisting of modified play activities, under various circumstances, are likely to have beneficial outcomes.

Heightened self-esteem by the child-clients may be achieved if both instructors and parents are encouraged to view the child's efforts to verbally acknowledge improvement in positive ways. Parental counseling may be necessary to help adjust their expectations, and to impress upon them the importance of emitting positive social responses imperative in enhancing the mental health of their child. Parents also may be helped to select specific sport skills in which instructional efforts may be beneficial. Often these skills include those in which the child has control over all components, rather than some sports skills in which the youngster must react to the unexpected and unpredictable actions of others. That is closed skills are preferable to open skills.

Programs consist of individual task-sessions that last from a few minutes to a quarter or an hour or longer. Two or three remedial periods spaced throughout the child's week are usually best, as is the spaced practice of given skills. Progressive part practice is often needed as an awkward child acquires a difficult skill. This method requires a teacher to begin with a simple part of the skill and gradually add components until the entire task is mastered. Over learning of skills is necessary to insure maximum retention, as is well motivated practice. Motivational efforts can employ extrinsic rewards to initially gain a child's attention and cooperation. However it should be attempted to phase out intrinsic rewards, and substitute as reinforcement the intrinsic satisfaction youngsters derive from mastering necessary motor tasks.

Developmental knowledge, coupled with social sensitivity should be required of personnel working with awkward children. Developmental knowledge permits effective sub-task analysis so that skills and levels of difficulty are appropriate to the child's developmental age. Developmentalists working with youngsters should be armed with backgrounds in both theory and also reflecting practical operations. A theoretical orientation alone will likely results in a therapist knowing *why* things should be done, but not knowing just *what* to do. A individual whose background includes only 'practical' operations will probably know things to do, but will have difficulties accommodating and assessing to practices, reacting effectively to individual differences. Furthermore an absence of theoretical background will likely result in personnel who do not know *why* they are doing what they are doing!

QUESTIONS FOR DISCUSSION

1. Discuss the concepts of narrow versus wide transfer width. Theories emphasizing which of the two types of transfer are likely to be more popular among parents of awkward children? Which transfer-model is likely to produce better results?
2. Discuss in specific terms how goals might be set for a child entering a program of skill development? Can you give an example of how might a specific short-term goal may be related a long term objective?
3. Discuss the idea of skill specific motor training, versus more general motor training as applied to youngsters of various ages? At what ages does skill specific practice appear most useful?
4. Discuss how one might measure the self-concept of a child entering a program of motor education? What specific strategies might be employed to enhance a child's self-concept in such a program?
5. How might a skill be taught, using a progressive part method of practice? Be specific.
6. How might rewards given too often, or inappropriately blunt performance? What principles can you derive for the administration an effective reward program within a clinic intended to enhance physical skills?
7. Discuss what teaching strategies should be employed, when working with a clumsy child, if general principles of skill acquisition are to be taught and are to transfer from task to task.
8. Discuss the ideas of skill families, and of levels of skilled performance discussed and diagrammed in the chapter. How may these ideas be implemented in a skill development program?
9. What considerations should be kept in mind when selecting and training personnel for a motor enhancement program?
10. In what setting are awkward children likely to be exposed to remediation and assessment? What do you believe are the advantages and drawbacks of the various settings listed in chapter?

Chapter 13
Prognosis for Change

INTRODUCTION

A question frequently asked by parents, whose youngsters evidence clumsiness is, "Can anything really be done to change my child's coordination?". At times this query is accompanied by statements like, "I was a clumsy child and nothing was done". Thus some caretakers, by this latter admission, seem infer that since he or she somehow survived a childhood of awkwardness, why shouldn't their child undergo the same discomfort and indignities?

Some medical specialists may also voice skepticism about the efficacy of remedial efforts when an awkward child has been diagnosed as evidencing the motor symptoms reflecting a minimal neurological handicap. The assumption is made that this problem is not improvable through training because the nervous system is not very plastic and modifiable. Similar to this viewpoint are professional opinions that the child will 'outgrow' the problem, and that thus remedial efforts are not likely to be successful.

Professionals formulating programs for awkward children should be prepared for these questions during parent conferences following evaluations. They should attempt, furthermore, to offer the best answers possible, by referring to best the available data and to expert opinion. Several variables should be taken into consideration when formulating an answer. These include the age and emotional state of the child, the degree of awkwardness present, and the skills in which improvement is needed.

Unfortunately there is not a great deal of literature illuminating the nature of possible changes in motor performance and related functions, resulting from remedial efforts. Most of available the data has come from investigations whose authors have focused upon modifying the performances of normal children through teaching and exercise. Also relatively plentiful are studies dealing with programs intended to change the physical capacities of more severely involved atypical populations, including cerebral palsied youngsters, the emotionally disturbed and the mentally retarded.

Little emphasis has been placed upon exploring the potential for eliciting change in movement capacities among populations of moderately awkward children. Also scarce are studies of the possible improvement that may be achieved among groups of poorly coordinated children exposed to remedial efforts designed change manual skills and self-care tasks. The few clinical descriptions available that reflect improvement in graphic behaviors in moderately and mildly dysgraphic-clumsy youngsters may be found in chapter 7. Promising, however, are several longitudinal studies that have sampled the motor difficulties measured in populations of awkward children, over significant periods of time. (Losse et al 1991) (Gillberg & Gillberg 1989).

There are general principles, however, that appear valid when considering the nature of possible changes in motor performance attributable to education and remediation. These guidelines include observations made by Benjamin Bloom (1956). He noted, after exploring the literature, that most marked changes, elicited through education, in performance, attitudes, and skills are likely to occur, when the remedial efforts are applied during the time of life these changes normally take place as the result of maturation.

Thus, Bloom concluded, if one wishes to mold and change political attitudes, these efforts will meet with the most success if applied between the ages of about seventeen and twenty-five, the time of life during which time these attitudes are usually in a state of flux. Likewise efforts to modify motor abilities and capacities, it may be hypothesized, are likely to be most successful earlier in life. Because between birth and about six to eight years of age, the neuromotor system is relatively pliable and plastic, and thus most amenable to modification. Similarly speech-language therapy may be most effective when applied between the ages of two to five or six years, during the time when language and speech functions normally mature.

There are other guidelines for predicting positive changes in perceptual-motor capacities. Included among these is the common finding that less severe problems evidenced by children, youth and adults are more modifiable, as are more severe problems occurring in childhood and adolescence. This principle seems to hold true when remedial efforts are applied to those with motor coordination deficits. Children and youth with marked forms of cerebral palsy are not as likely to exhibit positive, measurable changes as are those with mild to moderate coordination problems. Awkward children, just as true of the learning disabled, have been found to be greatly aided, by the presence of supportive and understanding parents present during the trials and tribulations they are likely to encounter throughout their childhoods, adolescence and early adulthood.

Surveying and interpreting the results of research literature dealing with the effects of remedial efforts, poses several problems. The information is both scarce, and scattered in a wide variety of journals both foreign and domestic, dealing with superior, normal and inferior physical ability groupings. Additionally it is difficult to attach precise meanings to such terms as *motor ability, physical incoordination, fitness motor learning, rehabilitation, perceptuo-motor dysfunction,* and to similar terms denoting both poor and adequate physical functioning. These and similar words are difficult to interpret because of the wide variety of measures of physical skills, fitness, motor learning, coordination, agility and performance employed to describe these qualities by interested scholars.

The research for valid 'change' information is also made difficult because there is an absence of well-controlled studies, employing populations of awkward children. Indeed there is a scarcity of research depicting the ways in which the movement capacities of *normal children and youth* may undergo possible modifications as the result of teaching.

The main purpose in this chapter is to review data from studies reflecting possible improvement, through education. The basic qualities examined in this context include skills requiring accuracy, coordination, agility, balance, ball skills and some manual tasks. Other reviews of literature about the possible improvement of self care skills and other manipulative skills, within developmentally delayed populations may be found in elsewhere (Cratty 1975) (Cratty 1989b).

Muscular fitness change are not covered thoroughly the following section. However, fitness and endurance capacities among the awkward youngsters probably, however, interact with levels of physical-coordination they likely evidence. The low fitness scores from learning disabled population reviewed in Chapter 9 (Cratty et al 1990), for example, probably reflect tendencies of poorly coordinated children to avoid recreational tasks requiring vigorous physical effort. This inclination to avoid physical activities in which poorly coordinated youngsters feel inferior, probably blunts basic strength and endurance capacities. Investigations of strength and endurance improvement in programs for children have been reviewed elsewhere, (Cratty 1989c). Information of this nature is also appears in an increasing number of studies to which the interested reader may refer. (Mero et al 1990) (Daniels 1971) (Eriksson et al 1974) (Macek 1971) (Mirald & Bailey 1981) (Vaccaro & Clarke 1978).

In the following section, a brief look will also be taken at data from studies exploring how medication may improve motor abilities. Although these data are scarce, there are both clinical observations and experimental findings suggesting that if attention and self-control are enhanced through medication, motor skill improvement may be a positive outcome.

RESEARCH STUDIES

The literature about skill improvement in children and youth is divisible into several categories. Studies in the United States during the 1930's and early 1940's usually reflected the collection of developmental norms, data that often included motor development sign-posts. During this same period several co-twin control studies were conducted, representing attempts to answer to the elusive question as to whether nature (inherited), or nurture (environmental variables, including teaching programs), are more likely to influences development.

The scholars conducting these latter investigations first surveyed the effects of training one of an identical twin pair, in one or more motor skills. They then attempted to determining whether the skill(s) taught to the trained twin exceeded the levels seen in the untrained twin, in the same tasks. (Minerva 1935) (McGraw 1935) (Hicks & Ralph 1931), (Werner 1974) (Gesell & Thompson 1934) (Hilgard 1932). If training resulted in superior performance, the teaching environment was credited with the changes measured. If, on the other hand, the physical abilities of untrained twin stayed even with those of his educated brother, arguments were made for the influence of maturation upon the qualities investigated.

During the first decades of the 20th century a few studies also appeared whose authors attempted to illuminate the effects of teaching of single motor skills to groups of children. Several different types of physical tasks were used, including ball skills and locomotor activities. These investigators, usually employed normal pre-school and school-age youngsters as subjects.

Studies evaluating the physical performance changes of college-age men and women appeared in the literature from 1930 to the 1960s. During and after both the First and Second World War, many were concerned about the poor physical fitness of the nation's youth, when they were evaluated as potential soldiers. These worries resulted in the institution of physical ability testing programs applied to entering college-university freshmen and women. Low scores posted in the initial testing sessions were signals that the student must enter special physical improvement classes whose content was intended to rectify performance and fitness problems. After the programs were completed, physical capacities and skill were re-assessed, to document the possible improvement that may have been taken place. For the most part positive outcomes were recorded (LaFuze (1951) (Broer (1951). The test batteries employed in these studies typically consisted of tasks requiring muscular fitness and strength, rather than reflecting the need to exhibit coordination and control.

From the early 1960's investigations have dealt with the possible effects of early infant stimulation applied to pre-school youngsters. This type of study was often part of the Head-Start movement which began during this time. The evidence obtained suggesting that remedial efforts instituted earlier in life were likely to be more beneficial, than interventions starting later in life. This trend for early childhood special enrichment has been given new life recently by the recent appearance of Federal Legislation in the United States (Public Law 99-457). This law which mandates that school districts engage in the early identification and education of infants, shortly after birth, suspected of displaying developmental delays.

Another trend in the literature during the last half of the 20th Century, included studies stimulated by appearance of numerous programs of motor ability initiated to elicit parallel changes in academic abilities. Studies and articles of this type first surfaced in the 1950's and they continue in the literature currently. While motor ability has been the training variable in these investigations, the primary the intent of many of the authors was to demonstrate that academic changes are certain outcomes of motor training.

Often those writing of these reports and conducting these investigations, were not equipped to conduct well-controlled studies. Their inexperience as researchers plus the cursory treatment of the data, often resulted in outcomes that were less-than-believable and of questionable validity. A helpful meta-analysis of data from 180 of these investigations was published in 1983. Its authors found that the motor programs researched did not elicit the hoped for improvement in academic skills, including reading, also that *motor abilities* of the subjects were not modified. (Kavale & Mattson 1983). These writings encouraged many teachers and parents to take closer looks at motor coordination in children. The interest engendered by these writings and the programs they spawned was not directed primarily toward improving physical skills, but was focused upon the possibility that one might quickly elicit changes in reading, and other academic capacities by administering a few simple perceptual-motor activities.

Another type of investigation found literature, since 1960's have been studies exploring the possible modifications of motor abilities among moderately to severely delayed populations of both adolescents and adults. Not only have the studies emphasized extending their physical skills, including essential self-care activities, but also upon improving endurance and fitness through exercise and training. The populations surveyed have included the mentally retarded, the emotionally disturbed, the visually impaired, the hearing impaired, and youngsters and adults with cerebral palsy.

A fourth issue recently covered in the available studies has revolved around the mechanisms and usefulness of endurance training for children and youth. Prior to 1970's information as to whether endurance training was harmful or helpful to pre-adolescent children was scarce indeed. However during the last two decades some tentative answers to both operational-programmic questions, queries about biophysiological issues are beginning to be formulated. (Mero et al 1990)

A fifth trend in the literature appearing the 1970's and 1980's, emphasized the effects of instructor-behaviors and teaching methods upon performance changes. Methodological issues such as whether teacher-directed, or child instigated instruction, are more effective were dealt with. Additionally influences of teacher-attitudes toward low and high functioning children were explored. These data have contrasted the outcomes of creative child-centered programs to programs closely controlled by teacher-directions.

During the 1960's researchers exploring hyperactivity in children tried to determine if classroom behaviors, and specific academic skills including printing and writing, were positively influenced by medication. This interest was accompanied by several attempts both by clinicians (Carpenter 1962) and experimentalists (Reeves and Wherry 1987). The results of these investigations are discussed later in the chapter.

Finally, and most promising, were the appearance in the 1980's of several longitudinal studies that have sampled the motor and social-emotional and academic behaviors of awkward children over time. The findings of these will be surveyed later. It is hoped that the are the precursors of others to follow. (Losse 1991) (Gillberg & Gillberg 1989)

The thorough illumination of important questions and tentative answers, contained within the historical trends listed, exceeds the limitations of this chapter. The following discussion is limited, therefore, to considering how some of this emerging data may impinge upon the question of whether programs containing physical tasks are likely to significantly modify the movement capacities of awkward children. The chapter content has thus been organized around the following main themes: (1) The effects of early stimulation upon motor capacities. (2) investigation of motor skill improvement of youngsters in early and middle childhood; and (3) movement capacity changes in atypical populations, including groups of awkward youngsters.

INFANT STIMULATION AND EARLY INTERVENTION: PROGRAM EFFECTS

Numerous studies of the effects of infant stimulation have been carried out during the past two decades. The content of these studies, however, contain only indirect implications for the improvement of physical awkwardness in children. Most of the time moderate awkwardness is not diagnosable until youngsters begin to walk, or until later within the fourth and fifth years of life. It is also difficult to find, studies of infant stimulation in which movement skills are the only objectives. Most of this work has focused upon helping a wide range of abilities including social and language skills, together with cognitive functions.

Most studies of subjects in early childhood, focusing upon the improvement of motor abilities, have concentrated upon youngsters with obvious handicaps including cerebral palsy, Down Syndrome, and spina bifida. (Harris 1987). These and similar conditions are diagnosable at the time or birth or shortly thereafter. In contrast some forms of physical awkwardness, dysgraphia for example, may not appear until the sixth or seventh year of life. Thus the awkward child has seldom been the focus of these types of investigations.

Delays in infant development first received attention at the end of the last century in Europe. In England during the late 1800's, for example, it was found that about 75% of all children born failed to reach the age of two. Data from New York City, early in this century, revealed that the death rate of infants from founding homes was

60% within the first year of life. (Bremmer 1971).

During the first decades of this century it was found that infants born into environments lacking adequate caretakers, accompanied by poor nutrition, and inadequate social-emotional stimulation, evidenced poor development that included delays in motor maturation (Dennis 1960) (Dennis & Najaria 1957). It has only been within the last twenty-five years that positive opinions about the potential role of early stimulation has encouraged the institution of intervention programs focusing upon potentially 'slighted infants'. The emphasis in these programs has been to instruct the parent or caretaker about how to best encourage motor, speech, cognitive, social and language skills. The programs have studied methods that would result in skills that would help young children to be successful later upon entering school.

Motor tasks are used in several ways within early intervention programs. Exploratory locomotor and manipulative behaviors are encouraged. Self-efficacy is promoted by helping children learn that they can accomplish things if they try hard enough. Social skills are encouraged within play environments, and thus the improvement of play skills is often an important objective. Manipulative skills are also encouraged so that the child may master self-care tasks, and acquire important graphic skills necessary for success in school. (Gray 1977) (Guinagh & Gordon 1976). (Cratty 1989). Both receptive and expressive language skills are also enriched. Typically these programs have employed contained combinations of activities, reflecting several objectives, and have included language games, arts and crafts, and playground skills.

The findings from these studies indicate that whether the program is conducted using trained teachers-clinicians, or with parents, is not as important as the duration of time devoted to the efforts at stimulation. Generally programs that persist for prolonged period of time, from two to three years, have been found to be more effective than those taking place for shorter periods of time. (Huntington 1979). Focusing upon younger children also seemed more productive of change than dealing with those in middle childhood.

The emotional tone of the program has often found to be more predictive of improvement of both motor skills and cognitive functions, than the precise content of the program. For example Birns and Golden (1972) discovered that the pleasure young children derived from task performance was predictive of later intellectual performance. Positive attitudes toward performance has been termed "competence motivation" by some (White 1959) and "pleasure in mastery" by others (Hendrick 1943). The data thus began to it clear that those formulating programs of early intervention should pay close attention to strategies designed to heighten the pleasure and feelings of success the youngsters experience as the result of their participation. (Brown 1981).

In recent years there have been an increasing number of studies conducted exploring how the movement capacities of several types of young handicapped children may be improved through intervention. These studies have surveyed the effects of various forms of physical rehabilitation and therapy applied to infants evidencing Down Syndrome, Spina Bifida, and to youngsters exhibiting various forms of cerebral palsy. However, the difficulty in locating groups of young clumsy children, together with problems in the early diagnosis of moderate awkwardness, have discouraged extensive efforts to scrutinize this sub-population during the early months and years of life. Rehabilitation programs when applied to the obviously motorically handicapped, however, generally have produced positive effects. (Harris 1987).

Taft (1981) a pediatric neurologist recommended, upon surveying the available evidence, that early intervention programs to improve motor competencies among young physically handicapped populations are useful in order to,

(1) improve parent-child relationships,

(2) to motive the child to attempt new and useful motor tasks,

(3) to assist the young child toward improved independence earlier in life, and

(4) to produce handicapped children who are likely to grow up emotionally healthier, than if their physical qualities skills are not attended to.

The same goals could be listed to support the importance of establishing programs involving the early identification and remediation of children who display moderate coordination problems early in life.

SKILL IMPROVEMENT IN EARLY AND MIDDLE CHILDHOOD

Two types of studies have dealt with the teaching skills to young, normal children. The first of these were a group of investigations whose writers intended to illuminate the relative contributions of nature (inheritance) versus nurture (education) to the production of movement skills. The second type of investigation were straightforward attempts to determine whether various kinds of skills encountered by young children were improvable through training. The skills studied often including those involving the larger muscle groups. Important self-care activities essential in early childhood were not scrutinized as closely.

The results of these studies have implications for those designing programs for younger awkward children. For example, if maturation seems to be more influential of skill improvement early in life, then many awkward children should be left alone to simply 'mature out' of their motor problems. On the other hand, if data from these training studies indicate that skills may improved more through education then remedial programs are justified. Unfortunately the results of the studies do not always offer data supporting clear-cut answers to these difficult questions.

Co-Twin Control Studies

The results of several co-twin control studies were reported in the 1930's. Their results constituted a way in which the then-popular controversy about whether nature or nurture were more likely to be the primary modifier of the maturing personality and of emerging abilities of infants and children.

The results of these efforts, however, offer little evidence for those taking either side of the argument as to whether inheritance or training molds physical abilities. For example, Hilgard (1932) found that the untrained twin quickly caught up with the trained twin in tasks involving locomotion and climbing. A study conducted at Yale University at about the same time (Gesell & Thompson 1934) produced similar results in tasks involving block manipulation and climbing; training effects were quickly overcome by the untrained twin. Minerva (1935) on the other hand found that while training helped one twin in complex throwing tasks, more basic locomotor functions were not significantly accelerated when the efforts of the trained twin were contrasted to his untrained brother. McGraw, (1935) however, found that in both tasks trained for, locomotion and climbing, superiority was registered by the twin exposed to enrichment, in contrast to the twin who was left alone.

Data from these co-twin control, studies plus correlative data I obtained in the late 1950's, suggests that basic locomotor activities may be less amenable to training and are more the result of inheritance, than are activities involving the upper limbs such as throwing, manipulation and the like. In a comparative study of skills exhibited by father-son pairs, high and positive correlations between fathers and their off-spring were recorded in both broad-jumping and sprinting. In contrast a bar-vault and throwing task evidenced no significant father-son correlations. It thus appeared that vigorous locomotor skills were more influenced by familial variables, while activities of the upper limbs were more molded by experience and training. This interesting inter-generational data were obtained when both father and son were college freshmen. The testing took place on the same facilities and was conducted by the same testers. (Cratty 1960)

During the next decades the popularity of co-twin control studies diminished, and they were replaced by others in which basic locomotion was trained in infants (Zelazo 1983). Investigations also appeared dealing with the effects of training upon skill changes in early, middle, and late childhood. These potential changes were also researched within populations of college and high-school age adolescents. The results from these studies also indicated that locomotor-type skills including climbing, running, and the like were more difficult to modify than those in which contain more learned elements such as throwing, manipulative activities and the like.

Skill Training in Early Childhood

Several investigators, in the 1930's explored the educability of various motor skills in populations of various ages. In a 1960 survey of the literature, however, only four investigations using younger children were cited (Mohr (1960). The skill most investigated was ball throwing, and the ages of the subjects varied from 2-6 years of age.

The results of these training studies were mixed. Hicks produced positive findings when training young children to hit a moving target (1931). These data indicated that improvement was due to what was termed 'general' instructions (teaching general principles) rather than to "specific" directions. Dusenberry (1952) using 56 children from three to seven years of age, also found improvement in throwing distance occurred after training sessions given within a five week period.

In contrast to these data, Miller (1957) found no improvement in throwing among first grade children trained during 26, 20 minute periods in a program lasting several weeks. A comparison of the methods employed in this, and in the previous study, does not readily reveal the possible causes for the different results obtained. Training of general principles, engaged in by Dusenberry, might have had more positive effects than the more skill-specific training engaged in by Miller. However different tasks were employed. Dusenberry training distance throwing, while Miller focused upon throwing accuracy.

Similar to the data from the co-twin control studies previously reviewed, the results of these training studies also indicated the improvement in locomotor skills may be more difficult to achieve than improvement of ball skills, and of similar activities. Dohrman (1964), for example elicited no significant improvement in kicking skills among eight-year olds, as the result of training. Halverson (1985) similarly found that skill in hopping, in children two to five years of age, was resistant to significant change as the result of practice.

The few available studies using young children often suffered from methodological short-comings. Many included only a hand-full of subjects Often the potentially influential variables were not well controlled, or were they clearly delineated. Hypotheses explored were often vague. For example, children described as unfit in one study (Tweit et al 1963) were found to imporve in a training program emphasizing attempts to improve the reaction time!

In still other studies sub-tests within test batteries, differing widely. Yet all purportedly evaluated general motor ability (Whittle 1961) (Henry 1956). Some batteries contained a predominance of tasks requiring bodily strength and speed, while others contained sensory-motor measures reflecting accuracy, coordination and kinesthetic abilities. This latter type of test battery, for example, was employed in a study by Masche (1970). He was able to improve skill in specific motor tasks, but failed to produce positive personality changes, among a group of second grade children exposed to a structured physical education program.

There are other studies in which physical training effects are studied among older youngsters exhibiting average and below average physical abilities. Whittle (1961) found that a regular and structured physical education program produced positive effects upon the motor ability of boys twelve years of age. Broer (1958) elicited similar changes among junior high school girls, based upon data from eight motor ability tests.

MOTOR SKILL CHANGES IN AWKWARD CHILDREN

Few Studies have been conducted with children-subjects diagnosed as evidencing physical coordination problems. One exception may be found in the physical education literature from Japan. In this study a small group of fifteen-year old girls with poor physical coordination were successfully trained to run a 50 meter hurdle race with increased speed (Tsutsui 1988).

An earlier, more comprehensive study used "neurologically impaired" children as a sub-population. It was completed in 1968 by G. Lawrence Rarick and his then doctoral student Geoffrey Broadhead (Rarick & Broadhead 1968). Their study explored the possible influence of several variables upon change in a number of physical abilities. Two major subjects populations were employed including a group of 206 "minimally brain damaged" boys and girls, placed within two age groups; one a younger group of six to nine year olds, and a second group ranging from ten to thirteen years of age. A second group consisted of 275 "Educable Mentally Retarded" children were divided into the same two age groups.

Several variations of instruction were applied in this study, thirty-five minutes daily, five days a week, for a twenty week period. These included one group taught whose members were physical education individually, and a second group instructed as a small class. Two control groups were also present. One of these remained in their regular physical education classes. The second control group was given art-instruction in order to control for the possible effects of special attention upon the changes recorded in the two experimental populations. These controls were included because in previous studies of this nature using retarded subjects (Corder 1966)(Lowe 1966)(Oliver 1958) it appeared possible that the positive changes obtained were due to special attention, rather than due to some combination of program instruction and/or content.

The motor performance tasks contained within the battery, applied before and after the programs were administered included tests of arm, abdominal and strength, tests of running speed and bodily agility, a softball throw and a 300 yard run. In addition measures of intelligence and emotional-social competencies were also obtained (Rarick and Broadhead 1968).

The results of Rarick's study were highly promising. For example it was found that significant changes in most of the motor performance tests were recorded by the experimental group exposed to an individualized program. The children labeled minimally brain damaged (who might be labeled hyperactive-learning disabled today) recorded significantly greater changes in motor abilities than did the retarded youngsters. The older male children with minimal brain damage improved more in overall motor abilities, than did the girls, or groups of younger children.

This study by Rarick and Broadhead, although the best available up to that time, contained several limitations (1968). For example the measures of intelligence were not usually employed. They consisted of a picture-vocabulary test and a drawing test., rather than well-standardized testing instruments such as the Stanford-Binet, or The Weschler Intelligence Scale for Children (WISC). Secondly the measures of motor performance did not include tasks requiring complex bodily coordination, target throwing, or balance skills. Thus, reasons for possible changes in coordination, among the minimally brain damaged subjects, were not completely illuminated. However, the data do strongly suggest, that a well designed program of individualized physical activity will produce positive performance gains, significantly greater than those produced simply by the imposition of special attention or by exposing a class to physical education activities taught in traditional ways. (Rarick & Broadhead 1968).

In 1972 my colleagues and I completed a study in which we contrasted the possible improvement in motor abilities measured in a group of twenty-eight awkward boys and girls (7-12 years of age) with whom were working at UCLA. Their scores were contrasted to motor abilities measured in a control group of learning disabled children from a local school district. The control group engaged in a regular program of physical education, while the experimental group came to the University twice weekly for one-hour programs of individualized work in motor skills and coordination. The program included work on drawing-printing skills and also contained the teaching of various gross motor skills. The children in both groups were evaluated initially, and at the end of a five month period. The scores of the trained subjects, were matched and contrasted by age and sex to those of the controls (Cratty et al 1972).

The data also offered some support for the efficacy of a special program of motor development. Overall the percent of improvement, as shown below (Table 13-1), was over 2.7 times greater by the experimental group, than was true among the control group when the average scores, reflecting percent of increase, from the battery of gross motor tests were contrasted. Additionally the mean scores from a figure drawing task also evidenced more improvement among the experimental subjects (14.4%), than was recorded in the data from the control group (1.1%).

Additionally the progress in various types of gross motor tasks depicted on (Table 13-2), revealed that the most marked improvement through training, occurred in balance, locomotor agility, and the catching of balls. Less improvement was noted in scores denoting

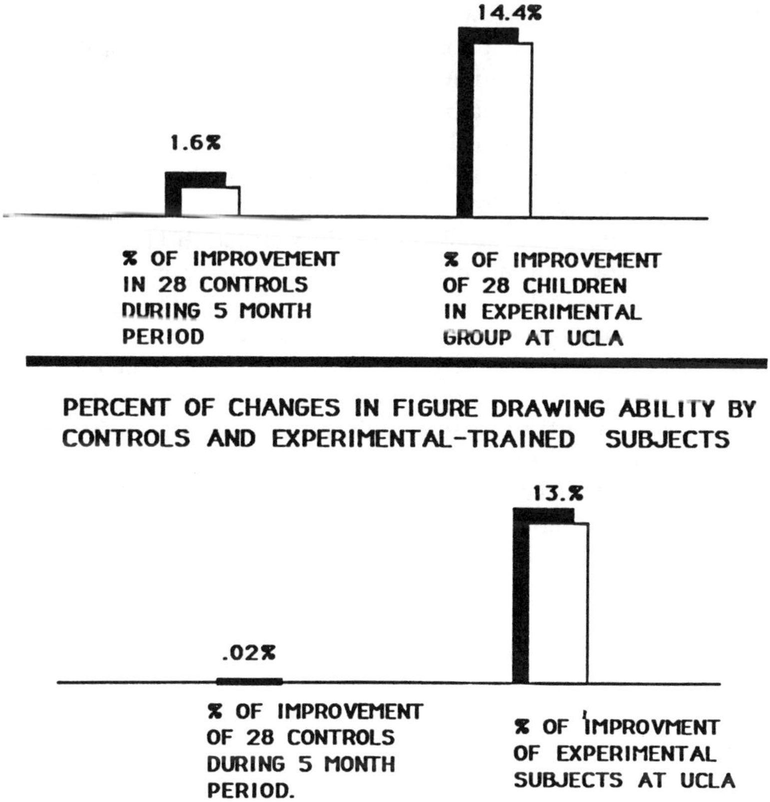

Table 13-1. Percent of change in overall gross motor functioning contrasting controls, with experimental-trained group

the identification of body parts, and in gross agility (ascending quickly from a back lying position, and copying a four-part movement of the total body). Encouraging was the finding that the ability to execute complicated geometric figures, adding one part at a time, was highly modifiable through training.

The data was also analyzed to determine within what age ranges the percent of improvement was most apparent. As can be seen (13-2. 13-3) the improvement among the fourteen younger children from 7-9 years, was more marked than among the fourteen children whose ages ranged from 10-12 years of age (Table 13-3).

The study suffered from several methodological problems including the use of a test battery that was not well normed, and controls whose physical abilities were not as deficient as those of the experimental subjects. However, there are indications in the data that it is *not inevitable* that positive changes in physical coordination will occur through maturation. The controls, even though exposed to a regular physical education program, *regressed* in some ability areas. Similar regression in physical attributes, as a function of disuse, has been found in more recent studies among the learning disabled (Cratty and Delrahim 1992).

A 'change' study was published in 1988 by Judith Laszlo (Laszlo et al 1988). The training methodology focused upon what were termed 'process variables'. These variables were conceptualized as consisted not only of motor qualities, but also as information obtained through several sensory channels including kinesthesis, and those involving visual-motor integration. The training consisted of non-visually practicing a small fluid-patterned maze, placed on a desk top. using a stylus.

Laszlo hypothesized that participation in training tasks that applied visual-perceptual stresses, visual memory, and drawing strategies, would elicit transfer to groups of motor skills in which these processes are important. Special evaluation tools were designed for these studies (The perceptual-motor abilities test, the PMAT (1985a), and the Kinesthetic sensitivity Test, KST 1985b). Teacher's ratings also were used both as screening instruments and to verify changes produced.

The outcomes of this study and of a previous investigation by this research group (Laszlo & Bairstow 1983) were positive. Thus these researchers postulated, as the result of their data, that their "process approach" was superior to focusing only upon the motor training of specific skills. Others, however, have been unable to replicate the

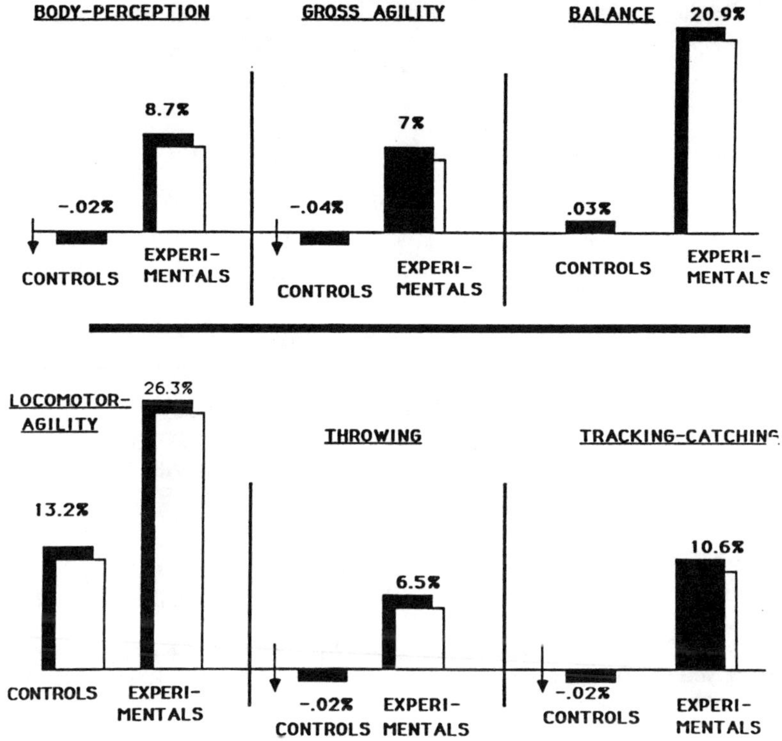

Table 13-2. Percent of change, by category in gross motor test battery, contrasting the scores of 28 controls with 28 subjects in experimental-trained group

findings emanating from the studies by Laszlo and her colleagues (Lord & Hulme 1987). The research has also been criticized as poorly designed, and containing too few subjects.

Furthermore it appears somewhat naive, to jump conceptually from the valid observation that various kinesthetic processes aid motor task performance, to the supposition that blindfolded maze practice is *the* tyype of kinesthetic practice needed to improve printing. In truth kinesthesis is a highly differentiated quality and ability, and furthermore is difficult to evaluate. (Cratty 1975) (Cratty 1961).

Within recent years both clinicians and researchers have suggested strategies for remediating dyspraxic symptoms in children (Gschwend 1988) (Gubbay 1975). Seaman and De Pauw, for example,

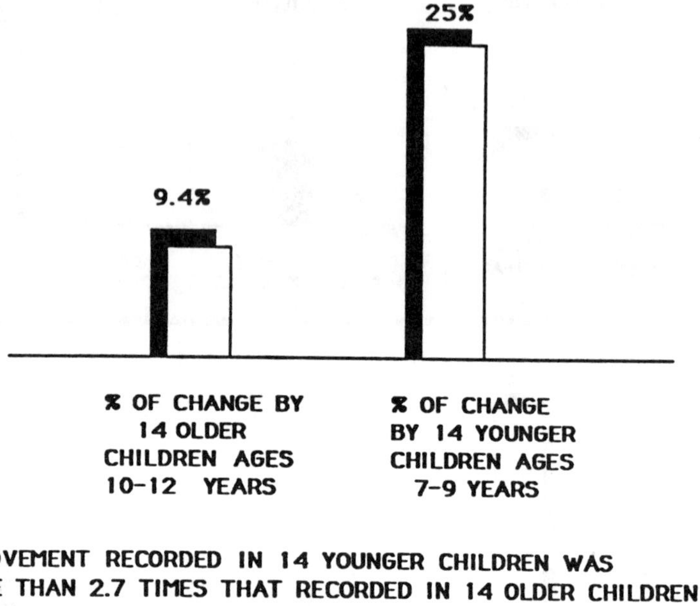

Table 13-3. Percent of change in gross-motor abilities by 14 younger children (7–9 years) contrasted to change in 14 older children (10–12 years) in experimental-trained group

listed twenty-one activities purporting to remediate fifteen signs dyspraxia in children. However their suggestions were not accompanied by research data substantiating their worth. (Seaman and DePauw 1982).

Gschwend (1988) also purposed a program for dealing with dyspraxia in children. This program included music and art therapy, playing chess, and other types of cognitive training labeled "will training". Gschwend's suggestions thus appear to constitute a more global approach to generalized cognitive-motor strategies than was true in the more skill-specific program suggested by Seaman and DePauw (1982).

The argument that improvement in several developmental parameters will inevitably take place because of maturation is advanced frequently. Usually those voicing this proposition further suggest that developmentally delayed children need simply be 'held-back' in school so that they may somehow "catch up". Simply holding a child back a grade, without the imposition of effective interventions, intended to remediate of both academic and coordination deficiencies, however, is not likely to elicit changes. In fact the available data reviewed here, strongly imply that the reverse may likely occur. The child who is retained with a group of less mature peers is likely to suffer a severe insult to his or her self-concept, making further remedial efforts more difficult. Moreover if remedial strategies are not applied intelligently during the time a youngster is retained in a school grade one year longer, the chances of both educational and physical improvement appear slight.

For example, in a recently completed study it was that significant improvement in upper-body strength was elicited by exposing learning disabled children to a fitness program. (Delrahim & Cratty 1991). In this same study marked improvement in strength was also found among sub-groups of learning disabled girls, and pre-adolescent boys and girls. Most interesting, however, was evidence that control populations who *did not* participate in training *recorded decrements* in fitness and strength, measured over time periods lasting from six to twelve months in duration.

Longitudinal studies which began to appear the late 1980's corroborated the persistence of coordination problems, along with social-emotional difficulties, among groups of motorically deficient youngsters. (Gillberg & Gillberg 1989) (Losse et al 1991). In the study by Losse (1991) for example, it was found that motor problems, reflected in the presence of motor soft signs, were present not only at the age of six when her thirty-two subjects were first evaluated, but were also seen in evaluations conducted ten years later. While some of the children surveyed over time had made progress, the majority had experienced stress from teachers, and also negative social pressure from peers during their childhood and adolescent years. Gillman and Gillman (1989) have also found that while some of their subjects had improved over time, many had continued to evidence coordination difficulties.

It is hoped that these recent longitudinal studies will inspire others. The data from these investigations, and from earlier studies, suggest that remediation of motor difficulties *may take place*, but only with the institution of effective, individualized programs, that are carefully staffed and planned. Moreover the information obtained in comprehensive effort by Losse and her colleagues in London, suggests that only with sustained and effective parental support are poorly coordinated youngsters likely to weather the social and academic 'storms' they are likely to encounter during their childhood and adolescent years. (Losse 1991)

It is becoming clear, however, that to elicit changes in motor and fitness functions of various populations of children precise program formulation is necessary, coupled with close supervision and good instruction applied by professionals possessing appropriate educational backgrounds. In the meta-analysis by Kavale & Mattson (1983) of data over 180 studies, in which programs were conducted by individuals with little or no background in motor development, revealed no significant changes in the motor coordination scores obtained from the 13,000 subjects involved.

MEDICATION AS AN INTERVENTION?

Several years ago in our Clinic, at UCLA, we evaluated a boy of about six years of age who evidenced dysgraphic symptoms. He did not enter our program, but returned a few months later for a follow-up evaluation. The improvement hand-eye coordination, reflected in his second drawings, was striking. When we asked his parent what had taken place between evaluations they stated that he had been exposed to medication intended to reduce hyperactivity. His improvement was marked, and reflected a two-year change occurring within just a three months.

Carpenter in an comprehensive clinical analysis of graphic skills in the learning disabled, also documented moderate to marked changes in printing and writing as the result of taking medication to reduce distractibility (Carpenter 1972). However he presented some evidence that retrogression in printing accuracy may occur in a limited number of children, either because of daily mood shifts, or because of unwanted side-effects emanating from medications. Generally the medication applied in these investigations are stimulants. Some postulated initially that stimulants act to activate important inhibiting centers of the brain, thus reducing activity level and lengthening attention span. Others have suggested more recently that medication results in neurotransmitters acting in more effective ways. (Cantwell 1992).

Dennis Cantwell recently described a summer camp program for learning disabled children in which baseball teams were medicated on alternate days to reduce hyperactivity and to lengthen improve attention. He related how each day, the medicated teams consistently won by a large score over the non-medicated teams. It was observed, he reported, that members of the non-medicated team were not attending to, or were they able to, intercept balls hit toward them. Members of the team medicated each day, in contrast, were able to first perceive and then to field both grounders and fly balls well. (Cantwell 1992). Thus the boys in this camp enjoyed winning baseball games, but only on alternate days!

In addition to clinical evidence, there have been several experimental studies conducted, whose authors have attempted to determine if the reduction of motor soft-signs, including indices of poor coordination, occurs after exposing children to medication intended to improve attention span and reduce hyperactivity. The findings from these studies have been mixed. Skekim and his colleagues conducted a study to determine whether soft-signs were reduced as the results of medication (3-methoxy-4-hydroxy-phenethyleneglycol, a norepinephrine metabolite). The study was not well controlled. The reduction of soft signs noted may have been due not only to the effects of medication, but and also because of the subjects matured during the relatively long time interval during which study was conducted. (Skekim et al 1979).

Lerer and Lerer (1976) studied the effects of methylphenidate upon forty hyperactive children who exhibited three or more soft-signs. Sixteen of the twenty children in the experimental group evidenced a reduction of soft-signs, in contrast to no reductions among children in the twenty-member control group. However the study suffered from several methodological problems including the use of a neurological evaluation of questionable objectivity, and the lack of adequate controls (Reeves & Wherry 1987).

In still another study of the effects of medication, McMahan and Greenberg (1977) found that some of the subjects, in both the experimental and control groups, evidenced a reduction in soft-signs. However in both experimental and control groups several of the forty-four hyperactive children in the study evidenced more soft signs at the conclusion of the experiment!

Wherry and Reeves (1987) and McMahan and Greenberg (1977) have highlighted the problems when trying to ascertain if medical interventions will reduce the presence of soft-signs, including determining valid indices of motor incoordination. The vexations they wrote about also included the lack of reliable measures of soft-signs, and the sometimes paradoxical effects of medications when applied to hyperactive children.

Further conundrums are seen in the data from a study by Ross (1982). They found that the medication they employed resulted in the childrens' teachers reporting them more manageable and educable. At the same time, however, significant changes in academic scores were not forthcoming. This kind of finding has also surfaced, when learning disabled children are medicated. These latter data point to the probability that, while medication usually improves attention and reduces hyperactivity, medication needs to be paired with intelligently applied remedial strategies and within well conceived program, in order for significant improvements in both academic and motor abilities to occur. Ross (1982) also expresses concerns about the use of medication in an extensive review of the topic. Both clinical observations and experimental data thus support the judicious use of medication in programs for hyperactive, poorly coordinated children, but only if paired with intellectually applied remediation.

It has been found among the youngsters in our clinic program that a judiciously medicated, hyperactive child becomes easier to work with in a remedial setting. It has been our observation also that these youngsters may also evidence immediate change in motor functions. The tasks evidencing improvement include both graphic skills and balance. It was assumed that the changes noted, and sometimes measured, are due to improved attention to the task at hand. However medication that produced less extraneous eye movements could have stabilized the balance efforts, when measured the second time after medication.

Wheery and his colleagues also noted, in a medication change study, that improved response time in learning tasks occurred in children who were given chemical help to control their hyperactivity (Wherry et al 1969). It is hoped that research in the future will further explore the efficacy of potentially useful medical accompaniments to traditional forms of motor therapy.

SUMMARY AND OVERVIEW

The limited evidence available suggests that, under optimum circumstances, some motor skills of young children are modifiable within limits. The more changes seem to occur in younger rather than in older populations. There are apparently optimum ages at which to apply a structured-instructional program in various motor skills. Between the ages of about four years and six or seven years seems best.

Changes recorded in investigations in which in ball throwing for distance and accuracy has been assessed, indicate that these qualities in normal, and among awkward, young children may be moderately improvable through training. In contrast locomotor activities (hopping, skipping and the like) appear to be more resistant to change through education in groups of young children. Available information also indicates that drawing and printing tasks also seem modifiable through the application of effective educational strategies that include specific motor practice of the tasks involved (Cratty & De Oliveira 1989a) (Cratty et al 1972) (Chapter 7).

In the few available studies of awkward children, the data indicates that coordination tasks, and related activities seem modifiable with training. Moreover remedial efforts may be assisted with the judicious application of medication when hyperactivity accompanies motor incoordination However, the presence of soft signs reflecting poor coordination may persist through childhood and into the teens. With effective interventions the changes that are recorded may occur in specific and useful "splinter skills." However, the underlying neurological deficits seem to remain. Finally interventions throughout an awkward youngster's life need to be accompanied by supportive behaviors emanating from family members, in order to reduce or eliminate undesirable social-emotional side-effects.(Losse 1991).

Also the available data indicates that *retrogression* in fitness and physical coordination may take place if effective remediation is not instituted (Cratty et al 1972) (Cratty & Dalrahim 1992). The best progress appears to take place when programs are carefully designed, and individual differences are provided for (Rarick & Broadhead 1968).

Information about the outcomes of remedial programs, intended to elicit change in motor qualities of children, is scarce. More research is needed to explore the influence of a number of variables including various kinds of instruction, the presence of severe versus moderate coordination problems, and the effects of motor training upon children of various ages. Additional longitudinal studies are important to carry out. This data will further reflect the nature of prolonged intervention programs applied over time.

QUESTIONS FOR DISCUSSION

1. During what years are changes in motor abilities likely to be elicited? What principle contained in the chapter explains your answer?

2. What kinds of studies were consulted for content for this chapter? Can you think of other types of journals that are likely to contain information on this topic?
3. What are co-twin control studies? What general and specific questions were they expected to answer?
4. Historically can you trace the interest in the manner in which remediation changes motor task performance?
5. What area of needed research were outlined in the chapter? What topics do you think need researching?
6. What can you say about the psychological and/or biochemical mechanisms that may make motor abilities modifiable through medication designed to reduce hyperactivity and inattention?
7. What kinds of motor tasks, was it suggested, are most amenable to modification through training? What kinds of tasks were hypothesized as less modifiable through training?
8. What does evidence from available longitudinal studies say about 'basic' changes in motor functioning of awkward children? Can you differentiate between basic changes due to training, in neuromotor functioning, and specific changes in splinter skills?
9. How would a program for children intended to bring about the most marked changes be constructed in an ideal way?
10. During the past century what social forces in the United States apparently encouraged university educators-researchers to become interested in exploring the manner in which fitness and motor abilities are modifiable in college-age students?

Chapter 14
Overview and Needed Research

OVERVIEW

Historical Perspectives

Before the beginning of this century the primary focus of scholars and physicians, interested in movement anomalies, was upon neurological problems whose presence were obvious, and whose causes came to be diagnosed straight forward ways. Literature dating back several hundred years, for example, has contained descriptions of the classic symptoms of cerebral palsy, of choreas, and of a variety of other dramatic movement aberrations.

It was not until the second and third decades of the 1900s that some began write and provide assessments for those evidencing subtle neurological deficits, often hidden until difficult tasks were attempted. Among these newly discovered problems was physical awkwardness. This more subtle kind of anomaly was first studied in older stroke patients. Later, others began to research poor coordination in maturing children.

In the 1920s information about the clumsy child syndrome becamc illuminated by two main groups. In one hand were professionals who focused upon straight-forward measures of motor performance, including proficiencies in tasks involving smaller muscle groups upon tasks seen primarily on the playground. This interest was typically evidenced by physical educators as they testing the motor abilities of normal children, and by developmentalists as they sought to establish age appropriate norms reflecting appropriate early motor abilities. Therapists also began to try to understand and assist self-care skills of various handicapped groups.

Upon evaluated motor performance quantitatively. The efforts of these groups revealed the presence of awkward children within normal populations. They found that uncoordinated children were more often boys, and that they constituted from five to over fifteen percent of populations from which the obviously physically, emotionally, and sensorially handicapped had been excluded. After a time the research of some focused upon attempts to determine if improvement in youngsters' coordination and skill could be elicited, both when printing and writing, as well as when attempting recreational-sports skills.

At about the same time some perceptive scholars within the medical community also became attracted to the presence of 'neurological soft-signs' found among groups of neurologically and behaviorally 'suspect' youngsters. These individuals were often, developmentally oriented pediatricians and pediatric neurologists. The 'soft-signs' they begun to study and measure, unlike the traditional and obvious signs of neurological involvement researched throughout past history, could not be easily attached to structural problems including quantifiable lesions or tumors.

These subtle signs of neurological dysfunction they studied, included motor coordination problems and other subtle movement anomalies. They also found that 'soft signs' were apparently more prevalent within groups of hyperactive, learning disabled, or psychiatrically unstable youngsters.

The primary purposes of these medical researchers included:

(1) attempts to effectively evaluate soft-signs. and

(2) trying to determine if causal relationships exist between their presence and other neurological-structural and behavioral problems.

The research emanating from these physicians, thus reflected an interest in qualitative aspects of motor incoordination, and related behaviors. In contrast the previous work by physical educators usually contained data resulting from the measurement of obvious quantitative components of motor performance, in tasks such as ball throwing, agility, running and balance.

As research continued, symptoms reflecting motor incoordination and associated symptoms (soft-signs) were studied within various categories of atypical infants children and adults. Developmental scales began to include more useful and valid norms for assessing motor development. Further the measurement tools began to contain *range* of time with which a given motor task is likely to emerge in a maturing youngster. Some of their earlier scales, in contrast, specified that a given motor task did not appear at a single month in the life of a child, some kind of abnormality was certainly indicated.

Some discussions in the book were about the ways in which incoordination occurs within youngsters evidencing progressive ataxias, different types of dystrophies, Tourette's Syndrome, genetic problems including Down Syndrome, and by those evidencing both major and minor signs of cerebral palsy. The main focus of this text, however, was upon the analysis and description of sub-syndromes, and symptoms seen within a broader range of children labeled clumsy, in the absence of other medical problems.

Sub-Syndromes

It has been pointed out that "the clumsy children syndrome" is multi-dimensional. The various sub-classifications of awkwardness discussed in the text included children who evidence unusual variations in muscle tonus, including either hypertonia or hypotonia. Another syndrome described, behaviorally and neurologically included an "dyspraxic-apraxic syndrome". This second sub-group, it was pointed out, is composed of children who cannot observe, plan and then execute complex tasks well.

Other sub-groups of awkward children analyzed included those evidencing unsteadiness and/or tremors, and children whose motor coordination problems may be attributable to possible defects in vision and visual perception. Specific dysgraphic sub-syndromes were also described both in Chapters 6, and 7. The possibility of a child exhibiting a combination of symptoms reflecting the presence of a 'mixed syndrome', was also discussed and interpreted.

Specific Symptoms

Within macroscopic syndromes, it was postulated there exist collections of both subtle and obvious symptoms. The movement qualities discussed included apraxia, asymmetries, unsteadiness and tremor, associated movements (synkinesia), perseveration, and impersistence in movement tasks, and also difficulties when attempting to integrate parts of actions into wholes.

Sub-groups within selected symptom classifications were also discussed. These included how various types of dyspraxia may cause children problems not only when tying shoes but also when walking around a classroom. Associated movements (synkinesia) of two types were discussed. These include those that spread out over the body's space. A second type, it was hypothesized, occurs within a time dimension. This second type is seen after some excited awkward children have vigorously completed a motor task (throwing a ball for example), and continue to exhibit excess and extraneous movements. After ball throwing some, for example, some youngsters may continue to flap their arms, exhibiting unusual movements resembling the wings of a bird in flight.

Impersistence in both actions and positions was also surveyed. Impersistence occurs as youngsters try to maintain static movements and also reflects the inability to persist in moving, cyclic actions. Perserveration, in contrast, involves the inability to change a movement program once it has begun. Thus a child who perserverates is one who often is seen to engage in a action in a kind of persistent and inappropriate manner, while apparently being unable to move to the next appropriate task.

Sensory-Perceptual Problems

Various sensory-perceptual problems that often accompany motor ineptitude discussed within several contexts. Chapter 8 was devoted to this important kind of information. A principle postulated was that there are a parallel sensory losses in areas of the body that also evidence signs of motor incoordination. The hypothesis that movement qualities and movement perceptions occur on concert, was reflected in discussions of how various bodily agnosias and dysnosias disrupt motor tasks essential in daily life. For example it was explained that poor sensory awareness in the hands is often accompanied both by the disinclination to climb, and may also result in children holding pencils in an awkward, fisted grips. By grasping a pencil with four fingers youngsters afflicted with moderate digital agnosias, are thus apparently able to augment sensory information about the location and movements of their writing implements.

The presence of general spatial agnosias, it was further pointed out, may prevent children from being aware of whether or not shirts are tucked in, or if there is food left on their faces after eating. Parallels were drawn between uncoordinated behaviors attributed to poor motor planning (dyspraxias) and to problems due to sensory losses (dysgnosias and agnosias). Further sensory motor difficulties dealt with include those making difficult the accurate movement of the child's total body through space. Relationships between various bodily agnosia, including trunkle agnosia, to similar dyspraxic symptoms were explored.

Social-Emotional Variables

In Chapter 10, and elsewhere in the text, relationships between social-emotional characteristics and motor ineptitude were discussed. It seems apparent that many, if not most, physically awkward children feel badly about their problems, and evidence signs of low self-esteems. The nature of their disability, similar to the hidden problems of the learning disabled, often causes awkward youngsters to be socially evaluated in harsh, unfair, and negative ways by those with whom they come in contact.

Awkward youngsters often seem to others, to be *purposefully* acting in confused and inappropriate ways, rather than evidencing problems over which they have little control. Thus the negative social feedback they receive often contributes to feelings of failure and incompetence. The clinical and experimental-scientific evidence, reviewed in Chapter 10, documented the chain of events that leading from poor coordination, to low self-esteem, to inappropriate social behaviors, to negative responses from parents, peers, and teachers, and finally to behaviors reflecting an even lower self-esteem exhibited by awkward youngsters.

The social problems uncoordinated children have with peers, parents, and teachers result in a variety of avoidance, and compensatory, strategies that were discussed in Chapter 10. These compensations, may include hyperverbalization, appearing either as a constant stream of comedic expressions, or simply in word-barrages designed to keep the task, and teachers, at arms' distance.

Compensations discussed also included avoidance strategies. These range from constant requests to help the classroom teacher, while other youngsters go to recess, to more serious types of regressive infantile behaviors. School phobia is also a symptom often seen among groups of awkward children.

Aggression expressed against classmates constitutes another compensation for frustrations experienced at play. Sometimes awkward children may evidence withdrawn passivity when encountering difficult task situations, constituting another type of compensation. Finally compensations were also discussed, that reflected a child's avoidance of activities by retreating into more academic pursuits for excessive periods of time.

Learning Disabilities

Learning disabilities were discussed within several contexts. On one hand various types of dysgraphia were described as types of specific learning disabilities (Chapter 7). It was pointed out also that dysgraphia was one of the last problems that may appear within the ability-profile of a maturing child. And dysgraphic symptoms may therefore follow the appearance of other normal motor behaviors and adequate communicative competencies. Relationships between expressive speech, and language, and written communication also represent links between academic and social functioning and dysgraphia. The emotional costs that a dysgraphic child must pay within highly structured classrooms, were discussed in several parts of the book including Chapter 7.

The presence of various types of motor problems within learning disabled populations was also illuminated, with recently obtained data (Chapter 9). It was pointed out that:

(1) While some sub-groups within learning disabled populations evidence various types of motor problem syndromes, other sub-groups are free of obvious coordination difficulties,

(2) That some symptoms causing motor difficulties, dyspraxia among others, may persist in learning disabled youngsters through adolescence and into adulthood.

(3) That simply addressing motor problems among the learning disabled is not likely to improve reading and mathematics competencies, and finally that

(4) Motor incoordination causes many learning disabled youngsters marked social and practical problems. Furthermore it was emphasized that signs of clumsiness among the learning disabled should be addressed with specific, and developmentally sound, remedial interventions.

From a practical standpoint, it was recommended that awkward, learning disabled children should be:

(1) be given direct help in modifying the type of motor problems with which they are afflicted. For example, they should be extended help enabling them to clearly print letters; and

(2) They should be helped to devise acceptable ways to compensate, or avoid direct confrontation, with difficult movement tasks.

They should be provided with shoes without laces that do not require tying, for example; and finally

(3) The demands on them should be modified, in line with their decreased capacities to engage in difficult motor tasks.

For example they should be introduced to various 'closed skills' such as running, swimming, and body condition, that do not require quick reactions to the unexpected and varied responses of others. In contrast continued demands to engage in 'open skills' such as those needed defensively in baseball, should usually be avoided. These latter skills are likely to cause undue stress and anxiety.

To give another example, demands for a great deal of written home work might be modified for dysgraphic-awkward children by substituting oral recitation or audio-taped reports for lengthy, written book reports and examinations. Finally it was emphasized that exposing the learning disabled to programs containing motor tasks should not be viewed as a simplistic strategy that is likely to remediate reading and other wayward academic problems.

Evaluation and Programming

Several chapters covered evaluation, prognosis, and program formulation (Chapters 6, 11, 12, 13). Evaluation programs and tests were surveyed together with possible components of evaluation programs. Judiciously applied motor performance tests, it was pointed out, results in a quantitative look at motor performance and coordination. In additional obtaining various qualitative measures, by assessing selected motor neurological soft-signs that may be present, adds an additional and important dimension to an evaluation program. Other parts of assessment programs might include measures of self-esteem (See appendix), as well as measures of graphic and manipulative competencies.

It was emphasized when formulating programs, that care should be taken to specifically address a variety of motor qualities and problems that might need improvement. It was pointed out also that only after precise evaluation, coupled with sound remedial strategies taking place within individualized programs, is positive change likely to result. Further it was emphasized that it is fallacious to expect transfer to occur from a few tasks practiced, to a broad group of motor performance needs. It was also stated that components of evaluation programs should correspond precisely both to stated objectives, and to the nature of content-skill areas that are addressed during remedial sessions.

A few studies have been conducted indicating that positively modifying specific motor skills and fitness qualities may be possible. Recent longitudinal evidence suggests, however, that the underlying neurological soft-signs tend to persist over time, and may continue to plague youngsters well into their teens. There are, however, clear indications that:

(1) To produce positive changes in a motor development among youngsters of various ages, individualized programs need to be carefully planned.

(2) Further the available information strongly suggests that simply allowing a child, or group of youngsters, to 'mature out of a problem', will likely result in regression in motor functions and capacities, rather than positive change.

(3) The research also indicates that the most change in motor abilities, as the result of an intervention program, will occur among younger children, and among those with less marked coordination problems.

(4) Finally contemporary evidence supports the notion that parental understanding and support are critical as the awkward child grows up and attempts to interact with society. Without this understanding and support poorly coordinated youngsters will likely evidence symptoms reflecting a variety of emotional and social difficulties.

NEEDED RESEARCH

Throughout the text references were made to needed research. Some of the suggestions pertained to exotic biochemical-medical interventions. Other recommendations focused upon psycho-social and motor behaviors. These latter suggestions often pertained to program considerations and improvement in evaluation tools. Many of the subjects discussed were formulated upon scanty data bases. Thus, acquiring additional evidence appears imperative, within most of the topic areas surveyed in the text.

Intervention Effects

There is an obvious need for studies about how changes in motor competencies might be elicited. Indeed the available data might lead one to question whether any positive and substantial changes may take place because of remedial efforts. The lack of solid evaluative tools makes difficult the confirmation of possible changes that may take place. Some motor soft-signs and symptoms of incoordination seem somewhat transitory, while others are apparently more persistent., and may remain diagnosable through the life of the child.

The capricious manner in which some subtle signs of poor coordination are appear and at times seem to diminish, coupled with the scarcity of well normed tests of motor performance, make both pre-program prognoses and post-program follow-ups somewhat tenuous undertakings. Thus it appears that the most critical research needs are for studies of possible changes brought about through intervention, together with investigations that could result in the formulation of better evaluative tools. Research of this second type should result in instruments that combine both qualitative and quantitative measures of motor competency.

Intervention studies need to focus upon the influence of several variables. For example, more studies need to explore just when, during a child's life, intervention efforts are likely to result in optimum positive effects. It is likely that the institution of intervention efforts directed toward the improvement of various abilities are age-specific.

It is reasonable to hypothesized, for example, that efforts at language enrichment may produce best results between the second to fourth years of life. Attempts to improve motor quantities also will likely vary from task-type to task-type. Locomotor training seems most effectively applied around the time of the first birthday, with early graphic skills most amenable to remediation between the fourth and sixth birthdays.

Other variables requiring exploration are those involving optimum levels of stimulation appropriate in various programs for application to various populations of motorically deficient youngsters. For example it becoming apparent that if moderate to low levels of motor, perceptual, verbal and cognitive stimulation accompany remedial programs applied to drug-stressed infants. These neonates and infants are likely to do better within a calm stimulus environment than if they are exposed to too much stimulation. Other types of developmentally delayed children, in contrast, may require levels of stimulation, involving various sensory modalities, that are above average levels.

The use of medication in programs for the learning disabled and hyperactive youngster, has had a long history. However this kind of assistance within programs focused upon the remediation or coordination problems is just beginning to be researched. The logical assumption that the efforts of movement educators are likely to prove more fruitful if they are working with a well-controlled youngster, needs to be explored further by researchers.

Additional work is needed to illuminate just what independent motor qualities and factors reside within the overall 'motor personalities' exhibited by populations of awkward children. Prior to the 1990s the factor analytic data available often was based upon tests of questionable validity and reliability. These studies also often suffered from sampling problems. At times the samples had been poorly defined, and at other times the subjects were too few in number. However, the data from several contemporary factor analytic studies (cluster analyses) conducted in the 1990's, and reviewed in the text, offer important precursors to other work which, hopefully, will follow (Miyahara 1992) (Hoare & Larkin 1991).

Studies focusing upon techniques and interventions that may be influential in changing behaviors and symptoms, specific to various sub-syndromes, are also needed. Hypothetically specific groups of interventions may be usefully applied to the hypotonic-floppy child, to the overly tense hypertonic youngster, to the apraxic, and to unsteady-ataxic children. Data from these investigations could result in programs that will better deal also with specific dysgraphic syndromes. Thus, when symptom-specific intervention programs become researched, formulated and are applied, it is probable that more positive behavioral changes will be forthcoming.

Intervening Variables

There is a pressing need for studies indicating how intervening variables may contribute to changes in motor performance and coordination. Statistically these studies might employ trend analyses, or pathway analyses. In this type of approach the course of a series of possible causal relationships, and how they interact, are traced. For example, one might explore first how improvement in motor task performance might positively contribute to an improved self-concept, which in turn might be shown to contribute to more effective classroom efforts, which finally is likely to result in even higher self-esteem. The use of successive correlations might illuminate this and other chains of events and variables.

A combination of program strategies, including movement therapies coupled with medication, may elicit positive modifications in coordination. However there are a number of intervening variables that may have created these positive findings. These variables include measures of improved self-concept, and/or the prolongation of attention span coupled with the reduction of hyperactivity. Both self-concept changes as well as closer attention to various tests (motor, perceptual and academic) by an awkward and medicated youngster will likely be accompanied by reductions of 'emotional overlay' as well as in positive changes in self-confidence. However the details of how these and other variables inter-act with remedial efforts need further study.

Evaluation Studies

Assessment instruments need to be constructed, combining objective measures of performance change, with more qualitative measures of concomitant neurological 'soft-signs' that often accompany incoordination. Additional factor analyses are called for using comprehensive, valid and reliable tests, and while using large representative and carefully selected subject populations.

A useful the outcome of this research should be the appearance of more useful test batteries, than are now available. These improved testing programs should include measures to identify not only motor problems, but also the type of social-psychological compensations a child is likely to employ when confronted with the necessity of performing physically. Information of this second type may be obtained from parent-questionnaires, by interviewing the child, by observing the youngster during other parts of the evaluation, as well as from the results of psycho-social tests including self-concept measures.

The formulation and use of new and comprehensive instruments should result in the identification of specific patterns, and profiles unique to each child. The overall result of the application of such instruments should illuminate relationships between the most pronounced sub-syndrome present (together with associated symptoms) coupled with the most prevalent social compensations employed by the youngster. Reference to each child's individual profile should lead toward the more effective program content. Program suggestions should also include the most useful reward system to employ, the length and frequency of sessions, and finally include suggestions about productive instructor behaviors. A chart depicting these interactions is located at the end of Chapter 11.

New Populations

Contemporary problems and trends in the United States and elsewhere dictate that specially designed programs for various types of afflicted children should be formulated. These new programs should be directed toward 'new' problem populations, including drug-stressed infants and youth, and those afflicted with HIV. For example the optimum amount of exercise to apply to youngsters infected with HIV should be explored.

This type of research should be based upon valid research evidence obtained from newly designed assessment instruments, focusing upon symptoms seen in infants afflicted with AIDS, other and behavioral anomalies, including the apparent outcomes of maternal substance abuse. Continuing to work with developmental scales formulated decades ago, or with those merely imitating the content of these earlier instruments, does not seem productive. When these earlier tools were formulated, infants did not evidence the tremors, choreas and tonus abnormalities present in the make-up of many unfortunate children whose symptoms were not seen until the 1980s.

It has been estimated that from four to five million children in the United States, now entering school, evidence problems reflecting prenatal exposure to maternal drug use. Their behaviors range from jittery non-attention, through vicious aggression, to disinterested-lethargy. These contrasting conditions result in their inability to dealt effectively with both pre-academic and academic lessons. A strong research emphasis is needed, focusing upon the formulation of better evaluative instruments, that in turn should result in more effective programs of early intervention.

Currently schools and school personnel are being stressed, financially and emotionally, with the influx of members these 'new populations' into kindergarten and first grade. As these often-aggressive youngsters become older, and hypothetically more difficult-to-handle, one can only speculate at the greater energy costs that must be paid by teachers, and shudder at the monetary costs that will be faced by tax payers.

Other "new" populations to be researched and planned for include those whose motor problems might have been unavoidably elicited by the application of contemporary medical interventions. For example leukemia in children is being placed under control. However, the medication and radiation used may damage critical areas of the brain that mediate imperative motor functions including graphic behaviors. The imposition of useful and life-saving strategies should be accompanied by parallel attempts to blunt the possible motor problems induced. These forms of "preventive enrichment" might include providing opportunities to engage in scribbling, finger-painting, and in drawing-printing tasks, and to engage in activities exercising gross motor functioning. This type of enrichment should probably engaged in prior to, during and after being exposed to radiation and/or to various chemical interventions employ to treat tumor-related disorders

In the decades ahead it is likely that tumors will be dealt with in specific and precise ways by the insertion of isotopes into the central nervous system that will search and destroy tumors without harming adjacent structures. However the present interventions may cause trauma to important cortical control centers. These harmful outcomes, may be partially blunted by symptom-specific efforts at remediation. This enrichment should be applied before, and after, the essential, but sometimes noxious, medical strategies that are currently employed.

Neural Bio-Chemical Research

There were a number of suggestions contained in the text (Chapter 3) focusing upon the importance of continuing biochemical and neural-developmental work of both a theoretical and applied nature. For example, the more effective use of medication intended to reduce hyperactivity and distractibility could result in a reduction of symptoms reflecting motor incoordination.

Another potentially important area of research deals with the manner in which the normally maturing nervous system seems to 'prune' itself by eliminating non-essential neural networks, and cells. This process of neural regression when completely understood, should result in the better understanding of children who may be hyperactive motorically and/or hyper-reactive sensorially. Moreover when the process and sub-processes may be chemically modified, helpful adjuncts should be formulated assisting in remedial programs for youngsters evidencing a variety of problems.

An Overview

Contemporary research efforts focused upon awkward children are likely to prove fruitful if they reflect cooperative efforts expended by medical experts in pediatrics, neurology and psychiatry together with experimental inroads produced by university neuroscientists. Moreover, and remedial personnel from education, special education, physical education, adapted physical education, and from occupational and physical therapy should attempt to communicate more clearly with each other. A closer inspection of the research literature, coupled with a more sophisticated grasp of what current research means, should somewhat blunt the appearance of various magic movement cures that periodically have dotted the 'scene' since the 1940s. When a heightened understanding of the nature of motor awkwardness, is gained by both medical and educational professionals, improved service will likely be made available to these children and their families. Obtaining a clearer grasp of what practicing movement tasks can, and cannot do, within remedial program, both by professionals and educators is essential. This knowledge passed on to families, should result in a reduction of the exposition of phantom promises for the outcomes of remedial movement activities that are currently and continually being advanced.

Contemporary movement therapists should be exposed to 'solid' and valid research findings, and helped to understand the meanings of these data. Indeed this text was an attempt to assist this process. When this expansion of understanding begins takes with increasing frequency, improved communication and heighten respect and cooperation are likely to be engendered between members of the medical community, behavioral and neurological scientists, and those in clinics and school settings concerned with applying useful remedial strategies.

QUESTIONS FOR DISCUSSION

1. Discuss how individuals' educational backgrounds interact with the type of research that might be undertaken.

2. How might a team approach be fruitful when trying to illuminate some of the questions posed in the chapter? Who might be members of such a team?
3. What intervening variables, located between remedial strategies and behavioral outcomes, were discussed in the chapter? How might researcher study variations in these factors, as influential of different kinds of outcomes from programs designed to remediate motor activities?
4. What further research seems needed in the identification of motor incoordination sub-types?
5. How might the current and future work on movement sub-types result in more useful remedial strategies being developed? Can you cite specific symptoms, strategies and behavioral outcomes when giving your answers?
6. What problems might be caused by a lack of congruence between stated goals, program content, and assessment sub-tests? In what ways might these problems be overcome? How might additional research assist to overcome these problems?
7. What research appears needed in the study of neurological-motor-soft signs? How, and by whom, might these signs be assessed within a comprehensive evaluation program? What specific and general information might be derived from evaluating these signs?
8. How might medication to control hyperactivity result in poorer motor and/or academic performance? What research topics, if explored, might avoid this kind of problem?
9. Discuss how the kinds of tests selected to be administered to awkward children, and then subjected to a cluster (or factor) analysis, will likely influence the nature of the groupings (clusters-factors) that emerge? How might the heterogeneity or homogeneity of the tests selected influence the factor-groups coming out of such an analysis?
10. What qualities and backgrounds, do you perceive as useful among personnel working with groups of awkward youngsters? Can you formulate a test battery, or assessment tools with which to assess these qualities? What research topics might illuminate the personal and professional qualities needed among workers within remedial program?

Glossary

accommodation, of the eyes: Simultaneous converging (conjugate) movements of the eyes as they come together to focus simultaneously upon distant objects, or when engaging in near-point fusion in classroom tasks.

adiadochokinesia: Inability, or difficulties, in producing rapid, alternating movements, often evaluated by requesting rapid pronation and supination of one arm-hand. Is believed to reflect cerebellar, and/or basal ganglia dysfunction.

aggregates: Collections of three or more figures grouped together, and drawn by children of from four to six years of age and older.

apraxia: The inability to execute a motor tasks requiring the integration of several parts, in the absence of obvious sensory difficulties, mental retardation, and/or other peripheral muscular-skeletal problems.

apraxic syndrome: A term used to denote one of the sub-syndromes found within the broader category *The Clumsy Child Syndrome*. Youngsters within this sub-group have problems with executing sequences of sub-actions within complex motor tasks.

agnosia: Refers to insensitivity to various kinds of sensory-perceptual information. The term may be attached to problems involving the lack of sensory awareness within one (or more) of several modalities, including vision, audition, and/or various types of kinesthetic, and tactile stimuli. The term Dysgnosia is used to denote dysfunctional sensory-perceptual abilities

agraphia: Inability to draw and/or to write and print letters, may be seen developmentally in the maturing child, or as the result of a cerebral stroke among more mature client-patients.

astereognosis: Inability to tactually obtain information about objects' form, shape, texture, size weight etc, without the use of visual information. Insensitivity to touch.

ataxia: Unsteadiness, tremor, and/or poor kinesthetic awareness, usually believed to be caused by cerebellar lesions. A type of movement quality classified under the broader term, cerebral palsy. Sometimes labeled cerebellar ataxia.

ataxia-telangiectasia: A type of progressive ataxia, characterized by atrophy of the cells within the cerebellum. Symptoms include hypotonia, choreas, and abnormal eye movements.

athetosis: A type of movement quality usually classified under types of cerebral palsy, marked by constant uncontrollable motion, writhings, and/or tremors, usually attributed to damage to the basal ganglia.

attention Deficit Disorder: (ADD) A group of symptoms marked by inattention, distractibility; If accompanied by motor impulsivity and hyperactivity it is sometimes labeled ADHA (Attention Deficit-Hyperactivity Disorder). Often accompanied by learning disabilities.

attention deficit-hyperactivity disorder (ADHA) Poor attention, accompanied by hyperactivity and distractibility.

Basal Ganglia: Circuits and nuclei, believed by some to mediate, formulate, and store motor programs. They are located just above the ventricles of the brain, and consist of four major portions, the putamen, caudate nucleus, globus pallidus, substantia nigra and sub-thalamas. The reticular formation and red nuclei are sometimes considered parts of the basal ganglia.

Benign hypotonia: A group of symptoms marked by below-average levels of resting muscle tone, involving a condition that is non-progressive (benign)

bio-underclass, of children: A term representing the large number of infants and children whose development has been delayed, or marred, by maternal use of abusive substances during gestation.

body agnosias: A group of conditions marked by symptoms that reflect the lack of tactual awareness of the body, of poor perception of limb position, and/or of faulty knowledge of the body's position in space.

buccofacial apraxia: Also termed *oro, or oral apraxia* and denoting the inability or difficulty in chaining together movements of the face and cranial muscles controlling speech.

cell migration: Microscopic, neural-developmental processes (most of which occur prenatally) involving the transportation and relocation of various types of neurons to form networks, structures, and connections to sensory end organs and to muscles.

central sulcus: The cortical fissure separating the sensory and primary motor cortex, located in the parietal area of the brain, and across which specific neural projections pass, connecting corresponding motor and sensory functions of various body parts.

cerebellar ataxia: A type of cerebral palsy reflecting symptoms that include poor balance and unsteadiness, often coupled with poor kinesthetic awareness, purportedly caused by a cerebellar lesion. May be seen in movements by either the upper or lower limbs, or on both parts of the body. Other symptoms can include inaccurate reaching and pointing, as well as the breakdown and dissolution of coordinated movements. May be of a mild or more severe nature, and can include either the upper or lower parts of the body, or involve the total body.

cerebellar syndrome: A type of sub-syndrome identified among children labeled as evidencing The Clumsy Child Syndrome. Specific symptoms can include poor refinement of movements, and unsteadiness seen in the gait and/or lack of precision when reaching for objects, and when pointing. Regular tremors and inaccuracies often occur when attempting to print and/or write letters, numbers and words.

cerebral palsy: A broad term representing a group of non-progressive conditions that are marked by atypical movement behaviors, and incoordination, due to central nervous system injuries and lesions. Various types are classified both according to the body part(s) involved, as well as with reference to the movement qualities seen, ie. ataxic, athetoid, spastic, mixed etc.

chorea: (from the Latin 'to dance'), Spasms, jerking motions sometimes appearing as neurological soft signs, or as symptoms of major neural pathologies. Choreas may appear in the limbs, the trunk and/or in the eye muscles.

choretiform: A term used to denote choreas, spasms, uncontrolled twitching. Choretiform movements are 'slight and jerky, and are characterized by short duration, and sudden occurrence. See *chorieform movements* below.

choreiform movements: Another term used to mean choreas, spasms, uncontrolled twitching. Choreiform movements are irregular, and occur arthymically in various muscle groups. They are of short duration and are clearly distinguishable from slow tonic athetoid movements. May appear as unimportant soft-signs not connected with major problems, or as accompaniments to major neural pathologies. (see also choreas, and choretiform movements above).

clonus, clonic reactions: A sign of increased muscle tone in the lower extremities due to the possible presence of a number of conditions including various forms of cerebral palsy, usually spasticity or athetosis. Clonic reactions may appear in the ankle and be seen when pressure to the ball of the foot is applied either when the child is in a supine position. When walking, clonic reactions may result in an uneven, unsteady gait. Clonic reactions are usually accompanied by hyperactive reflexes, and are often considered a clinical sign denoting faulty functioning of the cerebellum.

closed brain injury: A closed brain injury occurs when trauma to the cranium does not involve penetration. Damage can occur at point of impact, and/or at other points at which increased cranial pressures may occur. Damage may also occur, because of twisting or shearing actions, damaging surface neurons. Primary damage occurs at time of blow, and secondary damage may occurs later.

Clumsy Child Syndrome: A broad term applied to children whose coordination is not at levels usually expected for those of a similar chronological age. Usually absent are obvious signs of neuropathology. Also absent are pronounced sensory losses, mental retardation, or other peripheral muscular-skeletal abnormalities.

combines: A collection of two combined figures, seen as children begin to acquire drawing and graphic skills.

congenital maladroitness: A term that has been used to denote awkward children who were seen to lack adequate coordination.

conjugate movements: Movements of the eyes in which both eyes move in the same direction, such as saccades employed when scanning written material, and when tracking moving objects. Tracking movements also, are conjugate movements, and appear as slow tracking movements (ramps). Some micromovements are also conjugate, occurring when the eyes move in unison and in the same direction.

construction apraxia: A lack of ability to construct objects, using blocks, to print letters, and/or to engage in a number of self-care skills involving sequences, such as shoe-tying and dressing. May appear in the absence of sensory losses, mental retardation or obvious peripheral skeletal-muscular problems.

corpus callosum: The largest cross-hemispheric connection in the brain, consisting of axons that connect the cortex of the two hemispheres. Its axons unite similar regions on both hemispheres.

criteria referenced test: A test formulated using the available literature, rather than upon normative data specifically obtained for the test's construction.

dedifferentiation: Lack of sufficient nerve cells and networks, due to defects in microscopic developmental processes including cell migration.

demylination: Deficiencies in the formation of, or a wasting away of, the myelin sheath along the lengths of neurons, present in numerous neuropathological conditions, including progressive ataxias, multiple sclerosis, various peripheral nerve disorders, and conditions caused by chemical (ie. lead) poisoning.

developmental agnosias: Symptoms reflecting inadequate or poor sensory awareness, relative to various stimuli. They appear as maturation is taking place in infants, and children. Developmental body agnosias appear as the child demonstrates poor kinesthetic awareness, poor awareness of his/her body's position in space, and/or difficulties with tactual perception. Other agnosias may appear in the visual or auditory modes. See Dysnosias

developmental apraxia: Incoordination appearing as a child matures, reflected in the inability to perform motor tasks expected at various chronological ages. Some times used in the literature to mean totality of symptoms appearing in all awkward children.

developmental coordination disorder: A term used earlier in the literature to denote clumsy children, and to those evidencing developmental apraxia, used instead of "The Clumsy Child Syndrome".

developmental dysgraphia: Dysgraphia appearing as a child matures, appearing as difficulties are encountered when attempting to draw and to print letters, numbers and words at levels expected at specific chronological ages.

developmental expressive writing disorder: A term, used to denote developmental dysgraphia in children, employed in the classification system reflecting developmental disorders used by Psychiatrists and Psychologists in the United States

diadochokinesia: Refers to the ability to execute alternating reciprocal actions, such as quick pronation and supination of the hand-arm. (see adiadochokinesia). Usually interpreted as a sign of cerebellar dysfunction.

digital agnosia: Refers to a group of symptoms reflecting lack of sensitivity of the hands and fingers, when they are being touched, or when objects are handled.

dispractic: An adjective sometimes used to denote dyspraxia, the disruption of coordinated actions. (see dyspraxias below).

dis-use syndrome: A collection of symptoms reflecting the lack of opportunities, or unwillingness, to engage in vigorous and/or complex motor activities. May appear as poor muscle tone accompanied by postural problems, together with apparent awkwardness and/or lack of confidence in sport-skill situations.

Down Syndrome: Several types of conditions caused by chromosomal anomalies, associated with an extra Number 21 chromosome, or an effective trisomy for this chromosome by its translation to another chromosome, usually number 14 or 21/22. Symptoms include aberrations of sensory-motor functions, endocrine functions, as well as mental retardation

dressing apraxia: Difficulties encountered when trying to put on or take off clothing, a type of construction apraxia, reflecting poor sensory awareness of the body and also motor sequencing problems.

Duchenne's Type of Muscular Dystrophy: The most prevalent type of muscular dystrophy seen in childhood, muscle fibers appear enlarged, and large accumulations of fat cells appear between muscle cells. Skeletal-postural problems occur, together with myocardial degeneration, due to fatty infiltration. Transmitted in a sex-linked recessive manner, the symptoms appear in early childhood.

dynamic visual acuity: Ability to extract information from moving objects and/or stimuli.

dyscalculia: Inability to calculate, to do mathematics operations well.

dysnosia: Disturbance of awareness of limb and bodily sensations, has been evaluated by testing ability to replicate demonstrated limb movements, as well as by other methods. See *agnosia*

dysgraphia: Disruption of efforts directed toward writing, drawing and/or graphic arts.

dysjunctive movements: Movements of the eyes in which each moves in a different direction, such as when accommodating as each moves inward toward the nose.

dyslexia: Literally disruption of lexicon, difficulties in reading, sometimes used to mean reading problems accompanied by other signs of minimal neurological dysfunction.

dysmetrica: Difficulties when attempting to execute movements of precise lengths, associated with various other symptoms of cerebellar ataxia, dysmetria seen as a child over-reaches, or fails to reach accurately for objects place adjacent to him or her.

dyspraxia: Difficulties when attempting to perform coordinated movements, in response to demonstrations or to verbal directions.

dyspraxic syndrome, in dysgraphia: One of several sub-syndromes identifiable among the global dysgraphic syndrome, reflected in the inability to execute complicated letters well, or to sequence words in proper order within sentences.

Echolalia: Tendency for a child to continue echo what has just been said, or what has been heard in the past, in repetitive and in inappropriate ways.

Encephalitis: A neurological condition often triggered by measles, mumps and chicken-pox, marked by demyelination, as viral infections invade the nervous system. Now mostly treatable with vaccines.

extrinsic rewards: Rewards for performance, in various tasks, that are extraneous to the satisfaction the child may receive from performance. Extrinsic rewards can consist of maternal reinforcements, or social reinforcement.

factor analysis: A statistical tool which involves determining the presence of basic factors or qualities which may lie within a large number of tests or measures. Correlations of correlations, in order to obtain 'clusters' of scores identifying main traits or human qualities. More contemporary methods including, cluster analyses accomplish the same outcome.

factor-pure test battery: A test battery based upon factored evidence, so that each test evaluates a separate and independent quality or factor.

fading techniques: A technique used to teaching printing and writing skills in which letters are traced over, and then the guiding lines or dots are gradually faded out.

false negative, when evaluating: Falsely assessing that a child has no problem(s), when a problem(s) are indeed present.

false positive: Falsely diagnosing the presence of a problem, when no problem is present.

Fascioscapularhumeral Type of Muscular Dystrophy: A rare type of muscular dystrophy seen during the second to third decade, involving the face and shoulder girdle.

Fetal Alcohol Syndrome: A constellation of structural and behavioral problems triggered by maternal use of alcohol during pregnancy. Facial modifications together with hyperactivity are common symptoms.

figure-ground perception: The selecting out of a central figure, out of a background of information, may involve visual as well as auditory stimuli

finger opposition: A clinical test of manipulative ability, resulting from asking the child to touch each finger, in order to the thumb of the same hand. May be timed and scored for accuracy.

flooding Techniques: A term used in psychotherapy and in other forms of treatments for behavioral disorders, that involves asking or encouraging the client to engage in excessive amounts of the behavior (emotion, or thoughts) it is desired to eliminate or reduce.

formulation aphasia: A condition marked by hesitancy, or latency, seen as it is attempted to formulate a motor programs necessary when speaking, or when constructing a sentence or thought to be expressed verbally.

frustration-aggression hypothesis: The proposition that frustration causes aggression, and thus that most aggressive acts may be caused by frustrating circumstances.

Frederick's Ataxia: An inherited progressive ataxia marked by speech disturbances, skeletal-muscular problems, and cerebellar symptoms including poor coordination and unsteadiness. It is marked by progressive degeneration of the sensory cells in the dorsal ganglia, in the heart-lung system, and of peripheral nerves to the limbs and trunk

gamma efferent system: A neural feedback system associated with the reticular formation, thought by some to be responsible for the maintenance of resting muscle tone.

gaze characteristics: Individual differences in how a people's eyes come to rest upon a predetermined targets.

Gerstmann's Syndrome: A collection of symptoms that purportedly include digital agnosia, body image deficits, and acalculia, sometimes dyslexia is included in the grouping.

glial cells: The numerous 'supporting cells' within the nervous system. The most important of which are termed neuroglia (nerve glue). Glial cells hold and surround the neurons and supply them with some of their necessary chemicals. Early in development specialized *transport glial cells* move neurons to their final resting places.

Gower's Sign: An early symptom of muscular dystrophy seen as the child attempts to arise by locking his/her legs and then "walking" up the legs by using the arms. It reflects poor muscle tone and strength in the leg extensors, and other muscle groups that work against gravity.

grasp, pincer: A mature grasping action normally seen at about 4 to 6 months which involves grasping small objects by opposing the first finger and thumb

grasp, palmer: An immature grasping action which involves grasping objects with the palm, with the thumb aligned with the fingers, not facing them.

hard signs: Neurological symptoms and conditions having readily diagnosable causes, including structural lesions, tumors, encephalopathies, or signs of central nervous system involvement.

healed lesions: Lesions which may have been caused by early developmental traumas, such as small strokes when the neural structures are being vascularized, but which are diagnosable later in life.

helpless syndrome, in dysgraphia: One of the sub-syndromes seen in dysgraphic children, marked by an inability and/or unwillingness to grip the writing implement with a sufficiently strong grip, and by a disinclination to exert sufficient pressure to make distinct marks on paper when writing or printing numbers and letters. May be part of a larger psychological syndrome labeled *"learned helplessness"*.

Hemiplegia: A type of cerebral palsy marked by involvement on one side of the body, usually involving excess flexion in the upper limbs, and hyperextension reactions in the leg. Slight signs of hemiplegia are sometimes seen as symptoms among awkward children. Most hemplegics are involved on the right side, and symptoms may include speech problems.

heterotopic synkinesia: Associated movements, or overflow (synkinesia) reflected in unintentional movements mediated by portions of the central nervous system, (usually the motor cortex) that are adjacent to the area mediating intentional actions. For example, if a broad smile is intended (or requested), the eyes may be seen to squint, or when fingers are volitionally spread an unintentional smile may appear because portions of the sensory-motor cortex mediating these actions are adjacent.

hurry: A psuedo run seen in young children, prior to the appearance of true running. A *hurry* does not involve a 'lack-of-support" phase, as is seen in a true run, instead at least one foot remains on the ground throughout the act: a hurry thus is thus a fast walk.

hyperdifferentiation: The overproduction of nerves and neural networks, as the result of faulty neural regressive processes.

hypertonia: An excess amount of resting, residual muscle tone, present in mild, moderate and severe types of spastic cerebral palsy. May be accompanied by hyperactive reflexes.

hyperverbalization: The production of excess verbiage, often used to cover perceived inadequacies, or low self-esteem among both learning disabled and awkward children. Also used as to avoid uncomfortable performance situations.

hypotonia: Less than average amount of residual, resting muscle tone, may be progressive or benign depending upon causes.

hypotonic syndrome: One of the sub-syndromes within the clumsy child syndrome, characterized by lack of energy, low resting muscle tone (*hypotonia*), and poor coordination.

hypoxia: Insufficient oxygen content when breathing.

ideational apraxia: Difficulties when attempting to formulate a motor program, prior to executing the task. Characterized by an excessive long judgement-time, often measured as a prolonged reaction time, prior to task execution.

ideomotor apraxia: Difficulties in the ordering and sequencing of sub-movements contained within complex skills.

impersistence: Difficulties in maintaining a fixed position, or posture for reasonable periods of time.

infantilization: The results of parental or caretaker over protectiveness directed toward a child. Characterized by infantile behaviors less mature than those expected by a child of a given chronological age, including infantile speech, immature emotional behaviors, and poor skills.

inherited left-handedness: Left-handedness due to inherited traits, transmitted from left-handed relatives. In contrast, obligate left-handedness purportedly reflects some kind of cerebral incident modifying hand preference.

intrinsic rewards: Satisfactions received from mastery and fun when executing motor tasks (or other types of tasks), exclusive of external (extrinsic) social or material rewards.

insults (cerebral-neural): The results of trauma to components of the central or peripheral nervous system resulting in lesions, bruises, tears or other damage.

kinesthesis: Sensory information and the perceptions formed from nerve endings in muscles, tendons and joints resulting in awareness of limb position, body movement, and hand-finger activities.

kinetics, of drug use effects: The results, over time, of abusive substance use upon the fetus, or upon the substance abuser.

kyphosis: Winged and protruding scapulas, round shoulders caused by upper back weakness, and/or tightness of the chest (pectoral) muscles. Often accompanied by a forward head.

learned helplessness: A group of behavioral symptoms seen in some atypical children, reflecting the fact that they have been rewarded and have thus learned to exhibit behaviors at immature

learning disabled children: Youngsters evidencing academic learning problems, unaccompanied by mental retardation, sensory deficits, and/or marked emotional problems. They are commonly described as children working below their potentials in classroom tasks.

lesions: A wound or injury to the brain, a tear, or bruise, marked by the destruction of nerve cells, and/or injury to nerve centers.

Limb Girdle Muscular Dystrophy: A Dystrophy, muscular wasting, seen in the shoulder or pelvic region. The condition is relatively rare, and is believed due to the inheritance.

limb kinetic apraxia: Disruption in the manner in which sub-sequences of a complex motor skill are executed. i.e. holding the fork by the wrong end while eating, attempting to strike the wrong end of a match.

mandellas: Sun-like drawings appearing in the efforts by children in many cultures, characterized by radiating lines crossing a central circle.

manual-graphic syndrome: One type of sub-syndrome within the clumsy child syndrome: it may occur exclusive of problems involving the control of the larger muscle groups.

Minimal Cerebral Palsy: A term given to children with obvious neurological soft-signs, including learning disabilities, and motor incoordination. May reflect the belief that many forms of motor awkwardness hyperactivity and related disorders, are mild forms of cerebral palsy

mirror movements: Associated movements, or synkinesia, occurring on one side of the body while intentional actions are taking place in similar body parts, on the other side. Seen, for example, as finger opposition is engaged in with one hand, while the fingers on the other hand evidence involuntary movements.

mixed syndrome (of clumsy child syndromes): A syndrome composed of various symptoms from several of the sub-syndromes described in the text.

motor babbling: A term used to describe the nature of early scribbling, whose appearance resembles the random, but potentially useful sounds, voiced in infancy.

motor cortexes: (primary and secondary): Centers for the mediation of bodily movements. The primary motor cortex is located in the parietal lobe. The secondary motor cortex, located in the temporal lobe, and is believed by some to be involved in the mediation of speech and of graphic behaviors

Motor Deficiency Syndrome: A term used infrequently to denote clumsy children.

motor-free measures of visual perception: Measures of visual perception, excluding drawing tasks which often were used. These include making visual judgements, without the need to exhibit motor accuracy.

Motor Idiocy: A term used by the Russian Nicholas Oseretsky, in the 1920's to denote awkward children, and for whom he planned the first motor coordination tests.

motor planning: Praxic behavior, is a term that includes the perception of a demonstration, the correct interpretation of a direction, and then the subsequent translating of these perceptions into a coherent and acceptable action pattern. Usually denotes the planning and execution of a reasonably complex skill (see apraxia, and dyspraxia).

motor psychology: A term used to reflect the fact that numerous motor-kinesthetic measures were used by those initiating the first experimental psychology programs during the last century.

Moziac-type, of Down Syndrome: A rare type of Down Syndrome, characterized by chromosomal abnormalities within only a relatively small percentage of the body's cells (10-12%). Usually presents mixed symptoms that may include mild retardation and/or some motor involvement.

multi-component dysgraphia: Dysgraphia due to more than one cause, and characterized by several symptoms.

Muscular Dystrophy: Several types of inherited conditions characterized by a wasting and shrinking of the musculature of the body, seen in early childhood or adolescence.

Myotonic Dystrophy: A genetic condition, marked by the alteration of the muscle fibers, similar to that seen in muscular dystrophy, resulting in increases in fibrous and adipose tissue. First symptoms can include a tense appearance in face, and difficulties encountered when attempting to release objects held in the hands. Often appearing early in childhood, it is usually first seen as sysptoms reflecting general hypotonia.

narrow transfer width: The assumption that to reach specific objectives, transfer should be caused to occur by practicing rather specific and related content in educational programs, including programs of remedial motor education.

neural groove: The groove which forms early during gestation, composed of specialized cells, (*neurons*) from which the nervous system evolves.

neural regression: The process by which the nervous system is trimmed, or 'pruned' during its development, reflected in the elimination of unneeded neurons and neural networks.

Neuroleptic Drugs: Medications designed to alter the functions of the nervous system.

Neurological Schedules: Identifiable programs of neurological evaluation, sometimes aligned with medical clinics in which they were derived.

neurological overflow: Synkinesia, or associated movements, include involuntary movements occurring in conjunction with voluntary actions, but extraneous to intentional tasks. *Seee neuromotor overflow, below.*

neurological soft signs: Minor signs of neurological dysfunction for which diagnosable structural verification and substantiation is usually lacking. They include symptoms reflecting motor incoordination, associated movements and the like, and minor choreas.

neuro-motor overflow: Synkinesia, or associated movements, unintentional movements, which accompany volitional activity, of which the performer is often unaware.

normal athetosis, in infants: Arhythm and motor behaviors seen in infancy in the limbs, hands, and trunk.

nystagmus: Atypical, irregular, rhythmic eye movements .

obligate left-handedness: Left-handedness postulated as caused by some kind of minor or major neural-pathological incident, or accident.

opto-kinetic reflex: The reflex that permits the eye to perceptually 'stop" moving objects, and to extract information from them.

optic chiasm: A cross-shaped connection between the optic nerves, located below the base of the brain, where half the nerves from the eyes cross from one side of the brain to the other.

overlearning: Learning in excess of some stated or established criteria. Overlearning may contribute to the better retention of motor skills. ie. learning until 15 free throws are performed successfully, when it is desired to be able to perform 10 without a miss.

oral apraxia: Oral apraxia has historically involved two meanings, including problems in motor task performance when the task is requested, or described verbally; and the inability to chain together movements of the face, mouth and tongue, when attempting to formulate intelligible speech. See also *oromotor apraxia.* and *buccofacial apraxia.*

organogenesis: The generation and formation of organs, include formation of components of the central nervous system usually occurring developmentally during gestation.

oromotor apraxia: Apraxic symnptoms interfering with adequate speech articulation, involving difficulties in the programming of sequential movements of the tongue, and of other parts of the mouth and throat. *See oral apraxia and Buccofacial apraxia.*

overflow: Extraneous involuntary movements (synkinesias) occurring as adjuncts to the task, may occur in various portions of the time at the time of performance: or overflow may reflect temporal dimensions in the form of extraneous movements occurring after a task is performed.

parietal lobe: One of the four lobes on the surface of the cerebral cortex, just to the rear of the associational areas, containing the somatosensory cortex and primary motor cortex.

Parkinson's Disease: Caused by the degeneration of the nigrostriatal bundle in the basal ganglia, its symptoms include tremors, muscular rigidity, and problems when attempted to execute coordinated movements.

perceptual anticipation: The perceptual-visual "calculation" of the speed and distance traveled, and the later arrival point of moving objects, prior to their interception.

preseveration: The persistence in a task or motor program, past desired limits. Sometimes aligned with hyperactivity and distractability.

Pes Cavas: An unusually high longitudinal arch in the foot, marked by skeletal alterations. The condition sometimes occurs because of muscle imbalances caused by degenerative neurological problems. (progressive ataxias).

phylogenic: Qualities or functions that are traceable to evolutionary processes.

pincer grasp: Mature grasp characterized by precise opposition of the thumb and first finger

praxia: Refers to motor planning functions, the ability to respond correctly to a demonstration of, or verbal instructions, to execute a coordinated movement.

praxic abilities: Qualities reflecting the ability to see, or receive verbal directions, to execute a coordinated movement.

progressive ataxias: Syndromes, often reflecting cerebellar dysfunctions, as well as in other central and peripheral conditions in the nervous system, that are progressive and result in degenerative symptoms.

progressive hypotonia: Symptoms reflecting a loss of adequate levels of resting muscle tone.

progressive-part practice: A method of motor skill learning and practice involving the successive acquisition of an entire motor task, by the gradual acquisition of its parts.

pseudohypertrophy: Apparent increase in muscle size, without true muscle hypertrophy. Seen in as a symptom accompanying muscular dystrophy.

psychogenic factors: Psychological, emotional factors and conditions that may underlie changes in motor functions, and in other forms of unwanted or atypical behaviors.

reminiscence: Improvement in motor skill learning and performance as a function of spaced practice, of rest between practice sessions. Thus reminiscence implies motor skill improvement due to no practice, apparently leaving time for the nervous system to somehow integrate and incorporate previous practice.

response inhibition: Reduction of the tendency to respond, sometimes attributable sometimes to massed practice of skills or academic tasks, producing symptoms of psychological fatigue

restive behavior(s): Distractible, emotionally uneven behaviors, associated with learning disabilities and hyperactivity.

restive tremors: Tremors occurring when a limb, or hand, is at rest, usually when held against the body prior to extension or reaching activities.

Reticular Formation: A network of gray matter, within the central region of the brain extending from the medulla to the diencephalon. Sometimes designated as one of several sites controlling the inhibition or hyperactivation of motor activity.

right hemisphere syndrome: A collection of symptoms reflecting spatial-motor dysfunctions including poorly aligned lettering, excessive contact of people, and objects while walking, may also include metallic atonal speech.

saccades: Rapid jumps, or throws, the eyes make during reading, as well as when observing rapidly moving objects.

school phobia: A collection of symptoms indicative of the disinclination to attend school, appearing as morning nausea, temper tantrums, and the like.

Sciolosis: (from the Greek 'twisted') A lateral curvature of the spinal column, in the shape of a C, or S may appear at various levels within the spine, if attributable to muscular imbalance the condition is labeled 'functional' but if persisting over time, the condition may become 'structural' involving the change in shape (wedging) of the bones forming the spinal column. Severe sciolosis usually requires surgical correction, mild forms of functional sciolosis man be remediated through properly applied exercises.

self-care skills: Skills needed in daily life, including dressing, washing, brushing the teeth etc.

sensory cortex: Sometimes termed the somatosensory cortex, it is located in the parietal lobe behind the central sulcus adjacent to the primary motor area, receives sensory information from the surfaces, and movements of the body.

social modeling: The molding of behavior in response to, or when adjacent to, other people, involves 'social contagion'.

soft-signs: Minor symptoms denoting neurological dysfunctions for which no obvious pathological sign-posts may be determined. Includes signs of motor coordination and atypical movement qualities including associated movements, choreas, and the like.

somatoagnosia(s): A collection of syndromes and symptoms reflecting a lack of awareness of the location of the body in space, of limb positions and movements, as well as deficiencies in the tactual perception of the body's surfaces, and of the limbs, hands and fingers.

somatosensory cortex: The receptor area porterior to the central sulcus in the parietal lobe, mediates movement and bodily sensations. Receives fibers from the somatosensory system, and has direct neural connections to the adjacent primary motor cortex.

Spastic: A form of cerebral palsy marked by an excess of muscle tension and tonus, and a lack of adequate reciprocal innervation permitting controlled elongation of flexor muscles when extensor movements are desired and required.

spatial agnosia(s): A type of sensory loss that is reflected in confusions when the body is moving through space, with precision and/or in serial tasks.

specific learning disability: A specific learning problem, which may occur, or appear, independent of other signs of adequate, or superior, intellectual or academic abilities. A specific learning disability can include dysgraphia, acalculia, or other kind of problem.

spooning, of the hands: A type of synkinesia, or associated movement seen as the hands and arms supinate (rotate outward away from the body), sometimes appearing when the gait is stressed (the feet are turned outward) in neurologically 'suspect' children.

static acuity: The clarity and accuracy with which stable, non-moving, stimuli are seen. Also see *dynamic acuity*.

stereognosis: Refers to the ability to acquire information about objects, and shapes, tactually without the use of vision.

stereotypies: Normal rhythmic behaviors seen in infants, in various parts of the body during the first year of life, may involve hand, face, limb, and/or body movements.

stroke-related apraxias and dysgraphias: Problems in motor planning and graphic behaviors due to cerebral infarctions, involving minor or major ruptures of blood vessels in the central nervous system.

suspect infants: Infants whose appearance, birth histories, or atypical behaviors and symptoms suggest the presence of developmental problems and/or abnormal symptoms.

Syndrome: A collection, or group, of commonly associated symptoms.

Synkinesia: Unintentional movements that are outside the awareness of the individual and that, accompany, but are not necessary to the performance of a motor task and/or volitional actions. Also termed associated movements, or overflow. (see also overflow, associated movements, and heterotopic synkinesia).

Telangiectasia: (seee ataxia-telangiectasia)

tension syndrome(s): A sub-syndrome seen both among groups of awkward children, and among dysgraphic youngsters, characterized by excess of resting muscle tone, may reflect a mild form of spastic cerebral palsy.

terminal tremors: Tremors seen as movement are terminated, as when a reaching task is attempted and completed. Results in poor accuracy when attempting to contact objects, or when making pointing movements of the limbs and hands.

Tics: Jerking movements, spasms, or choreas occurring within various neuropathological syndromes, as well as to a lesser degree among normal youngsters. Sometimes appearing as unwanted noises or phrases (verbal tics) uttered by children with Tourette's syndrome.

Tourette's Syndrome: An inherited condition, characterized by the presence of both movement and often verbal tics, resulting in emotional instability and social censure. Accompanied by difficulties in performing motor tasks, and school work.

transport glial cells: A type of glial, supporting cell, assigned the jobs of transporting neurons to their final functional areas, or collecting them into neural centers, during the time the nervous system develops.

tremor syndromes: Unsteadiness, and movement inaccuracies, characterized by tremors among both dysgraphic and clumsy youngsters, sometimes forming identifiable sub-syndromes.

trunkle agnosias: Symptoms reflecting defects in the senses necessary when attempting to relocating and/or to move the body accurately in space, either in sequential movements, or when encountering people and objects.

trunkle apraxia: Symptoms reflecting the difficulties, encountered, when attempting to relocating and/or to move the body accurately in space, either in sequential movements, or when encountering people and objects.

Tumors: Uncontrolled pathological growth of cells, occurring in various portions of the body including the central and peripheral nervous systems. Damage to, and/or impairment of, motor functions may occur as the direct result of their presence, and because of treatment modalities used to control their growth.

unsupported step: A locomotor task, developmentally occurring between the emergence of jumping and hopping, and involving taking off with one foot, a non-support phase, and landing on the opposite foot.

vascular accident: The rupturing of a blood vessel, an infarction.

velocity resistant children: Children who are able to make accurate perceptual judgements about rapidly moving objects, who do not break-down perceptually when making judgements about objects moving at high speeds.

velocity susceptible children: Children who have difficulty making accurate perceptual judgements about rapidly moving objects, who break-down perceptually when required to make judgements about objects moving at high speeds. Youngsters who have difficulties make judgements about moving teammates, and balls in group games.

visual agnosias: Perceptual problems when dealing with visual stimulation, can include reading problems, lack of or poor letter or work recognition, inability to remember faces, and similar problems.

visual-motor disabilities: A term used to describe clumsy children with reference to the difficulties they may have associating visual information with motor output.

visual-motor incoordination: A term used to describe clumsy children with reference to problems many have putting together visual information with motor output, problems with visual-motor integration.

visual-perceptual clumsiness: A sub-syndrome within the clumsy child syndrome, referring to awkwardness caused by the presence of visual and/or visual perceptual difficulties.

vocal tics: Socially inappropriate words, phrases or noises, uttered repetitively by emotionally disturbed youngsters, and by those with Tourette's Syndrome.

wide-transfer width: Reflecting the hypothesis that transfer of training will occur from a few tasks contained within a program, to a wide range of tasks and objectives.

APPENDICES

Appendix I

Motor Development Check-List for Infants Stressed Prenatally with Maternal Cocaine Use

The following check-list was developed in 1989 to evaluate the unique motor problems unique to many drug-stressed infants. It has good inter-observer reliability but needs further work relative to its validity and to determine its potential usefulness in predicting later developmental problems.

Drug-Stressed Infants: Motor Development Checklist*

The scale has been formulated to assess tonus anomalies, tremor location, and other selected motor behaviors exhibited by infants subjected prenatally to maternal drug use.

Name ____________________ Patient no. __________ Sex __________

Date of administration: ____________ Date of birth ________________

Premature _______ Full-term _______ Weight at birth _______________

Drug(s), and amounts, reportedly used by mother during pregnancy:

____

____

When during pregnancy was drug use reported? ____________________

____

Father's history of drug use: ____________________________________

____

Status-title, of present caretaker: ________________________________

____

Name and title of individual using the scale: _____________________

____

Pertinent medical information:____________________________________

____

____

____

Other developmental scores and data (Apgar Score, etc.):

____

____

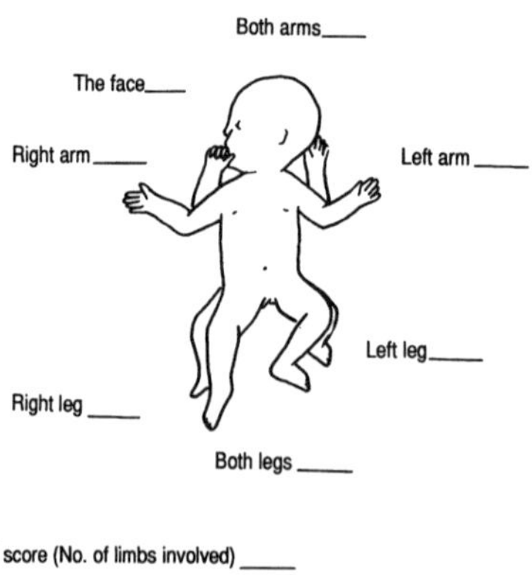

Fig-1. Tremors-location. (*Adapted from B.J. Cratty, 1979,* Perceptual and Motor Development in Infants and Children. *Englewood Cliffs, NJ: Prentice-Hall.*)

In this part of the evaluation the location of tremor-vibrations are noted. They are scored as present or absent (P or A) in each limb, in arms and legs as separate units, and in the total body, if tremors appear in both arms and legs simultaneously. The infant is disrobed and placed on his/her back for inspection of the presence of these tremors. Observations relative to the infant's general agitation level as well as the amplitude and frequency of the tremors should be included. Other observations should include the percent of time the tremors are seen throughout the day.

Notes, comments:

____

____

____

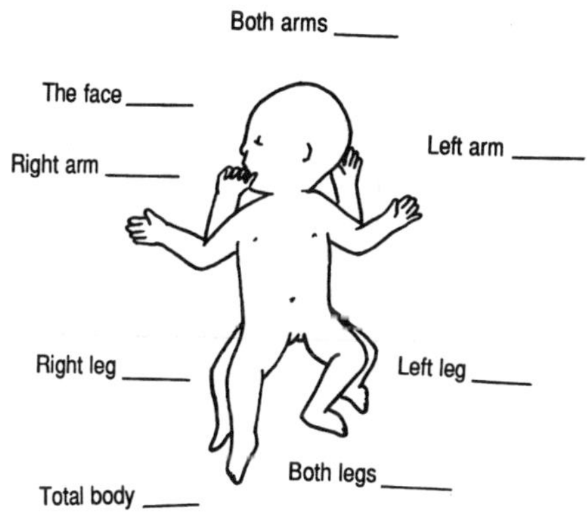

Fig-2. Irregular-jerking movements, spasms. (*Adapted from Cratty, 1979.*)

In this part of the evaluation, the presence and location of irregular jerking movements of a spasmodic nature are to be noted. Indicate next to the body part(s) whether these spasms are seen (3) often, (2) occasionally, (1) seldom, or (0) never.

Notes, comments: (When did these start, terminate?) ______________

______________________________ (Have they been associated with seizure or are they the forerunners of seizures?)

____

Miscellaneous comments______________________________

____

____

____

(cont)

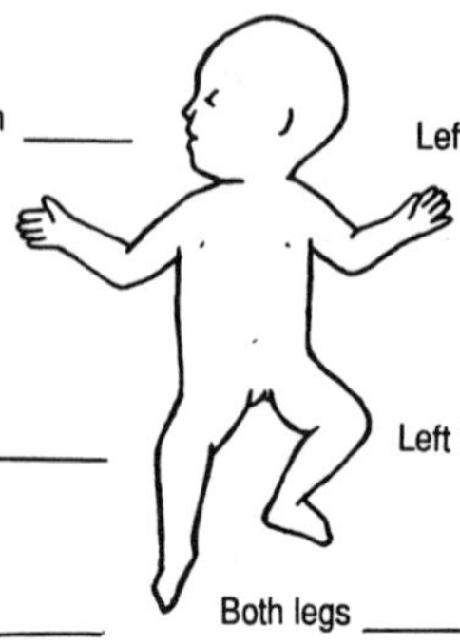

To detect tension in upper limbs of infants from birth to 8 months, place the infant on his/her back and gently attempt to move the arms simultaneously and bilaterally away from and then toward the body while holding the wrists. Note the amount of resistance encountered when attempting to move the arms-wrists away from the center of the body. To assess excess tension levels in the lower limbs, hold the ankles gently and attempt alternately to flex and extend the legs at the knees and hips. Note the amount of resistance given to the attempt to extend the legs-hips. Differentiate between tension exhibited by the left and right arms and between the left and right legs, if differences exist.

Score on a 5-point scale: 1 = marked hypotonicity, 2 = moderate hypotonicity, 3 = moderate, normal tension, 4 = excess tension, and 5 = marked hypertonicity. Score each limb separately and both upper and lower limbs as combined but separate units. Thus the lowest overall score that may be given (denoting normal tension) is 16, and the highest score obtained (most excess tension, marked hypertonicity) is 30.
Notes, comments: ____

____

Summary and Miscellaneous Developmental Data
Summary

1. Hypertonicity-hypotonicity scores: upper limb total __________. right arm __________, lower limb toal __________. left leg __________. right leg __________, total hypertonicity-hypotonicity score__________.

2. Location of tremors: total body __________, lower limbs __________. left leg only __________, right leg only __________. upper limbs only __________, right arm only __________, left arm only __________.

3. Previous totals, trends:
   Hypertonicity-hypotonicity ______________________________
   ____

4. Previous location, trends of tremors: ______________________
   ____

Developmental Data:

1. Ages at which the child: turned over front-to back unassisted ______________. sat without support ________. creeped __________. pulled to stand __________. walked unassisted ______________________________

2. Grasps object voluntarily (hand used?) __________________
   Uses both hands at midline of body on single object __________
   Releases small objefct with one hand ____________________

3. Miscellaneous data regarding speech, eating habits, social-emotional characteristics, etc.

____

____

____

____

(**Note*. Checklist from B. J. Cratty, Dept. of Kinesiology, UCLA.)

Appendix II

Test of Motor Planning (Praxic Behaviors)

The following tests were developed in the mid 1970s and have been employed with various modifications to average a typical group of children including the learning disabled, the deaf, and the retarded that have been cited throughout the text. They have been shown to have good test-retest and inter-observer reliability, but adequate norms are not available. At present they represent potentially useful for clinical screening potentially dyspraxic children, youth, and adults.

TEST OF LIMB PRAXIS

In the test of limb praxis the tester stands about 5 feet to the front and slightly to the left of the subject, and at the rate of one-a-second, moves from one position to the next, as shown. The test starts with the presentation of a single movement-position, and if the subject replicates the movement-position successfully a second is added, and then a third etc. The test proceeds in this manner until an error is committed (an error of ommission or commission), at which point additional series are presented, until a second error is committed. The score recorded is the longest series successfully replicated by the subject, and thus the scores range from 1–7

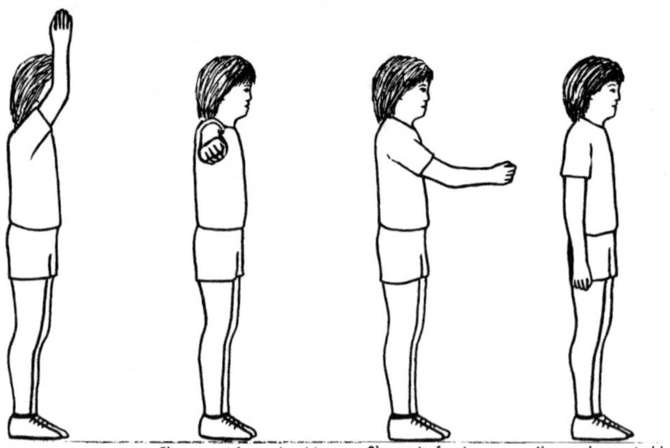

1) arm up 2) arm out from shoulder 3) arm to front 4) arm down at side

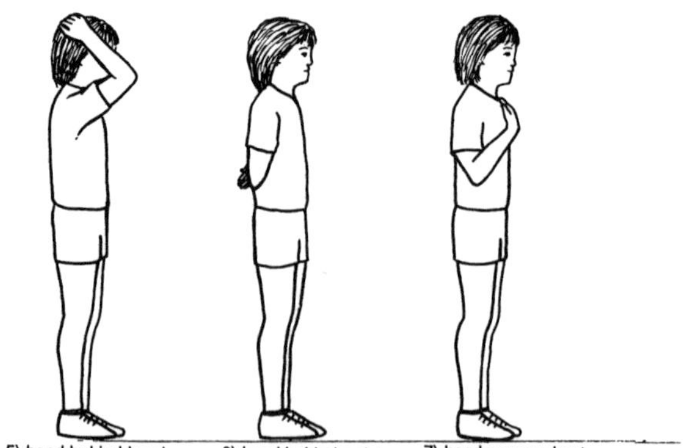

5) hand behind head 6) hand behind waist 7) hand across chest

TEST OF DRAWING PRAXIS

In the test of drawing praxis the tester sits at a table to the side of the subject's preferred hand. The tester then draws a single line, one a 2″ × 2″ piece of paper, and shows it to the subject for one second, and removes it from sight. The subject must then replicate it. If the subject is successful the next figure is drawn, in which a line is added. Successive figures are drawn by the tester, shown to the subject, and if the subject replicates them successfully the next more complex figure is drawn. The test proceeds in this manner until an error is committed (an error of ommission or commission), at which point additional figures are drawn, and presented for replication, until a second error is committed. The score recorded is the most complicated figure drawn successfully, consisting of from 1–7 lines; and thus the scores range from 1–7

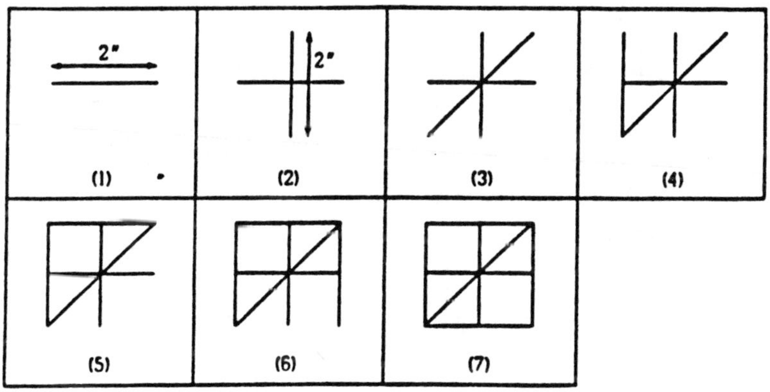

TEST OF HAND PRAXIS

In the test of limb praxis the tester sits at a table to the side of the subject's preferred hand. At the rate of one-a-second. The tester moves from one position to the next, as shown. Each hand position is moved to in a one-a-second rhythm, with hand rising about 12″ above the table in a rhythmic manner between positions assumed as the hand touches the table. The test starts with the presentation of a single movement-position, and if the subject replicates the movement-position successfully a second is added, and then a third etc. The test proceeds in this manner until an error is committed (an error of ommission or commission), at which point additional series are presented, until a second error is committed. The scroe recorded is the longest series successfully replicated by the subject, and thus the scores range from 1–7

1) fist, little finger down

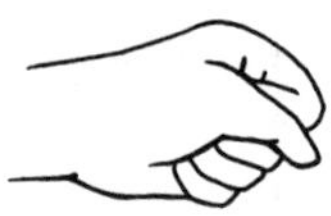

2) palm open, little finger down

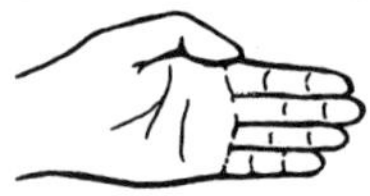

3) palm down, hand open

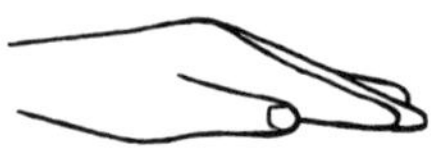

4) fist, palm down

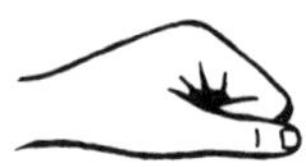

5) fist, palm up

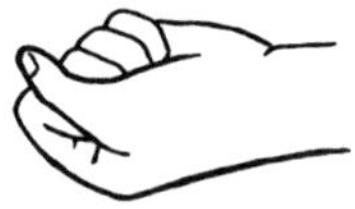

6) palm up and open

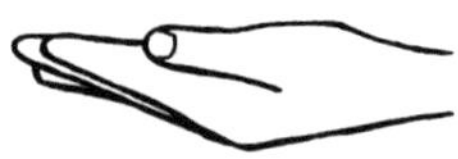

7) fist, thumb down

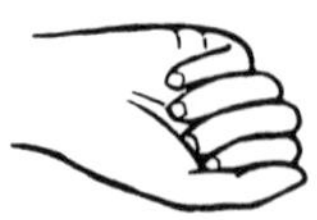

Test for Trunkle Praxis

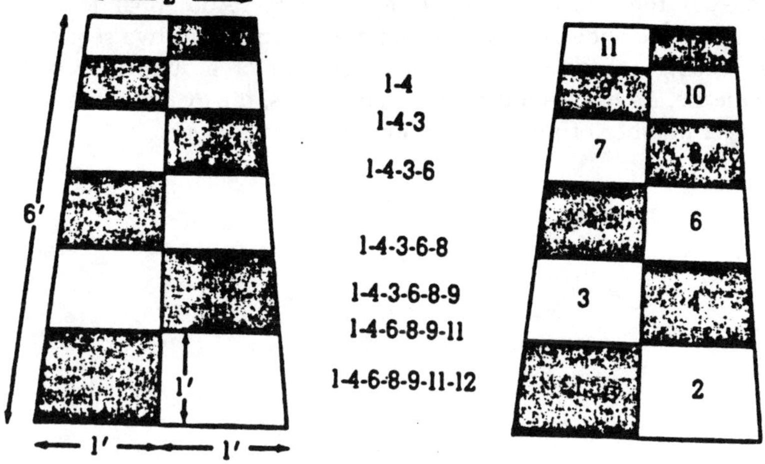

OVERVIEW

This test was added to the battery, in so far as the literature makes it clear that the serial positioning of the total body in space (trunkel praxia) ia a quality independent of other kinds of motor planning (using the hands etc). Our studies confirm this independence (Cratty and Samoy 1984). Unlike tests 31, and #2, however, the child-testee is not required to execute a new movement-position in each sequence, but is merely requested to remember the serial-location of where they jumped in a marked mat. Thus all seven movements are the same, jumping, with remembering locations providing the serial memory task. It is thus possible that this test may be more heavily dependent upon underlying verbal-cognitive coding, or cuing, than is true of the other tests in the battery. This tests like the others in battery is reliable, and may be reliably scored. Reliability reaches .8, and inter-tester agreement reaches 90% or better in pilot studies.

Administration and Scoring

The child is told that "Now we are going to play a jumping game. You should first watch me, and then you should watch where I jump, and then try to jump just where I have jumped on the mat. Any questions?" Next the tester, after positioning the child at the 4′

end of a matched marked as shown (see appendix) with 1′ × 1′ squares, jumps, using both feet together, in the first square. The child testee is then asked to replicate the jump. Additional locations (squares) are added one at a time, until the child fails two sequences (by failing to execute correctly a location of a jump in correct sequence. As has been true in the other tests, the overall score is the correct number of jumps taken in the correct squence.

Appendix III

Check-List for Assessing the Presence and Incidence of Infant Stereotypes

The following check-list has been employed in studies of drug-stressed infants as well as in studies of the emotionally disturbed and autistic.

NAME DATE

STEREOTYPIES	1	2	3	4	COMMENTS	GENERAL COMMENTS
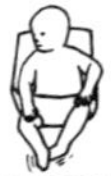 Foot-Rubbing						
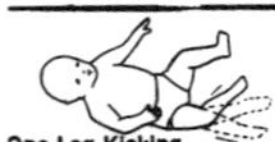 One Leg Kicking, Supine Position						
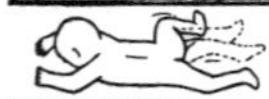 One Leg Kicking, Prone Position						
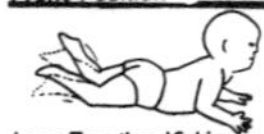 Legs Together Kicking						
ARMS/HANDS 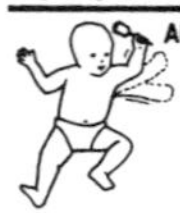 Arm-Waiving with or without Object						
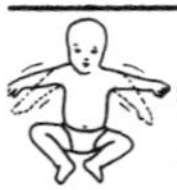 Sit-Bouncing Sitting Unsupported						
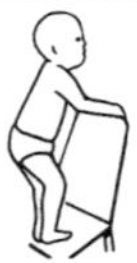 Standing						

NAME DATE

STEREOTYPIES	1	2	3	4	COMMENTS	GENERAL COMMENTS
KINDS 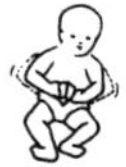 Banging Arms Together with or without Object						
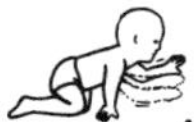 Arm Sway						
TRUNK 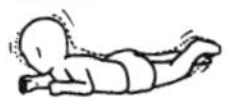 Foward-Back Rocking						
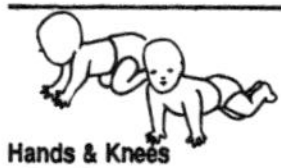 Hands & Knees Crawling						
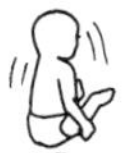 Foward Rocking Sitting Unsupported						
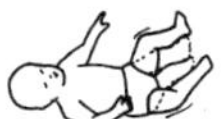 Alternate Leg-kicking Spine Position						

Appendix IV

Self-Concept Questionnaires

The following questionnaires have been employed in studies to determine how children feel about their skills, bodies, and performance capacities. The first scale was used in just one study with learning disabled children (1900, Cratty, Deoliverira, and Miyahara). The second is a modification of the component of the self-concept questionnaire originally developed by Ellen Piers and Dale Harris (1952), and has been used extensively over the years in a program for physically awkward children.

PHYSICAL ACTIVITY SURVEY

______________________________ ______________________________

Print Name Date

The purposes of this survey is to find out how you feel about games and exercise, and about yourself.

After each question circle the number that shows how you feel or what you believe. If you do not wish to answer any question, leave it out. If you do not wish to fill out the form, that is all right also. If you have any questions, ask them now, or while you are filling out the form.

1. I believe that my skills in games are.

Poor		About average		Very good
1	2	3	4	5

2. I believe that my body-build is

Too light		About right		Too heavy
1	2	3	4	5

3. If I have to play sports and games I am

Unhappy		OK		Very happy
1	2	3	4	5

The sports and exercise activities I like best are:

____

____

The physical activities I dislike are.

____

____

SELF-OPINION QUESTIONNAIRE

(Modified from the Piers-Harris)

Name ______________________________ Date ________________

Brothers-sisters, Ages: ____

(Score Yes-No responses, try to force response; also (H) for Hesitations) Place dash (-) after each low self-concept response.

1. Are you good at making things with your hands? ____________
2. Can you draw well? ____________
3. Are you strong? ____________
4. Do you like the way you look? ____________
5. Do children often say bad things to you? ____________
6. Do you have trouble making friends? ____________
7. Do you like school? ____________
8. Do you wish yo were different? ____________
9. Are you the last to be chosen in games? ____________
10. Do girls like you? ____________
11. Are you sad most of the time? ____________
12. Are you a good leader in sports and games? ____________
13. Are you clumsy . . . Do you drop things or trip often? ____________
14. Do boys like you? ____________
15. Do you play with younger children a lot? ____________
16. Is reading easy for you? ____________
17. Are you an important member of your class? ____________
18. Do your classmates think of you have good ideas? ____________
19. Do you get tired easily when you play? ____________
20. Are you happy most of the time? ____________

Total Low Self-Concept Responses ______

Bibliography

Abbir M. Douglas, H., & Ross. K. (1978) The clumsy child syndrome: observation in case studies referred to the gymnasium of the Adelaide Children's Hospital. *Medical Journal of Australia*, **1**, 65–69.

Abercrombie, M. L. J., (1964) Associated movements in normal and physically handicapped children. *Development Medicine and Child Neurology* **6**, 573–580.

Alberts C. L., & Landers D. M. (1978) Birth order, motor performance and maternal influence. *Research Quarterly*, **48**, 661–670.

Alexander, M. P. & Schmitt M. A. (1980) The aphasia syndrome of stroke in the left anterior cerebral artery territory. *Archives of Neurology*, **37**, 97–100.

Amber, J. (1989) "Cocaine Kinetics in Humans", Chapter 6 in Redda K. K., Walker, C. A. & Barnett G., (Eds) *Cocaine, Marijuana, Designer Drugs: Pharmacology and Behavior*, pp. 53–68, Boca Raton Florida, CRC Press.

Amuchie, P. (1979) *Relationships between measures of digital agnosia and finger, opposition*. Unpublished MS Thesis, Department of Kinesiology, University of California, Los Angeles.

Anderson, D. W. (1966) *Handwriting research: Movement and quality, in Research on Handwriting and Spelling*. In T.A. Horn Editor, Proceedings, National Council of Teachers of English, Champaign, Illinois.

Annell, A. L. (1949) Social problems in children of average or superior intelligence: A preliminary report, *Journal of Mental Science*, **95**, 901–909.

Apgar, V. (1953) A proposal for a new method of evaluation of the new-born infant, *Current Research in Anesthesia and Analgesia*, **32**, 260–267.

Armitage M. & Larkin D. (1991) *Laterality and coordination*. 18th ACHPER Convention, National/International Conference, Perth Australia.

Arnheim, Daniel D., & Sinclair, W. A., (1975) *The Clumsy Child: A program of motor therapy*, C. V. Mosby, St. Louis.

Askov E., Otto W, & Askov W. (1970) A decade of research in handwriting: progress and prospect. *Journal of Educational Research*, **64**, 3–25.

Ayres A. J. (1972) Types of sensory integration dysfunction among disabled learners, *American Journal of Occupational Therapy*, **26**, 13–18.

Badal J. (1888) Contribution of l'etude des cecites psychiques: alexie, agraphie, hemianopsie inferieure, trouble du sens de l'espace, *Arch d'opthal.*, **8**, 97–117.

Bailer, I., Doll L., & Winsberg, B. G. (1973) *Modified Lincoln-Oseretsky Motor Development Scale*, New York, New York State Monograph, State Department of Mental Health and Hygiene.

Barbeau A. (1982) "History of movement disorders and their treatment" in Barbeau A, (Editor) *Disorders of Movement*, Lippencott, Philadelphia Penna. pp. 1–29.

Basso, A., Luzszatti C & Spinler H. (1980) Is ideomotor apraxia the outcome of damage to well-defined regions of the left hemisphere? Neuropsychological study of CAT correlation. *Journal of Neurology, Neurosurgery and Psychiatry*, **43**, 118–126.

Battelle Developmental Inventory, (1986) Teaching Resources DML, Park New York.

Bayley N. A. (1935). *The development of motor abilities during the first three years*, Monograph, Berkeley, California Society for Research in Child Development 1–26.

Bayley N. A. (1969) *Bayley Scales of Infant Development*, Psychological Corporation, New York.

Beital P. A., & Mead, B. J. (1980) Bruinicks-Oseretsky Test of Motor Proficiency: A viable measure for 3–5 year old children, *Perceptual and Motor Skills*. **51**, 919–923.

Beller, E. K. (1959) Exploratory studies of dependency, *Transactions of the New York Academy of Science*. **1**, 414–426.

Benito, P. E. (1987) Development Gerstmann's syndrome: case report and review of the literature. *Journal of Development and Behavioral Pediatrics*., **8**, 229–232.

Benson, D. F. (1991) *Frontal dysfunction in ADHA and Dyslexia*, Proceedings, The Orton Society Convention, Portland Oregon.

Benson, D. F. & Geschwind N. (1968) Cerebral dominance, and its disturbances, *Pediatric Clinics of North America*, **15**, 759–769.

Benton, A. L. (1959) *Left-right discrimination and finger localization, development and pathology*, Heober-Harper Books, New York.

Berges, J. & Lezine I. (1965) The Imitation of Gestures, *Clinics in Developmental Medicine*, **18**, 1–122.

Birns, N. & Golden, A. (1972) Prediction of intellectual performance at three years from infant tests and personality measures, *Merrill-Palmer Quartery*, **18**, 53–58.

Bloom, B. S. (1956) *Taxonomy of Educational Objectives, Handbook I Cognitive Domaine*, David McKay Co, New York.

Bonnevier, J. A. (1968) A study of diadochokinesia in school children. *Acta Paedopsychiatrica*, **35**, 78–80.

Bowers, T. G. R. (1975) *Human Development*, New York, W. H. Freeman.

Bowlby, J. (1951) *Maternal Care and Mental Health*, Monograph World Health Organization, Geneva.

Brain, W. R. & Walton, J. N. (1969 *Brain's Diseases of the Nervous System, 7th Edition*, p 566, London, Oxford University Press.

Bradley, K. P. (1982) The effectiveness of construction praxis tests in predicting upper extremity dressing problems. *Occupational Therapy Journal of Research*, **2**, 184–185.

Brazelton, T. B. (1973) *Neonatal Behavorial Assessment Scale: Clinics in Developmental Medicine No 50*, Spastics International Medical Corporation, Philadelphia, Penna Lippencott.

Breitmeyer, B. G. & Ganz, L. (1976) Implications of sustained and transient channels for theories of visual pattern masking, saccadic suppression and information processing, *Psychological Review*, **83**, 1–36.

Bremmer, R. H. (1971) *Children and Youth in America*. Vol II, 1866–1932, Harvard University Press, Cambridge Mass.

Bremmer, M. N., & Gillman, S. (1966) Visuomotor ability in children – a survey, *Developmental Medicine and Child Neurology*, **8**, 686–703.

Brenner, M. W., Gillman, S., Zangwill, O. L. & Farrell, M. (1967) Visuomotor disability in school children. *British Medical Journal*, **4**, 259–262.

Broderick, Pia (1987) The drawing of squares and diamonds: A perceptual-motor task analysis. *Journal of Experimental child Psychology*, **43**, 44–61.

Broer, M. R. (1958) Effectiveness of a general basic skills curriculum for junior high school girls. *Research Quarterly*, **29**, 579–585.

Broer, M. R. (1955) Evaluation of a basic skills curriculum for women of low motor ability at the University of Washington, *Research Quarterly*, **26**, 15–27.

Brown, J. (1981) Effects of an integrated physical education/music program in changing early childhood perceptual-motor performance. Perceptual and Motor Skills, **53**, 151–154.

Brown, J. K. (1981) Learning Disabilities: A paediatric neurologist's point of view, *Transactions of the College of Medicine of South Africa*. December, 49–104.

Brown, J. W. (1972) *Aphasia, apraxia and agnosia: Clinical and theoretical aspects*, Charles C. Thomas, Springfield, Illinois.

Brown, R. M. (1989) "Pharmacology of Cocaine Abuse", Chapter 5, in Redda K. K., Walker, C. A. & Barnett G., (Eds) *Cocaine, Marijuana, Designer Drugs: Pharmacology and Behavior*, pp 39–52, Boca Raton Florida, CRC Press.

Bruck, M. (1989) Word recognition of skills of adults with childhood diagnoses of dyslexia. *Developmental Psychology*, **26**, 439–54.

Bruininks, R. H. (1978). *Bruinink's Oseretsky Test of Motor Proficiency*, American Guidance Service, Circle Pines, Minnesota.

Bryden M. P. (1982) *Laterality; Functional asymmetry in the Intact Brain*, New York, Academic Press.

Cantwell, D. (1992) Medication and Learning Disabilities, in B. J. Cratty (Ed.), *Experts talk with the parents of learning disabled children*, Landmark West School, Encino, California.

Case-Smith, J. (1989) Reliability and validity of the posture and fine motor assessment of infants, *Occupational Therapy Journal of Research*. **9**, 259–272.

Caramazza, A., Miceli, G., Villa, G. & Romani C. (1987) The role of graphemic buffer in the spelling: evidence of a case of acquired dysgraphia. *Cognition*, **17**, 58–85.

Carlson, M., Earls, F. & Todd, R. D., (1988). The importance of regressive changes in the development of the nervous system: toward a neurological biological theory of child development. *Psychiatric Development*, **7**, 1–12.

Carpenter, R. D. (1972) *Why Can't I Learn?*, Regal Books, Glendale, California.

Cermak, S. (1985) "Developmental Dyspraxia" in Roy, E. A. *Neuropsychological Studies of Apraxia and Related Disorders*, pp 225–243. North-Holland, New York.

Chandler, L. S., Andrews, M. S., & Swanson, M. W., (1980) *Movement Assessment of Infatns: Amanual*. Rolling Bay, Washington:

Chasnoff, I. J. (1986). "Perinatal Addition: Consequences of Intrauterine Exposure to Opiate and Nonopiate Drugs", in I. J. Chasnoff (Ed.), *Drug Use in Pregnancy: Mother and Child*, pp 52–63.

Chendru, F. & Gerschwind, N. (1972) Disorders of higher cortical function in acute confusional states, *Cortex*, **8**, 395–411.

Clements, S. D. (1966a) The child with minimal brain dysfunction, *Journal-Lancet*, **86**, 185–197.

Clements, S. D. (1966b) *Minimal brain dysfunction in children:* (USPHS Publication #141, US Government Printing Office. Washington D.C.

Clifford, J. & Bundy, A. C. (1989) Play preference and play performance in normal boys and girls with sensory integration dysfunction. *Occupational Therapy Journal of Research*. **9**, 3–15.

Cohen, D. J. (1988) *Tourette's syndrome and tic disorders*, Wiley, New York.

Cohen, J. J., Taft, L. T., Mahadeviah, M. S., & Birch, H. G. (1967) Developmental changes in overflow in normal and aberrantly functioning children. *The Journal of Pediatrics*, **71**, 39–47.

Colarusso, R. P., & Hammill, D. D. (1972) *Motor-free visual perceptual test*, Academic Therapy Publications. Novato, California.

Connolly, B., Morgan, S., Russell, F. F., & Richardson, B. (1980) Early intervention with Down's Syndrome. *Physical Therapy*, **60**, 1405–1408.

Connolly, K., & Stratton, P. (1968) Developmental changes in associated movements, *Developmental Medicine and Child Neurology*, **10**, 49–56.

Conrad, K. E., Cermak, S. R., & Drake, C. (1983) Differentiation of praxis among children, *American Journal of Occupational Therapy*, **37**, 466–473.

Cooke, R. (1984) Atlantoaxial instability in individuals with Down's Syndrome, *Mental Retardation*, **22**, 193–194.

Corballlis, M. C. (1983) Human Laterality, New York, Academic Press.

Corder, W. O. (1966) Effects of physical education on the intellectual, physical and social development of educable mentally retarded boys, *Exceptional Children*, **32**, 357–364.

Cornish, S. V. (1980) Development of a test of motor planning. *Physical Therapy*, **60**, 1129–1132.

Cowan, W. M., Fawcett, J. W., O'Leary, D. D. M., & Stanfield, B. B. (1984) Regressive events in neurogenesis, *Science*, **225**, 1258–1265.

Cratty, B. J. (1960) A comparision of fathers and sons in physical ability, *Research Quarterly*, **30**, 15–21.

Cratty, B. J. (1962) A comparsion of the learning of a fine motor skill to learning a similar gross motor skill, using kinesthetic cues, *Research Quarterly*, (of AAHPER) **33**, 212–221.

Cratty, B. J. (1967) *Perceptual and Motor Characteristics of Retarded Children and Youth*, The County Mental Retardation Services Board, Los Angeles, California.

Cratty, B. J. (1969) *Perceptual and Motor Development of Infants and Children 1st Edition*, MacMillan, New York.

Cratty, B. J. (1970a) *Movement and spatial awareness in blind children and youth*, Springfield, Illinois, Charles C. Thomas.

Cratty, B. J. (1970b) Chapter 1, The self-concept of children with coordiantion Problems pp 5–45, in Cratty, B. J., Ikeda, N., Martin, M.

M., Jennett, C., & Morris, M. *Movement Activities, Motor Ability and the Education of Children*, Charles C. Thomas, Springfield, Illinois.

Cratty, B. J. (1975a) *Physical Expressions of Intelligence*, Prentice-Hall Inc, Englewood Cliffs, New Jersey.

Cratty, B. J. (1975b) *Remedial Motor Activity for Children*, Lea and Febiger, Philadelphia, Penna.

Cratty, B. J. (1975c) *Motor Activity and the Education of Retardates* 2nd Edition, Lea and Febiger, Philadelphia.

Cratty, B. J. (1975d) *Movement Behavior and Motor Learning*, 3rd Edition, Lea and Febiger, Philadelphia, Penna.

Cratty, B. J. (1975e) Associated Movements, in, B. J. Cratty, *Remedial Motor Activity in Children*, p 134, Lea and Febiger, Philadelphia, Penna.

Cratty, B. J. (1979) *Perceptual and Motor Development of Infants and Children 2nd Edition*, Prentice-Hall Inc, Englewood Cliffs, New Jersey.

Cratty, B. J. (1985a) Chapter 8, Adjusting Arousal Level. in B. J. Cratty *Active Learning, 2nd Edition*, Prentice-Hall Inc, Englewood Cliffs, New Jersey.

Cratty, B. J. (1985b) *Active Learning*, 2nd Edition, Prentice-Hall Inc, Englewood Cliffs, New Jersey.

Cratty, B. J. (1987a) *From Scribbing to Printing*, I-Med, 1520 Cotner Ave, Los Angeles,CA 90025.

Cratty, B. J. (1987b) *Physical Development for Children, A Card File for Parents and Teachers*, Movement Consultants, 10827 Savona Dr, Los Angeles, California 90077.

Cratty. B. J. (1988) Physical Education for Creative and Gifted Children, *Gifted Children's Quarterly*, **11**, 79–91.

Cratty, B. J. (1989a) *Adapted physical activity in the mainstream 2nd edition*, Love Publications, Denver, Colorado.

Cratty, B. J. (1989b) *Perceptual and Motor Development of Infants and Children, 3rd Edition*, Prentice-Hall Inc, Englewood Cliffs, New Jersey.

Cratty, B. J. (1989c) "The beginnings of movement in the newborn: reflexes and stereotypies, Chapter 5, in B. J. Cratty, *Perceptual and Motor Development in Infants and Children, 3rd Edition*, pp 102–134 Prentice-Hall Inc. Englewood Cliffs, New Jersey.

Cratty, B. J. (1989d) "The Hands" Chapter 8, in B. J. Cratty, *Perceptual and Motor Development in Infants and Children, 3rd Edition*, pp 203–238, Prentice-Hall Inc. Englewood Cliffs, New Jersey.

Cratty, B. J. (1989e) Chapter 10 Physical Awkwardness, in B. J. Cratty, *Adapted Physical Activity in the Mainstream, 2dn Edition*, Denver, Love Publications.

Cratty, B. J. (1989f) *Conversations with caretakers of drug-stressed infants*, January to April 1989, Unpublished Notes, Department of Kinesiology, UCLA.

Cratty, B. J. (1989g) (Motor Planning Tests) in Chapter 12, The Awkward Child, in B. J. Cratty, *Adapted Physical Activity in the Mainstream, 2nd* Edition, Love Publications, Denver, Colorado. pp 206–224.

Cratty, B. J. (1989h) *Psychology in Contemporary Sport, 3rd Edition*, Prentice-Hall Inc, Englewood Cliffs New Jersey.

Cratty, B. J. (1989i) Chapter 26 Self-Control and Attention, in B. J. Cratty, *Adapted Physical Activity in the Mainstream, 2nd Edition,* Love Publications, Denver Colorado.

Cratty, B. J. (1989j) Chapter 25 Infant Stimulation, in B. J. Cratty, *Adapted Physical Activity in the Mainstream, 2dn Edition,* Love Publications, Denver Colorado. (pp 420–439).

Cratty, B. J. (1989k) Chapter 10 Mental Retardation, in B. J. Cratty, *Adapted Physical Activity in the Mainstream,* 2nd Edition, Love Publications, Denver Colorado. pp 169–184.

Cratty, B. J. (1989l) Exercise Effects and Performance Outcomes, Chapter 12, in B. J. Cratty, *Perceptual and Motor Development in Infants and Children 3rd edition* pp 314–336, Prentice-Hall Inc, Englewood Cliffs, New Jersey.

Cratty, B. J. (1990). Motor development of infants subject to maternal drug use: Current evidence and future research directions, *Adapted Physical Activity Quarterly,* **7**, 110–125.

Cratty, B. J. & Bergel, R. (1972) *Dynamic visual acuity: a development study,* Unpublished Monograph, Kinesiology Department, UCLA.

Cratty, B. J., Cratty, I. J., and Cornell, S. (1986) Motor planning abilities in deaf and hearing children, *American Annals of the Deaf,* **51**, 186–190.

Cratty, B. J., & DeOliveira, I. J. (1989a). *Rhythmic stereotypies of cocaine-exposed infants: Preliminary data and observations.* Unpublished Monograph. Department of Kinesiology, University of California, Los Angeles.

Cratty, B. J., & DeOliveira, I. J. (1989b) *Printing Behavior in Children: Seven Case Studies,* Unpublished Monograph, Department of Kinesiology, University of California, Los Angeles.

Cratty, B. J., Miyahara, M., & DeOliveira, I. J. (1991) Wahrnehmungs- und motorische Fahigkeiten von lernbehindereten Kindern Und Jugendlichen (Perceptual and Motor Abilities of Learning Disabled Children and Youth) *Motorik,* **14**, 173–184 (in German).

Cratty, B. J., and Gong, P. (1989) A test battery to evaluate motor planning (praxic behaviors), in *Motorik* (In Press).

Cratty, B. J., & Gibson, S. (1985) Studies in motor planning, impulsivity and attention in kindergarten children, *Motorik,* **8**, 51–58.

Cratty, B. J., Ikeda, N., Martin, M., Jennett, C., & Morris, M. (1972) *Movement activities, motor ability and the education of children,* Charles C. Thomas, Springfield, Illinois.

Cratty, B. J., Ikeda, N., Martin, M. M., Jennett, C., & Morris, M. (1972a) Changes in selected perceptual-motor attributes of children with moderate coordination problems, in Cratty, B. J., Ikeda, N., Martin, M. M., Jennett, C., & Morris, M. *Movement Activities, Motor Ability and the Education of Children,* Charles C. Thomas, Springfield, Illinois.

Cratty, B. J., & Omata, C. (1989) Motor planning abilities in retarded and in normal youngster, *Motorik* (In press 1989).

Cratty, B. J., & Samoy, E. (1984) Ein vergleisch praxischer verhaltensweissen bie gjarhiringen kindern, *Motorik,* **7**, 52–58.

Cratty, B. J., & Williams, H. G. (1968) A comparison of selected abilities in a twin pair, one sighted, the other blind, *Perceptual and Motor Skills*, **28**, 23–30.

Cruickshank, W. M. (1961) Bentzen, F. A. Ratzeburg, F. H., & Tannauser, M. T. A. *A teaching method of brain injured and hyperactivce children, Syracuse, New York Syracuse University Press.*

Da Costa, M. I. L. (1946) *The Ozeretsky Tests of Motor Proficiency. A translation from the Portuguese adaptation* (ed) Doll, E. A. Minneapolis, American Guidance Services, Inc.

Damasio, H., & Damasio AnR. (1989) *Leson Analysis in Neuropsychology* Oxford University Press, New York.

Daniels, J., & Oldridge, N. (1971) Changes in oxygen consumption of young boys during growth and running training, *Medicine Science Sports*, **3**, 161–165.

Dare, M. T., & Gordon, N. (1970) Clumsy children: a disorder of perception and motor organisation, *Developmental Medicine and Child Neurology*, **12**, 178–185.

David, I. S. (1985) *Motor sequencing strategies in school age children, Neurological Organization and Reading*, Charles C. Thomas, Springfield Illinois.

DeFonesca, V. (1985) conversation, Lisboa, Portugal, National Perceptual-Motor Conference.

Delrahim, M., Cratty, B. J. (1991) *The self-concept of boys ad girls with coordination problems*, Unpublished Study, Department of Kinesiology University of California, Los Angeles.

Dalrahim, M., & Cratty, B. J. (1991) Changes in motor abilities among learning disabled children exposed to a remedial program. Unpublished Study. Department of Kinesiology, UCLA.

Denckla, M. B. (1973) Development of speed in repetitive and successive finger-movements in normal children. *Developmental Medicine and Child Neurology*, **15**, 635–645.

Dencka, M. B., Rudel, R. G., Chapman, C., & Krieger, J. (1985) Motor proficiency in dyslexic children, with and without attentional problems. *Archives of Neurology*, **42**, 228–231.

Dennis, W. (1960) Causes of retardation among institutional children in Iran, *Journal of Genetic Psychology*, **96**, 47–59.

Dennis, W., & Najarian, P. (1957) Infant development under environmental handicap. *Psychology Monographs*, **7**, 1–77.

DeOliveira, I. J., & Cratty, B. J. (1991) A survey of Infants Exposed Prenatally to Cocaine Use, *International Journal of Rehabilitation Research*, **14**, 265–266.

Deren, S. (1986) Children of Substance Abuse: A Review of the Literature, *Journal of Substance Abuse Treatment*, **3**, 77–94.

DeRenzi, E., Fabrizia, M. D., Motti, M. D., & Nichelli, P. (1980) Imitiating gestures, a quantitative approach to ideomotor apraxia, *Archives of Neurology*, **37**, 6–10.

DeRenzi, E., Pieczoro, A., & Vignolo, L. (1968) Ideational apraxia: A quantitative study, *Neuropsychologia*, **6**, 41–52.

Deule, R. K., Feely, C., & Bonskowski, C. (1984) Manual apraxia in learning disabled children (Abstract) *Annals of Neurology*, **16**, 388.

Deule, R. K., & Robinson, D. J. (1987) Chapter 5, Developmental motor signs, in Tupper, D. E., *Soft Neurological Signs*, Grune & Stratton, New York. (pp 95–130).

Doll-Tepper, G. M. (1987) Effects of Physical Education on Children with Learning Disabilities, M. E. Berridge & G. R. Ward (Eds) *International Perspective on Adapted Physical Activity*, Human Kinetics, Champaign Illinois.

Dorhman, P. (1964) Throwing and kicking ability of eight-year-old boys and girls, *Research Quarterly*, **35**, 464–471.

Druker, P. (1978) *The finger position imitiation test.* Unpublished Master's Thesis, University of Southern California, Los Angeles.

Duane, D. D. (1991) Neurobiological correlates of reading, attention and nonverbal developmental disorders. *Proceedings*, The Orton Society Convention, November 7–10, Portland Oregon.

Dusenberry, L. (1952) A study of the effects of training in ball skills by children ages 3–7. *Research Quarterly*, **23**, 9–14.

Dvorak, K., Feit, J., & Jurankova, Z. (1978) Experimentally induced focal microgyria and status varrucosus deformis in rats, *Acta Neuropathol*, **44**, 121–129.

Dzenitis, A. J. (1966) Spontaneous atlanto-axial dislocation in a mongoloid child with spinal cord compression, *Journal of Neurosurgery*, **25**, 458–465.

Eichel, Valerie, (1986) *Stereotypies of Autistic Children*, Ph.D. Dissertation, Department of Kinesiology, University of California, Los Angeles.

Ellison, P. H., Browning, C. A., Larson, B., and Denny, J. (1983) Development of a scoring system for the Milani-Comparetti & Gidioni method of assessing neurologic abnormality in infancy. *Physical Therapy*, **63**, 1414–1423.

Eng, D. E., Koch, B., & Binder, H., (1979) *Infantile hypotonia: Diagnostic dilemma*. Monograph Children's Hospital, Department of Medicine and Rehabilitation. Washington D.C.

Erickson, E.N. (1950) *Childhood and Society*, New York, Norton.

Eriksson, B. O., Gollnick, P. D., & Saltin B. (1974) The effect of physical training on muscle enzyme activities and fiber composition in 11 year-old boys. *Activa Paediatics*, Belgium, 28 Monograph Supplement, 245–252.

Esenther, S. E. (1984) Development coaching of the Down's syndrome infants. *American Journal of Mental Deficiency*, **87**, 435–440.

Exner, S. (1881) *Unterschugen uber die Lokalisation der Funktion en in der Grossshirnride des Menschen*, W. Braumuller. Wein.

Faglioni, P., & Basso, A. (1985) Historical perspectives on neuroanatomical correlates of limb apraxia, in E.A. Roy (ed) *Neuropsychological Studies of Apraxia and Related Disorders*, Elsevier Science Publishers B.V. North Holland.

Filipek, P., & Kennedy, D. N. (1991) Chapter 6 "Magnetic Resonance Imaging: Its Role in the Developmental Disorders. In D. D. Duane, &

D. B., Gray eds. *The Reading Brain: The Biological Basis of Dyslexia,* York Press, Parkton Maryland, pp 133–160.

Fleishman, E. (1965) *The Measurement of Physical Fitness,* Prentice-Hall, Englewood Cliffs, New Jersey.

Fog, E., & Fog, M. (1963) Cerebral inhibition examined by associated movements. In M. Mac Keith & R. Mac Keith (Eds) *Minimal cerebral dysfunction.* Clinics in Developmental Medicine No 10, London: S.I.M.P. with Heineman.

Ford, F. R. (1966) *Diseases of the Nervous System in Infancy, Childhood and Adolescence,* 5th Edition, Thomas, Springfield.

Frankenburg, W. K., & Dodds, J. B. (1967) The Denver Developmental Screening Test, *Journal of Pediatrics,* **71**, 181–191.

Freischlag, J. (1973) Motor activities to teach handwriting to the poorly coordinated. *School and community,* **59**, 28–29.

Frost, M. (1988) Mechanism of structural and functional development in the thalamas: Retinal projections to the auditory and somatosensory systems in normal and experimentally manipulated hamsters. in *Cellular Thalmic Mechanism,* Eds. M. Bentivoglio & R. Spreafico, Amsterdam, Elsevier Scientific Publishing Co.

Frostig, M. (1958) *Developmental test of visual perception,* Palo Alto; Consult Psychologists Press.

Gerstmann (1927) Fingeragnosie und isolierte agraphie; ein neues syndrom, *Ztschr. Neurol. Psychiat.,* **108**, 152–177.

Gesell, A. (1925) *The Mental Growth of the Pre-School Child,* MTP Press Limited. New York.

Gesell, A., & Thompson, H. (1934) *Infant behavior: Its genesis and growth,* McGraw-Hill, New York.

Geschwind, N. (1975) The apraxias: Neural Mechanisms of disorders of learned movement. *American Scientist,* **63**, 188–195.

Geschwind, N., & Damasio, A. R. (1985) Apraxia 423–432, in Frederik's J.A.M. (ed) *Handbook of Clinical Neurology,* Vol 1. North-Holland Publishing Co, Amsterdam.

Getman, G. N. (1952) *How to develop your child's intelligenc, A research publication,* Luverne, Minnesota, G. N. Getman.

Gillberg, I. C., & Gillberg, C. (1989) Children with preschool minor neurodevelopmental disorders IV: Behaviour and school achievement at age 13, *Developmental Medicine and Child Neurology,* **31**, 3–13.

Gillberg, C. Rasmussen, P., & Walstorm, J. (1982) Minor Neurodevelopmental disorders in children born to older mothers, *Developmental Medicine and Child Neurology,* **24**, 437–447.

Gisel,E., & Pollock, N. A. (1988) Eating skills. A review of current assessment practices. *Occupational Therapy Journal of Research.* **8**, 38–50.

Glazer, S. M., & Curry, D.(1988) Word Programs: survival tools for children with writing problems. *Reading, writing and learning disabilities,* **4**, 187–199.

Golden, B., Gerney, M. (1986) The effects of direct teaching styles on motor skill acquisition of fifth grade children. *Research Quarterly of Exercise and Sport.* **57**, 215–219.

Goldenberger, M. (1986) The effects of direct teaching stules on motor skills acquisition of 5th grade children. *Research Quarterly of Exercise and Sport*, **57**, 215–219.

Goldstein, K. (1948) *Language and language disturbances*, New York, Grune and Stratton.

Goldstein, P. C., & Tupper, D. E. (1987) Chapter 3, Quantitative and Qualitative Measurement of Subtle Neurobehavioral Deficit. in Tupper, D.E. (Editor) *Soft Neurological Signs* pp 45–69, Grune & Stratton, New York.

Goodman-Edwards, B., Shelley, A., & Cermak Sharon, A. (1989) Integrating motor control and motor learning concepts with neuropsychological perspectives on apraxia and developmental dyspraxia. *The American Journal of Occupational Therapy*, **43**, 431–445.

Gordon, N. S. (1979) The Acquisition of Motor Skills, *Brain and Development*, **1**, 1–6.

Gray, S. (1977) *The family oriented visiting program. A longitudfinal Study*, Peabody College Monongraph, Nashville Tennesses.

Greer, J. V. (1990) The Drug Babies, Bulletin from the Council for *Exceptional Children*, **56**, 382–384.

Gschwend, V. G. (1988) Neuropsysiologisch Grundlagen der Bewegungstherapien. (Neurophysiological bases of movement therapy) Der Kinderazt, **19**, 1589–1597.

Gubbay, S. S. (1975) *The clumsy child: A study of developmental apraxic, and agnosic ataxia*, W. B. Sanders, Co, Philadelphia.

Gubbay, S. S. (1978) The management of developmental apraxia; *Developmental Medicine and Child Neurology*, **20**, 643–646.

Gubbay, S., Ellis, E., & Walton, J. (1965) Clumsy children: a study of apraxic and agnosic defects in children, *Brain*, **88**, 295–312.

Guinagh, B. J., & Gordon, I. J. (1976) *School performance as a function of early stimuation*. Final Report To Office of Child Development, Washington D.C.

Hacaen, H., & Rondot, P. (1985) apraxia as a disorder of a system of signs in E. R. Roy (Ed) *Neuropsychological Studies of Apraxia and Related Disorders*, Elsevier Science Publishers, BV (North Holland).

Hadders-Algra, M., Touwen, B. C. L., & Huisjes, J. J. (1986) Neurologically deviant newborns: Neurological and behavioural development at the age of six years, *Developmental Medicine and Child Neurology*, **28**, 569–578.

Hall, D. M. B. (1988) Clumsy Children, *British Medical Journal*, **296**, 375–376.

Halverson, L., & Williams, K. (1985) Developmental sequences of hopping over distance: a pre-longitudinal study. *Research Quarterly of Exercise and Sport*, **56**, 32–44.

Hamburger, V. (1980) Tropic interactions in neurogenesis: A personal historical account, *Annual Review of Neuroscience*, **3**, 269–278.

Hamburger, V., & Levi, M. R. (1949) Proliferation, differentiation and degeneration in the spinal ganglia of the chick embryo under normal and experimental conditions, *Journal of Experimental Zoology*, **111**, 457–501.

Hamburger, V., & Oppenheim, R. W. (1982) Naturally occurring neuronal death in vertebrates, *Neuroscience Comments*, **1**, 39–55.
Hammond, W. A. (1871) *A treatise of the diseases of the nervous system*, 1st Ed, Appleton-Century Crofts, New York 876 pp.
Haron, M., & Henderson, A. (1985) Active and passive touch in developmentally dyspraxic and normal boys. *Occupational Therapy Journal of Research*. **5**, 101–112.
Harris, S. B. (1987) Early intervention for children with motor handicaps. Chapter 5 in Guralnick, M. J., & Bennett, F. C. (eds) *The effectiveness of early intervention for at-risk and handicapped children*. Academic Press, Harcourt Brace, New York. pp. 175–212.
Harter, S., & Pike, S. (1981) *The Pictorial Scale of Perceived Competence and Acceptance of Young Children*, Monograph, University of Denver.
Head, H. *Aphasia and kindred disorders of speech* (1926) Cambridge: Cambridge University Press.
Heiden, J. S., Small, R., Caton, W., Weiss, M. & Kurtz, T. (1983) Severe head injury: Clinican assessment and outcome. *Physical Therapy*, **63**, 1946–1951.
Heilman, K. M., Rothi, L. J. and Valenstein, E. (1982) Two forms of ideomotor apraxia, *Neurology*, **32**, 3240–346.
Henderson, S. E. (1987) the assessment of 'clumsy children', old and new approaches, *Journal of Child Psychology and Psychiatry*, **28**, 511–527.
Henderson, S. E., & Hall, D. (1982) concomitants of clumsiness in young school children, *Developmental Medicine and Child Neurology*, **24**, 448–460.
Henderson, S. E., May, D. S., & Umney, M. (1989) An exporatory study of goal-setting behaviour, self-concept and locus of control in children with movement difficulties, European Journal of Special Needs, **4**, 1–14.
Henderson, S. E., & Stott, D. H. (1977). Finding the clumsy child: Genesis of a test of motor impairment. *Journal of Human Movement Studies*, **3**, 38–48.
Hendrick, I. (1943) The discussion of the instinct to master. *Psychoanalytic Quarterly*, **12**, 561–565.
Henry, F. M. (1956) Motor learning when performance levels are heterogeneous. *Research Quarterly*, **27**, 176–181.
Henry, F. M., & Nelson, G. A. (1956) Age differences and inter-relationships between skill and learning in gross motor skills of ten and fifteen year old boys. *Research Quarterly*, **27**, 162–175.
Henschen, S. F. (1922) *Klinische und anatomische beitrage zur pathologie des gehirns*, Stockholm, Nordiske-Bokhandein.
Hertiz, M. E., & Shapiro,T. (1987) Chapter 4. The assessment of Nonfocal Neurological Signs in School-Aged Children, In Tupper, E. E. (Editor), *Soft Neurological Signs*. pp 71–94. Grune and Stratton, New York.
Hicks, J. A. (1931) *The acquisition of motor skill in young children*. University of Iowa Studies in child Welfare. No 5, 9–30.
Hicks, J. A., & Ralph, D. W. (1931) The effects of practice in tracing the Porteus Diamond Maze, *Child Development*, **2**, 156–158.

Hilgard, J. R. (1932). Learning and maturation in preschool children, *Journal of Genetic Psychology*, **41**, 36–56.

Hoare, D., & Larkin, D. (1990) Assessment and Classification using the McCarron Neuro Developmental battery (abstract) *International Journal of Neuroscience*, **51**, 114.

Hoare, D., & Larkin, D. (1991) Coordination Problems in Children, No, No 18 State of the Art Review, National Sports Centre, Australian Sports Commission, Canberra, Australia.

Hoare, D., & Larkin, D.(1991) Kinaesthetic abilities of clumsy children, *Developmental Medicine and Child Neurology*, **33** (8) 671–678.

Hock, B. (1968) Promotive medicine and the phenomenon of health, Archives of Environmental Health, 16, 269–278.

Hopft, H. C., Schlegal, H. J., Lowitszsch, K. (1974) Irridiation of voluntary activity on the contra-lateral side in movements of normal subjects and patients with central motor disturbances, *European Neurology*, **12**, 142–147.

Horitz, H. R., Ellis, H. M. & Sternberg, P. W. (1982) Programmed cell death in nematode development, *Neuroscience Comments*, **1**, 56–65.

Hoskins, T. A., & Squires, J. E. (1973) Developmental assessment: A test for gross motor and reflex development. *Physical Therapy*, **53**, 117–125.

Hsu, E., Bardfield, S., Cratty, B. J., and Garfinkel, A. (1989) Cinematographical methods to assess associated movements in children. *Adapted Physical Activity Quarterly*, **6**, 255–267.

Hubel, D. J. H., Wiesel, T. M. N., & Le Van, S. (1977) Plasticity of ocular dominance columns in moneky striat cortex, *Philosophical Translation Research Society of London*, **278**, 377–409.

Hulme, C., Biggerstaff, A., Morgan, G., and McKinlay, I. (1982) Visual kinaesthetic and cross-modal judgements of length by normal and clumsy children, *Developmental Medicine and Child Neurology*, **24**, 461–471.

Hulme, C., Biggerstaff, A., Morgan, G., & McKinlay, I. (1984) Visual, kinaesthetic and cross-modal judgements of length by clumsy children: A comparision with young normal children. *Child care; health and development*. **10**, 117–124.

Hulme, C., Smart, A., & Moran, G. (1982b) Visual perceptual deficits in clumsy children. Neuropsychology, **30**, 475–481.

Huntington, D. S. (1979) Support programs for infants and children, J. D. Orfsky (ed) *Handbook of Infant Development*, New York, Wiley & Sons.

Huttenlocher, P. R. (1979) Synaptic density in the human frontal cortex. Developmental changes and effects of aging, *Brain Research*, **163**, 195–205.

Huttenlocher, P. R., de Courten, C., Garey, L. J., & Vander Loos, H. (1982) Synaptogenesis in the human visual cortex-evidence for synapse elimination during normal development, *Neuroscience Letters*, **33**, 247–252.

Iloeje, S. O., (1987) Developmental Apraxia among Nigerian children in Enugu,Nigeria, *Developmental Medicine and Child Neurology*, **29**, 502–507.

Jankovic, J. (1986) Recent advances in the management of tics, *Clinical Neuropharmacology*, **9**, 100–110.

Jebson, R. G., & Taylor, N., Threiscaman, R. B., Troter, M., & Howard,L. P. (1969) An Objective and Standardized Test of Hand Function *Archives of Physical Medicine and Rehabilitation*, **50**, 311–319.

Jerusalem, F., & Bischoff, A. (1972) Ataxia Teleangiectatica: Elekrtronenmikroskopische. Biopsie-befunde des nervus suralis vib 2 *Fallen, Z. Neurol*, **202**, 128–a135.

Kalverboer, A. F., de Vries, H. J., & van Delten, T. (1990) Social behaviour in clumsy children as rated by parents and teachers in A. F. Kalverboer, (Ed) *Developmental Biopsychology*, 257–268, Michigan, The University of Michigan Press.

Kavale, K., & Mattson, P. (1983) One jumped off the balance beam: Metanalysis of perceptual-motor training. *Journal of Learning Disabilities*, **16**, 166–173.

Kellogg, Rhoda (1969). *Analyzing children's art. Palo Alto,* National Books.

Kelso, J. A. S., & Tuller, B. (1981) Toward a theory of apraxic syndromes, *Brain and Language*, **12**, 224–245.

Keogh, J. F., Sugden, D. A., Reynard, C. L., & Calkins, J. A. (1979) Identification of clumsy children: comparisons and comments, *Journal of Human Movement Studies*, **5**, 32–41.

Kephart, N. C. (1956) *the slow learner in the classroom*, Charles E. Merrill, Columbus Ohio.

Kimura, D. (1976) the neural basis of gesture qua language, In H. Whitaker & H. A. Whitaker (eds) *Studies in Neuolinguistics*, V 1, Academic Press, New York.

Kimura, D. (1982) Left-hemispher control of oral and brachial movements and their relation to communication. *Philosphical Transactions of the Royal Society of London*, **298**, 135–149.

Kinnealey, M. (1989) Tactile functions in learning disabled and normal children. Reliability and validity considerations. *Occupational Therapy Journal of Research*. **9**, 3–15.

Knuckey, N. W., Apsimon, T. T., & Gubbay, S. S. (1983) Computerized axial tomography in clumsy children with developmental apraxia, and agnosia, *Brain & Development*, **5**, 14–19.

Kools, J. A., & Tweedie, D. (1975) The development of praxis in young children. Perceptual and Motor Skills, **40**, 11–19.

Koontz, C. C. (1974) The Koontz Developmental Program, Western Psychological Services, Los Angeles.

Kumor, K. M., Sherer, M. A., & Cascella, N. G. (1989) "Cacaine Use in Man: Subjective Effects, Physiologic Responses and Toxicity, Chapter 8 in Redda, K. K., Walker, C. A., & Barnett G., (Eds) *Cocaine, Marijuana, Designer Drugs: Pharmacology and Behavior*. pp. 83–92. Boca Raton Florida, CRC Press.

Lacey, D. J. (1986) Diagnosis of Tourette syndrome in childhood, *Clinical Pediatrics*, **23**, 433–435.

LaFuze, M. (1951) A study of the learning of fundamental skills by college women of low motor ability. *Research Quarterly*, **22**, 149–159.

Larkin, D., & Hoare, D. (1991) The movement approach: A window into the understanding the clumsy child. in J. J. Summers (Ed.) *Approaches to the study of motor control and learning*, 413–439 Amsterdam, North Holland.

Laszlo, J. I., Bairstow, P. J. (1980) The measurement of kinesthetic sensitivity in children and adults, *Developmental Medicine and Child Neurology*, **22**, 454–464.

Laszlo, J. I., Bairstow, P. J. (1983) Kinaesthesis: Its measurement, training, and relationships to motor control *Quarterly Journal of Experimental* Psychology, **35**, 411–421.

Laszlo, J. I., Bairstow, P. J. (1985a) Perceptual-motor behaviour: Developmental Assessment and Therapy. Holt, Rinhart and Winston, London.

Laszlo, J. I., Bairstow, P. J. (1985b) Kinaesthetic sensitivity test. Rinehart and Winston. London.

Laszlo, J. I., Bairstow, P. J., Bartrip, J., & Rolfe, U. T, (1988) Clumsiness or perceptuo-motor dysfunction? in *Cognition and Action in Skilled Behaviour*. A. M. Colley & J. R., Beech, (editors) Elsevier Publishers, BV, North Holland.

Laszlo, J. I., & Bairstow, P. J. (1986) *Perceptual-Motor Behaviour* Holt, Rinehart & Winston, New York.

Lehmkuhl, G. (1984) Ideomotorische un ideatorische Apraxie im Kindesalter. (Ideomotor and ideotory apraxia in childhood), *Acta Paedopsychiatrica*, **50**, 97–110.

Lerer, R. J., & Lerer, M. P., (1976) The effects of methylphenidate on the soft neurological signs of hyperactive children. *Pediatrics*, **57**, 521–525.

Lesny, I. A. (1980) Developmental dysgraphia-dysgnosia as a cause of cogenital children's clumsiness, *Brain and Development*, **2**, 69–71.

Lesser-Katz, M. (1982) Some effects of maternal drug addition on the neonate, *The International Journal of the addictions*, **17**, 887–896.

Levine, M. D., Meltzer, L. T., Busch, B. (1983) The pediatric early examination. Studies of neurodevelopmental examination for 7 and 9 year old children, *Pediatrics*, **71**, 894–903.

Levitt, P., & Rakic, P. (1980) Immunoperoxidase localization of glial fibrillary acidic protein in radial glial-cells and astrocytes of the developing rhesus-monkey brain. *Journal of Comparative Neurology*, **193**, 815–840.

Levy, D. M. (1943) *Maternal Overprotection*, Columbia University Press, New York, New York.

Lord, R., & Hulme, C. (1987a) Perceptual judgements of normal and clumsy children, *Developmental Medicine and Child Neurology*, **29**, 250–257.

Lord, R., & Hulm, C. (1987b) Kinaesthetic sensitivity of normal and clumsy children, *Developmental Medicine and Child Neurology*, **29**, 720–723.

Losse, A., Henderson, S. E., Elliman, D., Hall, D., Knight, E., & Jongman, M. (1991) Clumsiness in children-Do they grow out of it? A 10-year follow-up study, *Developmental Medicine and Child Neurology*, **33**, 55–68.

Lowe, B. J. (1966) *The effects of physical conditioning on the cognitive functioning of educationally sub-normal boys*, Monograph, Birmingham University, Birmingham England.

Lubs, H. A., Duara, R., Levin, B., Jallad, R., Lubs, M. L., Rabin, M., Kushch, A., & Gross-Glenn, K. (1991) Chapter 4 "Dyslexia sub-types: Genetics Behavior and Brain Imaging". in D. D. Duane, & D. B. Gray eds. *The Reading Brain: The Biological Basis of Dyslexia*, York Press, Parkton Maryland, pp 89–118.

Luria, A. R. (1966) Higher Cortical Functions in Man, Basic Books, Consultants Bureau, New York.

Lynch, K. B., & Bridle, M. J. (1989) The validity of the Jebson-Taylor Hand Function Test of Daily Living, *Occupational Therapy Journal of Research*, **9**, 316–318.

Manni, J. L., Martin, R., and Sewell, T. (1977) Imitation of Gestures Technique A Preliminary Report on a pre-school test of visual-motor integration. *Perceptual and Motor Skills*, **44**, 1067–1073.

Marcie, P., & Hacaen, H. (1979) Agraphia: writing disorders associated with unilateral cortical lesions. in K. M. Heilman & E. Valenstein (Eds). *Clinical Neuropsychology*, New York, Oxford University Press.

Margolin, D. D. (1984) The neuropsychology of writing and spelling: semantic, phonological, motor, and perceptual processes, *Quarterly Journal of Experimental Psychology*. **36**, 459–490.

Martinek, T. J., Johnson, S. B. (1979) teacher expectations: effects on dydatic interaction and self-concept in elementary school children. Research Quarterly of Exercise and Sport. **50**, 60–70.

Masche, K. A. (1970) Effects of two different programs of instruction on motor performance of 2nd grade students, *Research Quarterly*, **41**, 406–411.

McGraw, M. B. (1935) *Growth: A study of Johnny and Jimmy*, Appleton-Century, New York.

McInerney, M. F., McLaughlin, T. F., & Truhlicka, M. (1982) Increasing eye contact and instruction following behavior with a three-year-old Down's syndrome child with parents as therapists, *Journal of Special Education*, **18**, 71–80.

McKinlay, I., & Gordon, N. (1986) Motor Learning Difficulities: Clumsy Children, Chapter 8, pp 183–202 in Gordon, N. & McKinlay I, (eds) *Children with neurological disorders Book I, Neurologically Handicapped Children: Treatment and Management*, Blackwell Scientific Publications, Palo Alto.

McMahan, S. A., & Greenberg, L. M. (1977) Serial neurologic examination of hyperactive children, *Pediatrics*, **59**, 384–587.

Menkes, J. H. (1974) *Textbook of Childhood Neurology*, Lea and Febiger, Philadelphia, Pennsylvania.

Mercer, L., & Bloch, M. (1983) Residuial sensorimotor deficits in the adult head-injured patient. *Physical Therapy*, **63**, 1988–1981.

Mero, A., Kauhanen, J. H., Peltola, E., Vuorimaa, T., & Komi, P. V. (1990) Physiological performance capacity in different prepubescent athletic groups, *The Journal of Sports Medicine and Physical Fitness*. **30**, 57–66.

Meyer-Probst, B., Heider, B., Cammann, G., & Engle, H. (1980) Erfahrungen mit dem Dyspraxie-Test (nach Lesny) (Experience of the dyspraixa test of Lesny) Psychiatrie, Neurologie Und Midizinische Psychologie, **32**, 46–52.

Miceli, G. Silveri, M. C., Caramazza, A. (1985) Cognitive analysis of a case of pure dysgraphia. *Brain and Languages*, **25**, 187–196.

Milani-Comparetti, A., & Gidoni, E. A. (1967) Pattern analyses of motor development and its disorders. *Developmental Medicine and Child Neurology*, **9**, 631–636.

Milani-Comparetti, A., & Gidoni, E. A., (1987) *Motor Development Screening Manual*, Meyer Children's Rehabilitation Institute, University of Nebraska Medical Center, 44 So 44th St, Omaha, Nebraska.

Miller, G. (1989) Addicted infants and their mothers., *Zero to Three*, **9**, 20–23.

Miller, J. L. (1957) Effects of instructions on the development of throwing for accuracy of first grade children. *Research Quarterly*, **28**, 132–137.

Minerva, A. N. (1935) Psychomotor education and general development of pre-school children: Experiments with twin controls. *Journal of Genetic* Psychology, **46**, 433–454.

Mirald, R. I., & Bailey, D. A. (1981) Longitudinal comparision of aerobic power in active and inactive boys aged 7–17 years, *Annals of Human* Biology, **8**, 405–414.

Miyahara, M. (1992) Sub-types of learning disabled children and youth, based upon measures of gross motor functioning. Unpublished study, Department of Kinesiology, UCLA.

Miyahara, M., Cratty, B. J., & Goldman, R. M. (1990) Praxic behaviors among learning disabled Children and youth, Submitted to *Journal of Movement Behavior.*

Mohr, D. R. (1960) The contributions of physical activity to skill development. *Research Quarterly*, **31**, 321–350.

Morris, A. F., Vaughn, S. E., & Vaccaro, P. (1982) Measurements of neuromuscular tone and strength in Down's Syndrome children. *Journal of Mental Deficiency Research*, **26**, 41–46.

Morris, D. (1985) Conversation with Director of Motor Development Program for Children, California State University, Pomona, California.

Murphy, J. B., & Gliner, J. E. (1988) Visual and motor sequencing in normal and clumsy children. *Occupational Therapy Journal of Research*. **8**, 89–103.

Myers, P. I., & Hammill, D. D. (1990) *Learning Disabilities: Basic Concepts, Assessment Practices, and Instructional Strategies*. Pro-Ed, Austin Texas. p 439–441.

Myklebust, H. R. (1973) *Developmental disorders of written language: studies of normal and exceptional children*, Grune and Stratton, New York.

Nichols, P. L. (1987) Minimal Brain Dysfunction and Soft Signs: The Collaborative Perinatal Study. In Tupper, D. E. (editor) *Soft Neurological Signs* pp 179–200. Grune & Stratton, New York.

Noica, A. (1912) Etude sur les mouvements associes, *Ecephale* **7**.

Noterdaeme, M., Amorosa, H., Ploog, M., & Sheimann, G. (1987) *Quantitative and Qualitative aspects of associated movements in childrenwith specific developmental speech and language disorders and in normal pre-school children*. Max-Planck-Institut fur Psychiatrie, Munchen, Germany.

Obersteiner, H. (1881) On allochiria; a peculiar sensory disorder, *Brain*, **4**, 153–163.

Ogle, J. W. (1867) Aphasia and agraphia, *Report of the Medal Research Council of Saint George's Hospital*. **2**, 83–122.

O'Hare, A. E. Brown, J. K. (1989a) Childhood dysgraphia: Part 1 An illustrated clinical classification, *Child: Care, Health and Development*. **15**, 79–102.

O'Hare, A. E., Brown, J. K. (1989b) Childhood dysgraphia: Part 2: Study of Hand Function. *Child: Care, Health and Development*. **15**, 151–166.

Oliver, J. N. (1958) The effect of physical conditioning exercises and activities upon the mental characteristics of educationally sub-normal boys. *British Journal of Educational Psychology*, **28**, 155–165.

Orlick, T. (1978) *The Cooperative Sports and Games: Challenge Without Competition*. Book, Random House, New York.

Orpet, R. R. (1972) *Frostig Movement Skill Test Battery*. Consulting Psychologists Press, Palo, Alto, California.

Orton, S. T. (1925) "Word-blindness" in children. *Archives of Neurology*, **14**, 582–615.

Orton, S. T. (1937) *Reading, writing, and speech problems in children*, Norton Co, New York.

Oseretsky, N. A. (1931) *Methoden der untersuchung der motorile*, Heft 57. Beihefte Zur Zeitschrift Fur Angewandte Psychologie, Barth, Leipzig.

Oseretsky, N. A. (1948) A metric scale for studying the motor capacity of children, (in Russian), *Russian Journal of Clinical Psychology*, **12, 37–47.**

Otto, W., Askov, E., and Cooper, C. (1969). "Legibility ratings for handwriting samples, a pragmatic approach", in *Remedial Teaching,: Research and Comment*, Otto W., Koenke, K., Editors, Houghton Mifflin, Boston.

Paine, R. S. (1968) Syndromes of 'minimal cerebral damage,' *Pediatric Clinics of North America*, **15**, 779–801.

Phillips, M., & Summers, D. (1954) Relationships of kinesthetic perception to motor learning. *Research Quarterly*, **25**, 456–469.

Piaget, J. (1954) *Origins of Intelligence*, New York, Basic Books.

Pieper, A. (1966) *Neurological Organization in Infancy*, Academic Press, New York.

Piers, E. V., & Harris, D. B. (1964) Age and other correlates of self-concept in children, *Journal of Educational Psychology*, **55**, 91–95.

Poeck, K. (1982) Two types of motor apraxia. *Archives of Neurology* **2**, 361–368.

Poeck, K. (1986) The clinical examination for motor apraxia *Neuropsychologia*, **24**, 129–134.

Prechtl, H. F. R. (1987) Chapter 11 in Tupper, D. E. (editor) Soft Neurological Signs. pp 247–254. Grune & Stratton, New York.

Prechtl, H. F. R., & Stemmer, C. (1962) The choreiform syndrome in children, *Developmental Medicine and Child Neurology*, **4**, 119–127.

Purvis, D., & Lichtman, J. W. (1985) *Principles of Neural Development*, Sunderland Mass Sinauer Associates Inc.

Purvis, D., & Lichtman, J. W. (1980) Elimination of synapses in the developing nervous system, *Science*, **210**, 153–157.

Raibert, M. H. (1977) *Motor Control and Learning by the State-Space Model*, Ph.D. Thesis, Artificial Intelligence Laboratory, Massachusettes Institute of Technology. AI-RI 439, Cambridge Mass.

Rakic, P. (1971) Neuron-glial relationship during granule cell migration in developing cerebellar cortex. A golgi and electronmicroscopic study in the Macacus rhesus. *Journal of Comparative Neurology*, **141**, 283–312.

Rakic, P. (1977) Prenatal development of the visual system in rhesus monkey, *Philosophical Translation Research Society of London*, **278**, 245–260.

Rakic, P. (1981) Neural-glial interaction during brain development. Trends, *Neuroscience*, **4**, 184–187.

Rarick, G. L., & Broadhead, G. L. (1968) *The effects of individualized versus group oriented physical education programs on selected parameters of the development of educable mentally retarded, and the minimally brain injured children*. Unpublished Monograph, University of Wisconson, Madison, Wisconson.

Rarick, G. L. & Dobbins, D. A. (1975) Basic components in the motor performance of children from six to nine years of age, *Medicine and Science in Sport*, **17**, 105–110.

Rarick, G. L., Dobbins, D. A., & Broadhead, G. A. (1976) *The motor domains and its correlates in educationally handicapped children*, Prentice-Hall Englewood Cliffs, New Jersey.

Rasmussen, P., Gillberg, C., Waldstorm, E., & Svenson, B. (1983) *Developmental Medicine and Child Neurology*, **25**, 315–333.

Raychev, R., Pentscheva, S., Rainov, W., Valtscheva, M., Bojinov, S. (1984) Neuropsychologische aspekte uber die storungen der hoheren functionen der hirnrinde bie kindern mit sprachfehlern, *Psychiatry, Neurology, with Psychology*, **11**, 639–647.

Redda, K. K., Walker, C. A., & Barnett, G. (1989) *Cocaine, Marijuana, Designer Drugs: Pharmacology and Behavior*, Boca Raton Florida, CRC Press.

Reeves, J. C., & Wherry, J. S. (1987) Chapter 10, Soft Signs in Hyperactivity, in Tuper, D. E. (Ed) *Soft Neurological Signs*, Grune & Stratton, New York.

Regehr, S. M., & Kaplan, B. J. (1988) Reading disability with motor problems may be an inherited sub-type. *Pediatrics*, **82,** 204–210.

Rie, E. D. (1987) Chapter 9 Soft Signs in Learning Disabilities, in Tupper, D. E. (Ed) *Soft Neurological Signs*, Grune & Stratton, New York. (pp. 201–224).

Rie, E. D., Rie, H. E., Steward, S., & Rettemnier, S. (1978) An analysis of neurological soft signs in children with learning problems. *Brain and Language.*, **6**, 32–46.

Rodier, P. M., (1980). Chronology of neuron development: Animal studies and their clinical implications. *Developmental Medicine and Child Neurology*, **22**, 525–545.

Roeltgen, D. P., Heilman, K. M. (1985) Review of agraphia and a proposal for an anatomically based neuropsychological model of writing. Applied Linguistics, **6**, 205–229.

Rose, B., Berger, B., & Larkin, D. (1991) *A study of perceived competence, global self-worth and neuromuscular development,* (absract) Proceedings of the 18th ACHPER National/International Conference, Perth, Australia.

Rosenbloom, L., & Horton, M. E. (1971) The maturation of fine prehension in children. *Developmental Medicine and Child Neurology,* **13**, 3–8.

Ross, D. M., & Ross, S. A. (1982) *Hyperactivity: Current Issues, Research and Theory,* New York, John Wiley and Sons.

Rossett, H. L., & Sander, L. W. (1979) Effects of maternal drinking on neonatal morphology and state, in J. D. Osofsky (Ed) *The handbook of infant development,* New York Wiley.

Roy, E. A. (1978) A new look at an old-syndrome: *Journal of Movement Studies,* **4**, 191–210.

Roy, E. A. (1985) *Neuropsychological Studies of Apraxia and Related Disorders,* North-Holland, New York.

Rutter, M., Graham, P., & Yule, W. (1970) A neuropsychiatric Study in childhood. *Clinics in Developmental Medicine* Nos 35–36, Lippencott, Philadelphia.

Saida, Y., & Miyashita, M. (1979) Development of fine motor skill in young children aged 2–6. *Journal of Human Movement,* **5**, 104–113.

Satterfield, J. H., Cantwell, D. P., & Saul R. E. (1973) Response to stimulant drug treatment in hyperactive children. Prediction from EEG and neurological findings. *Journal of Autism and Childhood Schizophrenia,* **3**, 36–48.

Scamman, R. E. (1927) First seriatim study of human growth, *American Journal of Physical Anthropology,* **10**, 239–233.

Schain, R. J. (1972) *Neurology of childhood learning disorders,* Baltimore, Williams and Wilkins.

Schnabl-Dickey, E. A. (1978) Relationships between parents' child rearing attitudes and the jumping and throwing performance of their pre-school children, *Research Quarterly,* **48**, 382–390.

Schlling, D., Poppen, R. (1983) Behavioral relaxation, training and assessment, *Journal of Behavioral Therapy and Experimental Psychology,* **14**, 99–107.

Seaman, J. A., & Depauw, K. P. (1982) The New Adapted Physical Education, A Developmental Approach. Mayfield Publishing Co, Palo Alto, California.

Shapiro, A. K., & Shapiro, E. (1988) *Gilles de la Tourette's Syndrome,* Raven Press, New York.

Shapiro, A. K., & Shapiro, E. (1986) Semiology, nosology and criteria for tic disorderes, *Revue Neurologique,* **142**, 824–832.

Short, H., & Crawford, J. (1984) Last to be chosen the awkward child, *Pivot,* **2**, 32–36.

Silva, P. A., & Ross, B. (1980) Gross motor development and delays in development in early childhood: assessment and significance, *Journal of Human Movement Studies,* **6**, 211–226.

Skekim, W. O., Dekirmenjian, H., & Chapel, J. L. (1979) Urinary MHPG excretion in minimal brain dsyfunction and its modification by d-amphetamine. *American Journal of Psychiatry*. **136**, 667–671.

Sloan, W. (1955) The Lincoln-Oseretsky Motor Development Scale, *Genetic Psychology Monograph*, **51**, 183–252.

Sovik, N. Oddvar, A., & Thygensen, R. (1987). Relation of spelling and writing in learning disabilities. *Perceptual and Motor Skills*, **64**, 219–236.

Small, L. (1982) *Minimal Brain Dysfunction*, The Free Press, New York.

Smith, J. A. (1956) Relationship of certain physical abilities and traits to motor learning in elementary school children. *Research Quarterly*, **27**, 220–228.

Smith, O. W., & Smith P. C. (1966) Developmental studies of spatial judgements by children and by adults, *Perceptual and Motor Skills*, Monograph Supplement, **22**, 3–73.

Smythe, T. R., & Glencross, D. J. (1986) Information processing deficits in clumsy children. *Australian Journal of Psychology*, **38**, 13–22.

Solley, W. H. (1957) Ratio of physical development as a factor in motor coordination. *Research Quarterly*, **28**, 295–304.

Speece, D. L. (1987) Information processing sub-types in learning disabled readers, *Learning Disabilities Research*, **11**, 243–357.

Spitz, R. A. (1945) Hospitalization, A study of its manifestations in the first year of life, *Psychoanalytic Study of the Child*. **1**, 53–74.

Sprague, R. L., Wherry, J., & Davis, K. (1969) *Psychotropic drug effects on learning and activity level in children*. Paper presented at the Gatlinburg Conference on Research and Theory in Mental Retardation.

Steinthal, L. (1871) *Abriss der spatchweissenschaft*, Berlin.

Stott, D. H., & Marston, N. C., & Neill, S. J. (1971) *The Bristol Social Adjustment Guides*, 4th Edition, Educational Testing Services, San Diego.

Stott, D. H., Moyes, F. A., & Henderson, S. E. (1972) *Test of Motor Impairment Guelph*, Ontario, Canada, Brook Educational Publication Co.

Stott, D. H., Moyes, F. A., & Henderson, S. E. (1984) *Test of Motor Impairment*, Henderson revision, The Psychological Corporation San Antonio, Texas.

Strauss, A. A., & Lehtinen, C. E. (1947) *The Psychopathology and Education of the Brain-Injured Child*, Gruen and Stratton. New York.

Strauss, A., & Werner, H. (1939) Deficiency in the finger schema in relation to arthmetic disability (finger agnosia and acalculia) *American Journal* of Orthopsychiatry, **8**, 719–725.

Sugden, D., & Wann, C. (1987) The assessment of motor impairment in children with moderate learning disabilities. *British Journal of Educational Psychology*, **57**, 225–236.

Swanson, H. L., Cochran, K. F., & Ewers, C. A. (1990) Can learning disabilities be determined from working memory performance? *Journal of Learning Disabilities*, **23**, 59–67.

Szamari, P., & Taylor, C. D. (1984) Overflow movements and behaviour problems: Scoring using a modification of Fog's test. *Developmental Medicine and Child Neurology*, **26**, 297–310.

Szeto, H. (1988) Paper presented at the conference dealing with fetal drug exposure Sponsored by the National Institutes on Drug Abuse and the Behavioral Teratology Society, Washington D.C.

Taber's Cyclopedic Dictionary. (1973) Thomas, C. L. (editor) 12th Edition, Davis, Philadelphia.

Taft, L. A. (1981) Intervention programs for children with cerebral palsy, in C. E. Brown (ed) *Infants at risk: assessment and intervention,* pp. 73–82. Johnson & Johnson Baby Products, Boston.

Taft, L. T., & Barowsky, E. I. (1989) Clumsy Child, *Pediatrics in Review,* **10**, 247–253.

Talmadge, E. W., & Collins, G. A. (1983) Physical abilities after head injury: A retrospective study, *Physical Therapy*, **63**, 2010–2017.

Temple, G. (1988) Developmental dyslexia & dysgraphia, persistence in middel age, *Journal of Communication Disorders,* **21**, 189–192.

Thams, P. F. (1955) *A factor analysis of the Lincoln-Oseretsky motor development scale.* Unpublished Doctoral Dissertation, University of Michigan, Ann Arbor, Michigan.

Thelen, E. (1979) Rhythmic stereotypies in normal human infants. *Animal Behavior*, **27**, 699–715.

Thelen, E. (1981). Kicking, Rocking and Waving – Contextual Analysis of Rhythmic Stereotypies in Normal Human Infants: *A Ecological Perspective. Developmental Psychology*, **17**, 237–257.

Thelen, E. (1985). Developmental origins of motor coordination: Leg movements in human infants. *Developmental Psychobiology*, **18**, 1–22.

Thelen, E., & Fisher, D. M. (1983). The organization of spontaneous leg movements in newborn infants. *Journal of Motor Behavior*, **15**, 353–453.

Thelen, E., Kelso, J. A. S., & Fogel, A. (1987). Self-organizing systems and infant motor development. *Developmental Review*, **7**, 39–65.

Thelen, E., Skala, K., & Kelso, J. A. S. (1987) The dynamic nature of early coordination: Evidence from bilateral leg movements in young infants. *Developmental Psychology*, **23**, 179–186.

Touwen, B. C. L. (1987) Chapter 14 The meaning and value of soft signs in the behavioral sciences. in Tupper, D. E. (editor) *Soft Neurological* Signs. pp 281–296. Grune & Stratton, New York.

Touwen, B. C. L., and Prechtl H. F. R. (1970) *The Neurological examination of the child with minor nervous system dysfunction*, London, Clinics in Developmental Medicine, Heinemann.

Towbin, A. (1970) *Central nervous system damage in the premature related to the occurrence of mental retardation.* Proceedings from Fourth Multidisciplinary Conference on the Etiology of Mental Retardation. National Institutes of Health, Lincoln, Nebraska.

Towbin, A. (1987) Neuropatholic Correlates. In Tupper, D. E. (editor) *Soft Neurological Signs*, (pp. 157–178), Grune and Stratton, New York.

Tsutsui, K., Honda, A., Amano, Y. (1988) Children who cannot jump over hurdles well, *Physical Education*, (Japan), **36**, 53–55. (In Japanese).

Tupper, D. D. (1986) Neuropsychological screening and soft signs. In Orbzut, J. E., & Hynd, G. W. (Eds) *Child Neuropsychology*, Vol 2 Clinical Practice, pp. 139–186. Academic Press, Orlando Florida.

Tupper, D. E. (1987). *Soft Neurological Signs.* Grune & Stratton, New York.

Tweit, A. H., Gollnick, P. D., & Hearn, G. B. (1963) Effect of training program on total body reaction time of individuals with low fitness. *Research Quarterly*, **34**, 528–535.

Ulrich, B. D. (1987) Perceptions of physical competence, motor competences, and participation in sport. Their inter-relationship in young children. *Research Quarterly of Exercise and Sport*, **58**, 57–67.

Vaccaro, P., & Clarke, D. H. (1978) Cardio-respiratory alterations in 9–11 year old children, following a season of competitive swimming, *Medicine Science and Sports*, **10**, 204–207.

Vailas, A. C., Matsuda, J. J., Zernicke, R. F., Vittorio, A. P., Angiola, P. M., Maynard, J. A. (1986) Structural and mechanical adaption of immature bone to strenuous exercise, *Journal of Applied Physiology*, **41**, 2028–2034.

Van Rossum, J. H. A., & Vermeer, A. (1990) Perceived competence: A validation study in the field of motoric remedial teaching. *International Journal of Disability, Development and Maturation*, **37**, 71–81.

Vandenberg, S. G., & Streng, J. (1984) "The genetics of abnormal behavioral development in E. S. Gollin (Ed.) *Malformations of Development: Biological and Psychological Sources and Consequences*, Academic Press, New York pp. 315–350.

Villafana, T. (1988). Fundamental physics of magnetic resonance imaging. Radiologic *Clinics of North America*, **26**, 701–715.

Yamadori, A. (1986) Shikkou kenkyuu no genkyo (Trends in apraxia research. *No Shinkei (Brain & Nerve)* **38**, 27–33.

Waber, D. P., Mann, M. B., & Merola, J. (1985) Motor overflow and attentional processes in normal school age children. *Developmental Medicine and Child Neurology*, **27**, 491–497.

Walton, J. N. (1961) Clumsy children, *Spastic Quarterly*, **10**, 9–21.

Walton, J. N. (1963) Clumsy children in, *Minimal Cerebral Dysfunction*, Bax, M. and Mac Keith, R. (Eds) London, Spastics Society of London.

Walton, J. N. (1966) *Essentials of neurology, Pitman, London.*

Walton, J. N., Ellis, E., & Court, S. D. M., (1962) Clumsy Children, a study of developmental apraxia and agnosia, *Brain*, **85**, 603–612.

Waterland, J., & Hellenbrandt, F. A. (1964) Involuntary patterning associated with willed movement performed against progressively increasing resistance. *American Journal of Physical Medicine*, **43**, 13–30.

Watson, R. T., Fleet, W. S., Gonzales-Rothi, L., & Heilman, K. M. (1986) Apraxia and the supplementary motor area. *Archives of Neurology*, **43**, 787–792.

Werner, P. (1974). Education of selected movement patterns of preschool children, *Perceptual and Motor Skills*, **39**, 795–798.

White, R. (1959) Motivation reconsidered; the concept of competence, *Psychological Review*, **66**, 297–333.

Whittle, H. D. (1961) Effects of elementary school physical education upon aspects of physical, motor and personality development. *Research Quarterly*, **32**, 249–260.

Wiesel, T. N. (1982) The postnatal development of the visual cortex and the influence of environment, *Nature*, **299**, 583–592.

Williams, H. (1968) *The perception of moving objects by children*, unpublished monograph, Department of Kinesiology, UCLA.
Wolff, P. H., Gunoe, C. E., & Cohen, C. (1983) Associated movements as a measure of developmental age. *Developmental Medicine and Child* Neurology, **25**, 417–429.
Wolff, P. H., & Cohen, C., & Drake, C. (1984) Impaired motor timing control in specific reading retardation, *Neuropsychology*, **22**, 587–600.
Wolff, P. H., & Michael, G. F., & Drake, C. (1990) Rate and timing precision of motor coordination in developmental dyxlexia, *Developmental Psychology*, **26**, 349–359.
Wright, F. G., Blough, R. R., Chamberlin, A., Ernest, T., Halstead, W. C., Meier, P., Moore, R. Y., Nauton, R. F., & Newell, F. W. (1972) A controlled follow-up study of small prematures born from 1952 throgh 1956. *American Journal of Disabled Children*, **124**, 506–521.
Zelazo, P. R. (1983) The development of walking; new findings, old assumptions. *Journal of Motor Behavior*, **15**, 99–137.
Zernicke, R., Gregor, R. J., & Cratty, B. J. (1982) Balance and visual perception in children, *Journal of Mouvement Behavior*, **12**, 28–32.

Index

B

C

D

T